# Nutrition and Lifestyle for Pregnancy and Breastfeeding

## Sir Peter Gluckman

University Distinguished Professor, Professor of Paediatric
and Perinatal Biology, Liggins Institute,
University of Auckland

## Mark Hanson

Director, Academic Unit of Human Development and Health,
Director, Institute of Developmental Sciences, and British
Heart Foundation Professor of Cardiovascular Science,
University of Southampton and NIHR Nutrition Biomedical
Research Centre, University Hospital Southampton

## Chong Yap Seng

Acting Executive Director, Singapore Institute for Clinical
Sciences, Agency for Science, Technology and Research,
Department of Obstetrics & Gynaecology, Yong Loo Lin
School of Medicine, National University Health System,
National University of Singapore

## Anne Bardsley

Research Associate, Liggins Institute,
University of Auckland

## OXFORD
UNIVERSITY PRESS

# OXFORD
UNIVERSITY PRESS

Great Clarendon Street, Oxford, OX2 6DP,
United Kingdom

Oxford University Press is a department of the University of Oxford.
It furthers the University's objective of excellence in research, scholarship,
and education by publishing worldwide. Oxford is a registered trade mark of
Oxford University Press in the UK and in certain other countries

© Oxford University Press 2015

The moral rights of the authors have been asserted

First Edition published in 2015

Impression: 1

Published in the United States of America by Oxford University Press
198 Madison Avenue, New York, NY 10016, United States of America

British Library Cataloguing in Publication Data
Data available

Library of Congress Control Number: 2014943264

ISBN 978–0–19–872270–0

Printed in Great Britain by
Clays Ltd, St Ives plc

# Preface

**A healthy life depends on a healthy start to life**

Over the last few years there has been exciting progress in our understanding of what creates a healthy start to life. We now know that many aspects of embryonic, fetal, and infant development are affected by somewhat subtle aspects of parental health and behaviour. In this way, health—or conversely the risk of disease—is passed from one generation to the next, via processes operating independently of inherited genetic effects. This is important, because it means that parents, supported by their families and health care professionals (HCPs), can take many positive steps to promote the health of their children, even before those children are born.

As our scientific knowledge in this area has developed, it has become clear that the impact of parental lifestyle and behavioural choices extends beyond fetal development to influence the whole future life of the offspring. Small changes in the developmental environment created by parental health and behaviour before birth, and the circumstances of life over the first few years after birth, leave persistent echoes on the child's biology, operating both through what are called *epigenetic* processes and through learning.

The implications of new discoveries in this 'life-course biology' and the importance of the concepts of developmental plasticity are both exciting and profound for many clinical specialties, including obstetrics, midwifery, and paediatrics, and also for child psychology and the social sciences. These disciplines now have a critical role to play in future health promotion and preventative medicine. This also means that the content and nature of the information exchanged between HCPs and parents-to-be needs to change.

While the general principles of ensuring a healthy start to life may seem obvious, much of the emerging knowledge from the scientific community has not been disseminated widely or reliably. Moreover, it is important to consider a broader period of development than many of us realize—extending from well before conception though into late childhood and adolescence—and that both the mother and father can do things that make a healthy start to life more likely. But what advice should be given to parents-to-be? They want specific, clear information, but the confusion of messages available to both them and HCPs presents a real challenge.

We wrote this book in response to the frequent requests we receive from HCPs for clear guidance on what to recommend to young couples or parents-to-be about the nutritional and lifestyle choices likely to lead to the best pregnancy outcome and healthy growth and development of their child. These requests arise whenever we interact with such HCPs, whether informally, in response to our papers and books, or at scientific meetings. The precise questions vary, often relating to diet before pregnancy or in lactation, physical activity, stress, environmental toxin exposure, etc., but underlying them all is the same problem: while there is universal recognition of the importance of giving clear advice, there is no single, simple resource to which HCPs can turn to get the information upon which such advice depends.

While we hope that this book will help HCPs to advise prospective parents, we are well aware that there are many other sources of information to which such parents-to-be will turn. In fact, there are *too* many sources, especially on the internet and through a variety of media, as well from peers, formal and informal support groups, or clubs. These are often accessed before, or instead of, resorting to a HCP for advice.

All too often these disparate sources do not agree, even on fundamental issues with important health consequences. Sometimes the advice from informal sources is based more on folklore than science, but most prospective parents have no way of assessing its accuracy or quality. Faced with this overload of conflicting information, it is not surprising that some parents do not make the best choices about lifestyle. With this in mind, we have tried to make this book as user-friendly as possible while providing in-depth sources to support our conclusions, recognizing that it will provide a source of information for some parents as well as for their HCPs.

So what makes us so sure that we know the answers? To be honest, sometimes we don't. Throughout the book, we have therefore tried to be clear about our level of confidence in the information we present. In some cases, the data are unambiguous and a clear consensus exists, so there is no problem in being prescriptive. In others, when there is no such consensus, we have tried to be transparent about giving our view on the weight to be placed on what is sometimes confusing evidence. In still other situations, the evidence must be interpreted in context—for example, what might be appropriate weight gain in pregnancy for a woman of average BMI in the USA may not be appropriate for a woman of average BMI in India. Finally, there are situations where, frankly, we do not know the answers: the underlying issues can be explained and considered, but action may not be appropriate until further research is completed.

We also need to be clear at the outset in stating what this book is **not** about. It is not a self-help guide to pregnancy; it is not a textbook on the biology of human development; and it is not a guide to the complications or diseases associated with pregnancy and their management. There are many other books that serve those purposes.

What this book is intended to provide is a manual for a wide range of HCPs—from community health workers, hospital doctors, and midwives, to public health practitioners—about the importance of a healthy lifestyle for prospective parents. It sets out the essentials of current knowledge about this issue in a form that we hope can be easily accessed and can serve as a resource for informed discussion with the public and parents-to-be. We hope that this book will empower the HCP to take a major role in health promotion and disease prevention at this critical period in the life course, a time when parents are anxious to do the best for their family but are confused about the steps to take. In addition, we make no apologies for the extensive referencing. Given the confusion in the popular and technical literature, and the complications arising because of commercial claims, we think it necessary to provide access to the evidence to make clear the basis on which statements or recommendations are being made and to indicate further reading.

# Acknowledgements

We acknowledge the enormous effort of Dr E. Saputra (Department of Obstetrics, National University of Singapore), who undertook the literature searching that underpins many chapters of this book. We thank the many research associates in our laboratories in Auckland, Singapore, and Southampton, with whom we have worked over the years and who have provided many of the insights reflected in this book. We are grateful to our colleagues Philip Baker, Philip Calder, Mary Chong, Terrence Forrester, Jerrold Heindel, Francisco Mardones, John Newnham, and Sian Robinson for reviewing sections of the book.

# Contents

Abbreviations *xvii*

How to use this book *xviii*

## Section 1 **Fundamentals of healthy nutrition and lifestyle**

**1** The importance of nutrition and lifestyle to healthy development *3*

Developmental origins of health and disease *3*

Nutrition: providing the building blocks of development and the fuel for metabolism *5*

The importance of physical activity *10*

Avoidance of risky exposures *11*

Opportunities and challenges *12*

**2** Conceptual background to healthy growth and development *15*

Development is affected by early environment *15*

Developmental plasticity *18*

Other forms of developmental response *25*

Taking a 'life-course' approach *25*

## Section 2 **Nutritional requirements for pregnancy and breastfeeding**

**3** Practicalities: understanding nutrient recommendations *29*

Nutritional advice and caveats *29*

Dietary reference intakes *29*

Food labelling *30*

**4** Macronutrients and fibre requirements during pregnancy *33*

Macronutrient transfer to the fetus *33*

Macronutrient balance during pregnancy *33*

Recommended macronutrient and fibre intakes during pregnancy *37*

Our recommendations for macronutrient and fibre intake during pregnancy *38*

**5** Polyunsaturated fatty acids in pregnancy and breastfeeding *40*

Polyunsaturated fatty acids are essential for fetal and infant development *40*

Dietary sources of polyunsaturated fatty acids  *41*

Polyunsaturated fatty acid status in pregnancy and lactation  *41*

Effects of polyunsaturated fatty acids on health  *42*

Agency guidelines on polyunsaturated fatty acid intake  *45*

Our recommendations for polyunsaturated fatty acid intake during pregnancy and lactation  *45*

**6** Vitamin A in pregnancy and breastfeeding  *47*

Vitamin A functions  *47*

Vitamin A deficiency  *48*

Vitamin A in pregnancy  *49*

Vitamin A in lactation and infancy  *51*

Sources and metabolism of vitamin A  *52*

Risks of excess vitamin A during pregnancy  *52*

Agency guidelines for vitamin A intake  *53*

Our recommendations for vitamin A intake during pregnancy and lactation  *56*

**7** Vitamin B$_1$ (thiamine) in pregnancy and breastfeeding  *57*

Thiamine functions  *57*

Indicators of thiamine status  *57*

Thiamine deficiency  *58*

Thiamine in pregnancy  *59*

Thiamine in lactation and infancy  *59*

Thiamine sources  *60*

Effects of excess thiamine  *60*

Agency guidelines for thiamine intake  *60*

Our recommendations for thiamine intake during pregnancy and lactation  *61*

**8** Vitamin B$_2$ (riboflavin) in pregnancy and breastfeeding  *62*

Riboflavin functions  *62*

Indicators of riboflavin status  *63*

Riboflavin deficiency  *63*

Riboflavin in pregnancy  *64*

Riboflavin in lactation  *64*

Riboflavin sources  *65*

Risks of excess riboflavin  *65*

Agency guidelines for riboflavin intake  *65*

Our recommendations for riboflavin intake during pregnancy and lactation  *66*

**9** Vitamin B$_3$ (niacin) in pregnancy and breastfeeding  *67*

Niacin functions  *67*

Indicators of niacin status  *67*

Niacin deficiency  *68*

Niacin in pregnancy and lactation  *68*

Niacin sources  *68*

Risks of excess niacin  *69*

Agency guidelines for niacin intake  *69*

Our recommendations for niacin intake during pregnancy and lactation  *70*

**10** Vitamin B$_6$ (pyridoxine) in pregnancy and breastfeeding  *71*

Vitamin B$_6$ functions  *71*

Indicators of vitamin B$_6$ status  *72*

Vitamin B$_6$ deficiency  *72*

Vitamin B$_6$ in pregnancy  *72*

Vitamin B$_6$ in lactation and infancy  *74*

Vitamin B$_6$ sources and metabolism  *74*

Risks of excess vitamin B$_6$  *75*

Agency guidelines for vitamin B$_6$ intake  *75*

Our recommendations for vitamin B$_6$ intake during pregnancy and lactation  *76*

**11** Vitamin B$_7$ (biotin) in pregnancy and breastfeeding  *77*

Biotin functions  *77*

Indicators of biotin status  *77*

Biotin deficiency  *77*

Biotin in pregnancy  *78*

Biotin in lactation  *78*

Biotin sources  *78*

Risks of excess biotin  *79*

Agency guidelines for biotin intake  *79*

Our recommendations for biotin intake during pregnancy and lactation  *80*

**12** Vitamin B$_9$ (folate) in pregnancy and breastfeeding  *81*

Folate functions  *81*

Indicators of folate status  *83*

Folate deficiency  *83*

Folate in pregnancy  *84*

Folic acid genetics  *87*

Folate interactions with vitamin $B_{12}$ and choline  *87*

Food folate sources  *88*

Food fortification with folic acid  *88*

Risks of excess folate  *89*

Agency guidelines for folate intake  *90*

Our recommendations for folate intake during pregnancy and lactation  *93*

**13** Vitamin $B_{12}$ (cobalamin) in pregnancy and breastfeeding  *94*

Vitamin $B_{12}$ functions  *94*

Indicators of vitamin $B_{12}$ status  *95*

Vitamin $B_{12}$ deficiency  *95*

Vitamin $B_{12}$ in pregnancy and lactation  *97*

Vitamin $B_{12}$ sources  *98*

Risks of excess vitamin $B_{12}$  *99*

Agency guidelines for vitamin $B_{12}$ intake  *99*

Our recommendations for vitamin $B_{12}$ intake during pregnancy and lactation  *100*

**14** Choline in pregnancy and breastfeeding  *102*

Choline functions  *102*

Indicators of choline status  *102*

Choline deficiency  *103*

Choline in pregnancy  *103*

Choline in lactation  *104*

Choline and epigenetic mechanisms  *105*

Choline sources  *105*

Agency guidelines for choline intake  *105*

Our recommendations for choline intake during pregnancy and lactation  *106*

**15** Vitamin D in pregnancy and breastfeeding  *107*

Vitamin D functions  *107*

Vitamin D deficiency  *108*

Vitamin D in pregnancy  *110*

Vitamin D and fertility  *114*

Vitamin D sources  *114*

Vitamin D supplementation  *116*

Risks of excess vitamin D  *117*

Agency guidelines for vitamin D intake  *118*

Our recommendations for vitamin D intake during pregnancy and lactation  *120*

**16** Vitamin K in pregnancy and breastfeeding  *122*

Vitamin K functions  *122*

Indicators of vitamin K status  *122*

Vitamin K deficiency  *123*

Vitamin K in pregnancy and lactation  *123*

Vitamin K sources and metabolism  *124*

Risks of excess vitamin K  *125*

Agency guidelines for vitamin K intake  *125*

Our recommendations for vitamin K intake during pregnancy and lactation  *126*

**17** Vitamins C and E and other antioxidants in pregnancy and breastfeeding  *127*

Antioxidant functions  *127*

Antioxidants in pregnancy  *127*

Dietary antioxidants  *129*

Vitamin C  *131*

Vitamin E  *134*

Supplementation trials of vitamins C and E in pregnancy  *137*

Summary and recommendations for antioxidant intake  *140*

Our recommendations for antioxidant intake during pregnancy and lactation  *140*

**18** Calcium in pregnancy and breastfeeding  *141*

Calcium functions  *141*

Indicators of calcium status  *142*

Calcium in pregnancy  *142*

Calcium in lactation  *146*

Prevalence of calcium deficiency  *147*

Calcium sources  *148*

Risks of excess calcium  *149*

Agency guidelines for calcium intake  *149*

Our recommendations for calcium intake during pregnancy and lactation  *150*

**19** Iodine in pregnancy and breastfeeding  *152*

Iodine functions  *152*

Indicators of iodine status  *152*

Iodine deficiency in pregnancy  *153*

Iodine in lactation  *155*

Iodine supplementation in pregnancy  *155*

Iodine sources  *157*

Areas of concern for iodine availability  *158*

Risks of excess iodine  *158*

Agency guidelines for iodine intake  *159*

Our recommendations for iodine intake during pregnancy and lactation  *161*

**20** Iron in pregnancy and breastfeeding  *162*

Iron functions  *162*

Iron homeostasis  *162*

Indicators of iron status and deficiency  *163*

Iron in pregnancy  *163*

Iron deficiency in pregnancy and infancy  *164*

Infant iron requirements  *166*

Iron supplementation during pregnancy  *166*

Iron sources and metabolism  *168*

Risks of excess iron  *169*

Agency guidelines for iron intake  *170*

Our recommendations for iron intake during pregnancy and lactation  *173*

**21** Magnesium in pregnancy and breastfeeding  *174*

Magnesium functions  *174*

Indicators of magnesium status  *175*

Magnesium deficiency  *175*

Magnesium in pregnancy  *176*

Magnesium supplementation in pregnancy  *179*

Magnesium in breast milk  *180*

Sources of magnesium  *180*

Risks of excess magnesium  *181*

Agency guidelines for magnesium intake  *181*

Our recommendations for magnesium intake during pregnancy and lactation  *183*

**22** Potassium in pregnancy and breastfeeding  *184*

Potassium functions  *184*

Potassium in pregnancy  *185*

Potassium sources  *185*

Agency guidelines for potassium intake  *185*

Our recommendations for potassium intake during pregnancy and lactation  *186*

**23** Selenium in pregnancy and breastfeeding  *187*

Selenium functions  *187*

Indicators of selenium status *187*

Selenium and fertility *188*

Selenium in pregnancy *188*

Selenium sources *190*

Risks of excess selenium *190*

Agency guidelines for selenium intake *190*

Our recommendations for selenium intake during pregnancy
and lactation *191*

**24** Copper in pregnancy and breastfeeding *192*

Copper functions *192*

Indicators of copper status *192*

Copper deficiency *192*

Copper in pregnancy, lactation, and infant feeding *193*

Risks of excess copper *193*

Copper sources *194*

Agency guidelines for copper intake *194*

Our recommendations for copper intake during pregnancy
and lactation *195*

**25** Zinc in pregnancy and breastfeeding *196*

Zinc functions *196*

Indicators of zinc status *196*

Zinc deficiency *196*

Zinc in pregnancy *198*

Zinc in lactation and infant feeding *199*

Zinc sources and bioavailability *200*

Risks of excess zinc *201*

Agency guidelines for zinc intake *201*

Our recommendations for zinc intake during pregnancy
and lactation *202*

**26** Manganese in pregnancy and breastfeeding *204*

Manganese functions *204*

Indicators of manganese status/exposure *204*

Manganese in pregnancy *205*

Manganese sources *206*

Risks of excess manganese *206*

Agency guidelines for manganese intake *206*

Our recommendations for manganese intake during pregnancy
and lactation *207*

**27** Prebiotics and probiotics in pregnancy and breastfeeding *209*

Prebiotic and probiotic functions *209*

Probiotics and the immune system—the 'hygiene hypothesis' *210*

A potential role of probiotics in the prevention of gestational diabetes mellitus *210*

Our recommendations for prebiotic and probiotic intake during pregnancy and lactation *211*

## Section 3 **A healthy lifestyle for a healthy pregnancy**

**28** Pre-conception maternal body composition and gestational weight gain *215*

The impact of maternal pre-conception bodyweight *215*

Gestational weight gain *216*

Agency guidelines for weight gain during pregnancy *218*

Active management of gestational weight gain *219*

Our recommendations for pre-conceptional maternal body composition and gestational weight gain *220*

**29** Exercise and physical activity in pregnancy *221*

Exercise and physiological changes in pregnancy *221*

Cultural factors influencing exercise during pregnancy *221*

The benefits of exercise for expecting mothers *222*

The effects of moderate maternal exercise on the offspring *223*

The potential risks of exercise during pregnancy *224*

Agency guidelines on exercise for pregnant women *225*

Our recommendations on exercise for pregnant women *226*

**30** Foods, exposures, and lifestyle risk factors in pregnancy and breastfeeding *227*

Deciphering the messages about foods and exposures to avoid during pregnancy *227*

Foods to avoid during pregnancy and lactation *228*

Maternal behaviours that affect pregnancy outcomes *241*

Our recommendations concerning foods, exposures, and lifestyle risk factors during pregnancy and lactation *247*

**31** Cultural and traditional food practices in pregnancy and breastfeeding *248*

Pregnancy-related diet, food practices, and 'taboos' *248*

Fasting and dieting during pregnancy *250*

Postpartum food practices and beliefs *251*

Summary and recommendations concerning cultural and traditional food practices during pregnancy and lactation *252*

**32** Traditional and herbal remedies in pregnancy and breastfeeding *253*

The use of complementary medicine during pregnancy and lactation *253*

Indications for the use of herbal remedies during pregnancy *253*

Summary and recommendations for the use of traditional and herbal remedies during pregnancy and lactation *255*

**33** Maternal stress in pregnancy and breastfeeding *257*

The stress response during pregnancy *257*

Stress and conception *258*

Stress and pregnancy outcomes *258*

Stress hormones and lactation *259*

Stress and the offspring sex ratio *260*

Summary and recommendations for managing maternal stress during pregnancy and lactation *260*

**34** Effects of maternal age on pregnancy outcomes *261*

Advanced maternal age in pregnancy and breastfeeding *261*

Pregnancy and lactation during adolescence *263*

Summary and recommendations concerning maternal age during pregnancy and lactation *264*

**35** Paternal factors that affect conception and pregnancy *266*

Paternal pre-conception nutrition and lifestyle *266*

Paternal factors and pregnancy outcomes *270*

Our recommendations concerning paternal factors in pregnancy *272*

**Section 4 A management guide—from before conception to weaning**

**36** Guidelines for the pre-conception period *277*

Advice for a healthy pre-pregnancy state *277*

Recommended nutrition and supplementation prior to conception *278*

Weight status and exercise prior to conception *284*

Pre-conception exposures *284*

Diabetes control prior to conception *285*

Recommendations for a pre-conception diet *286*

**37** Guidelines for pregnancy  *287*
　　Guidelines for early pregnancy  *287*
　　Guidelines for middle and late pregnancy  *289*

**38** Guidelines for breastfeeding and weaning  *293*
　　Benefits of breastfeeding  *293*
　　Nutrition for lactation  *294*
　　Dieting during lactation  *299*
　　Exposures during lactation  *300*
　　Infant formulas  *302*
　　Weaning and complementary foods  *306*

　　References  *311*
　　Index  *399*

# Abbreviations

| | | | | |
|---|---|---|---|---|
| %DV | per cent daily value | | NCD | non-communicable disease |
| 25(OH)D | 25-hydroxyvitamin D | | NICE | National Institute for Health and Clinical Excellence |
| AA | arachidonic acid | | | |
| AAP | American Academy of Pediatrics | | NIP | nutrition information panel |
| ACOG | American Congress of Obstetricians and Gynecologists | | NSAID | nonsteroidal anti-inflammatory drug |
| AI | adequate intake | | NTD | neural tube defects |
| ALA | alpha-linolenic acid | | PAH | polycyclic aromatic hydrocarbons |
| alpha-TE | alpha-tocopherol equivalents | | PIH | pregnancy-induced hypertension |
| BMC | bone mineral content | | | |
| BMD | bone mineral density | | PL | pyridoxal |
| BPA | bisphenol A | | PLP | pyridoxal-5'-phosphate |
| CpG | cytosine–guanine dinucleotide | | PROM | premature rupture of membranes |
| DDT | dichloro-diphenyl-trichloroethane | | PTH | parathyroid hormone |
| | | | PUFA | polyunsaturated fatty acid |
| DFE | dietary folate equivalent | | RA | retinoic acid |
| DHA | docosahexaenoic acid | | RAE | retinol activity equivalent |
| EAR | estimated average requirement | | RBC | red blood cell |
| EPA | eicosapentaenoic acid | | RCOG | Royal College of Obstetricians and Gynaecologists |
| FAD | flavin adenine dinucleotide | | | |
| FMN | flavin mononucleotide | | RDA | recommended dietary allowance |
| GDA | guideline daily amounts | | | |
| GDM | gestational diabetes mellitus | | RNI | reference nutrient intake |
| GI | glycaemic index | | ROS | reactive oxygen species |
| Gla | gamma-carboxyglutamate | | sTfR | soluble transferrin receptor |
| HCP | health care professional | | T4 | thyroxine |
| IF | intrinsic factor | | THF | tetrahydrofolate |
| IOM | Institute of Medicine | | THR | thyroid hormone receptors |
| LA | linoleic acid | | THS | thyroid stimulating hormone |
| LRNI | lowest recommended nutrient intake | | UIC | urinary iodine concentration |
| | | | UL | tolerable upper intake level |
| MTHFR | methylenetetrahydrofolate reductase | | UTI | urinary tract infection |
| | | | VAD | vitamin A deficiency |
| NAD | nicotinamide adenine dinucleotide | | | |

# How to use this book

The book is written in four sections.

**Section 1** provides a general introduction to the science underpinning the impact of parental behaviour and particularly the effects of nutrition on pregnancy and offspring health.

**Section 2** details our knowledge of macro- and micronutrients on the mother and her fetus. It provides a reference manual for advice on specific nutrient intakes before and during pregnancy and lactation.

**Section 3** reviews aspects of parental lifestyle that might impact on the fetus and pregnancy outcomes. This includes safe and unsafe foods, exercise, and exposure to potential toxins. It also reviews weight guidelines for pregnancy.

**Section 4** takes the information in the prior sections and presents the health care professional with a checklist of advice according to the stage of pregnancy.

# Section 1

# Fundamentals of healthy nutrition and lifestyle

Although most prospective parents focus efforts during pregnancy on trying to make the right decisions about what to eat, what not to eat, and what else to do or not do, their sources of information are largely informal and often inconsistent, furthering their confusion and anxiety. Moreover, these questions often arise only after pregnancy is diagnosed, despite increasing evidence that nutrition and lifestyle matter not only during an established pregnancy, but also prior to and soon after conception. This section reviews the concepts and emergent science to explain how relatively subtle changes in parental behaviour can affect the outcomes of pregnancy, and why there are echoes of such influences across the whole of life of the offspring.

# Chapter 1

# The importance of nutrition and lifestyle to healthy development

## Developmental origins of health and disease

No one would be surprised by the statement that the healthy growth of the fetus and infant depends on the mother's nutrition, and can be influenced by her lifestyle. Clearly, the components that will form the growing body of the baby must come from the food that the mother consumes or, if from her own body, they will probably have to be replaced. Just as maternal nutrient intake has a positive impact on fetal growth and development, excessive alcohol consumption, smoking, or exposure to environmental toxins, infectious agents, or drugs may have detrimental effects: well-known examples include fetal alcohol syndrome, deafness of the child resulting from measles infection during the first half of pregnancy, and the limb deformities from thalidomide.

What is less well known is that such effects are extreme examples of a spectrum of processes that operate in all pregnancies and during infancy. This concept has evolved over the last few decades, as a result of very extensive research in many settings around the world. It has been conceptualized in several ways, one of which has become particularly influential—the 'developmental origins of health and disease' paradigm. This is the concept that the early development of each individual, starting from the time of conception, sets the scene for their future health and the risk of certain diseases from which they may suffer later. This topic has been the subject of many reviews and books [1–7].

There are two important aspects of this concept which should be explained at the outset, because they have implications for understanding and applying much of the information in this book. The first is that the development of the embryo (up until about 12 weeks of gestation), fetus, and infant is far from automatic. At a previous time when scientists believed that development was simply a process of assembling biological components sequentially on the basis of a genetic programme, there seemed little scope for the developing individual to play much of a role in the process any more than a car on the assembly line of a factory can control its manufacture. However, this is now known to be incorrect; while it is true that there are genetic programmes for the assembly of tissues, organs, and the layout of the body's components, the developing organism's own biology has very significant control over how those processes operate. For example, it can alter the number of filtering units it will form in its kidneys, the number of muscle cells in its heart, and the number of fat cells in its body and, once formed, these numbers will essentially be set for life.

The 'decisions' that the developing fetus makes about these numbers are embedded in its biology and are based on information it receives from its mother and, through her, about the wider environment, in terms of nutrition and physical activity, but also about stress and other aspects of lifestyle. These biological decisions are to a large degree final, so they have long-term consequences for health and disease. Research has begun to reveal how these processes operate physiologically, highlighting the importance of this period in our lives when our innate biology exerts far more control over our destiny than was previously thought.

The second aspect is related to the first. It used to be thought that, because of an apparently fixed genetic programme of development, the fetus would take whatever it needed from its mother and would be seriously underdeveloped if for some reason this was not available. However, just as it is now clear that the developing fetus can make 'decisions' about its development, so the mother is involved in a 'dialogue' with it about such decisions. Greater demand for a particular nutrient, for example, may be met by physiological changes in the mother and the placenta to supply it; or by a signal to the fetus that these demands are excessive in terms of the mother's nutrition, body composition, etc., and so the demand should be tempered and development altered accordingly. There is far more active cooperation between the mother and her fetus or infant than we used to think—and sometimes there is competition between them too if their conflicting demands cannot be met. When there are twins or triplets, the plot thickens still further.

We emphasize that these processes are completely natural or physiological and that they operate in all pregnancies, not just in those with particular problems. The processes are part of normal human biology and operate across a wide spectrum of development. This is reassuring, but it also presents both parents and health care professionals with some problems. For example, it is not always possible to give a fixed recommendation about the daily intake of a micronutrient. It should be possible to suggest a *range*, but the precise level will depend on many other factors that may interact and probably cannot be measured. The best advice is by necessity only an approximation; it is nonetheless valuable and important for future health.

# Nutrition: providing the building blocks of development and the fuel for metabolism

From an ecological perspective, humans are a generalist species; that is, humans can live in a wide range of environments across the globe rather than being confined to a relatively small niche environment, as are many other species. It is therefore perhaps not surprising that we are omnivorous and both can and want to consume a wide range of dietary components. Good fetal and infant nutrition, whether derived from the mother via the placenta before birth or ingested by mouth after birth, consists of the macronutrients protein, carbohydrates, and fats needed for building the fundamental components of the body, and micronutrients such as vitamins and trace elements that are essential structural components and cofactors in metabolic processes.

During development the need for nutrients is correspondingly increased in order to provide for growth, but the role of energetic macronutrients and micronutrients in providing the key factors to support basal metabolic processes must not be ignored. Examples would include the need for adequate trans-placental flow of glucose to support the energetic demands of the fetal brain, heart, and other organs, and the provision of thiamine (vitamin $B_1$) as a cofactor for oxidative decarboxylation of pyruvic acid and alpha-ketoglutaric acid as part of the energetic pathway. The daily nutrient requirements of the fetus are the subject of section 2 of this book.

## Essential vs non-essential components of nutrition

Essential nutrients are those that cannot be endogenously synthesized. Inadequate intake of these nutrients will lead in the longer term to deficiencies that will be associated with ill health or disease. A well-known example is vitamin C, a deficiency of which causes scurvy. Humans and our relatives the great apes must ingest vitamin C from the diet (primarily from fruit and vegetables), although interestingly this is not true of other primates, which can synthesize vitamin C endogenously. It appears that at some point in our evolutionary past, when abundant fruit and vegetable intake was a feature of our diets, the ability to synthesize vitamin C was lost due to a loss-of-function mutation in a synthetic enzyme [8].

Similar considerations apply to 9 of the 21 amino acids, which are therefore essential dietary components in humans. However during development, when nutrient requirements for growth are large, some nutrients become conditionally essential. This is the case for the amino acid glycine, an important component of one-carbon metabolism, for which fetal requirements in late gestation

**Table 1.1** Essential and conditionally essential amino acids in fetal development

| Essential | Conditionally essential | Non-essential |
| --- | --- | --- |
| Histidine | Arginine | Alanine |
| Isoleucine | Cysteine | Aspartate |
| Leucine | Glutamine | Serine |
| Lysine | Glycine | |
| Methionine | Proline | |
| Phenylalanine | Taurine | |
| Threonine | Tyrosine | |
| Tryptophan | | |
| Valine | | |

are large enough for it to become an essential nutritional component. Table 1.1 lists the essential and conditionally essential amino acids for the human fetus. Similarly there are essential polyunsaturated fatty acids, alpha-linolenic acid (an omega-3 fatty acid), and linoleic acid (an omega-6 fatty acid), but other fatty acids become conditionally essential during development; this includes docosahexaenoic acid, which is also an omega-3 fatty acid.

## What is a 'balanced' diet?

One of the challenges of nutritional science is that food is not just the composite of nutrients within it. The availability of nutrients is dependent on the food chemistry, its digestibility, the action of the gut microbiota, and gastrointestinal physiology. Thus, while it is easy to consider the post-absorptive requirements of the body in physiological terms, it is more complex to consider the nutritional requirements of the individual. Even where micronutrients are given as supplements, it is important to be aware of the potential interplay between those supplements and food. For example, phytates that are found in whole grains or unleavened bread can interfere with the absorption of calcium and other micronutrients.

It is important to note that diet and nutrition are not synonymous. A balanced diet means that all the nutritional requirements of metabolism, growth, immune function, etc. are being met. While variations in dietary intake in the short term can be tolerated through the use of body stores, in the longer term an unbalanced diet will lead to poor health and disease. For vitamin C, the half-life for levels in the body is about 20 days, so the effects of severe deficiency will be expected to appear after about 2–3 months if intake is zero, as found in sailors on long-distance voyages in the past.

A diet may be unbalanced either because of a deficiency or excess of macro- or micronutrients. Many micronutrients have complex dose/response relations. Too little can lead to a deficiency disease, but too much can lead to toxic effects. In some cases, such as for vitamin A, there is a relatively narrow safe band of exposure during development. Folic acid provides a good example, as low folate status in a pregnant woman during early gestation is associated with neural tube defects and other congenital anomalies in her fetus. However, sustained intake of very high levels of folic acid in adults is associated with greater risk of some forms of cancer (e.g. colon cancer) [9]. There is thus a healthy range for folate status. In other cases, such as for vitamin D, recent research suggests that previous recommendations for pregnancy may have been set at too low a level. These issues are discussed at length in section 2, where we analyse the specific micro- and macronutrient needs of pregnant and breastfeeding women and dissect a complex and sometimes confusing literature and a confusion of guidelines.

Similar considerations apply to macronutrients. Consumption of fat is needed for the provision of the essential polyunsaturated fatty acids, but excessive fatty food intake is associated with obesity and cardiometabolic disease. Both excess and deficient carbohydrate intakes during pregnancy can impact the mother and fetus. Very high protein intakes during pregnancy are associated with fetal growth restriction [10] (see chapter 4).

## Fundamentals of metabolic control

The body's metabolic processes are generally tightly regulated so that supply meets demand, and this control operates at several points along the metabolic pathway. For example, lower levels of blood glucose lead to hepatic gluconeogenesis to meet demand; when blood glucose levels rise following a meal, the rise in insulin secretion by the beta cells of the pancreas and the fall in glucagon secretion by the alpha cells lead to increased glucose uptake by tissues such as skeletal muscle, thereby providing a stimulus to carbohydrate metabolism or deposition, such as storage as glycogen. Carbohydrate metabolism interacts with other aspects of metabolism, such as the effects of fatty acids on the Krebs cycle, and these processes in turn interact with other body homeostatic mechanisms. Often this involves endocrine processes, for example, the regulation of appetite by leptin and GLP1 or the control of body fat stores.

Contrast this with the fetus, which cannot undertake gluconeogenesis until very late in pregnancy when liver enzymes mature and therefore depends on the supply of glucose across the placenta. When this is inadequate, fetal growth is restricted to conserve energy for cardiac, brain, and adrenal gland function. When it is excessive the excess glucose is stored as fat—hence the macrosomia seen in infants of diabetic mothers.

Despite small fluctuations on a day-to-day basis, it is clear that metabolic control is finely tuned, as body weight remains remarkably constant over long periods of time. Recent work investigating the underlying mechanisms has demonstrated how we, and indeed many other animal species, defend our protein requirement target more vigorously than we do other nutrient requirement targets. As Fig. 1.1 shows, if humans consume a diet of low protein content for a period of time, they increase their total food intake to achieve their preset protein target at the expense of ingesting excess carbohydrate and fat. This so-called protein leverage process [11] may explain why certain diets predispose to obesity. There is also increasing evidence that appetite control and food and taste preference is set early in life for life. This can be influenced by the flavours in the foods that mothers eat in pregnancy and during lactation and by the nature of weaning [12, 13].

Aspects of metabolism change across the life course, as does body composition. A key component of the metabolic adaptation to pregnancy is the development of mild insulin resistance and changes in appetite control in the mother [14, 15]. Both are induced by placental hormones including placental lactogen and growth hormone [15]. This mild insulin resistance is postulated to ensure enhanced and reliable transfer of glucose to the fetus while the mother's metabolism becomes more dependent on lipids [16]. Thus, as pregnancy progresses, insulin sensitivity decreases in the maternal peripheral tissues, which results in

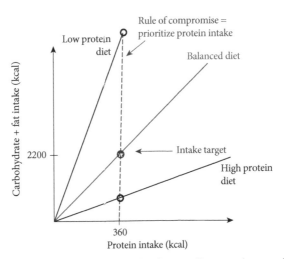

**Fig. 1.1** The protein leverage hypothesis. The diagram illustrates human dietary patterns, wherein protein intake is prioritised over intake of carbohydrates and fat. If the diet contains a low proportion of protein, the total food intake will increase (i.e. excess carbohydrate and fat will be consumed) in order to reach a target protein intake. Adapted from S. J. Simpson and D. Raubenheimer, Obesity: the protein leverage hypothesis, *Obesity Reviews*, Volume 6, Issue 2, pp.133–142, Copyright © 2005 with permission from John Wiley and Sons, DOI: 10.1111/j.1467–789X.2005.00178.x

the mild hyperglycaemia and insulin resistance associated with normal pregnancy. However, in women who are already prone to insulin resistance because of obesity or developmental factors, this physiological tendency to insulin resistance becomes exaggerated and the result is gestational diabetes mellitus (GDM).

GDM has been reported to affect 4–7 per cent of pregnancies in Caucasian women, and the incidence is somewhat higher (8–15%) and rising rapidly in Asian women, to over 25 per cent in some urban populations [17–19]. This is a particular concern because women who develop GDM are at a high risk of subsequently developing type 2 diabetes mellitus. Furthermore, their offspring have a high risk of developing obesity, impaired glucose tolerance, hypertension, and dyslipidaemia [20]. Uncontrolled hyperglycaemia in pregnancy is associated with some fetal abnormalities, for example, abnormalities of the heart [21], and carries a risk for the newborn of neurological damage from neonatal hypoglycaemia [22]. Maternal glucose intolerance that is milder than that in overt diabetes mellitus can also lead to adverse outcomes; [23] indeed, maternal glucose control has been shown to correlate with maternal, perinatal, and neonatal outcomes in a continuous linear association across both normal and pathological ranges [24]. New guidelines published by the International Association of the Diabetes and Pregnancy Study Groups therefore suggest a lower threshold for diagnosis of GDM [25].

Human metabolism even changes as we develop in early life. For example, the fetal heart depends on the supply of glucose for its metabolism, but within a short period after birth, it switches to the utilization of fatty acids [26]. There are long-term functional implications for this switch, as it occurs at the point at which the number of cardiomyocytes is effectively set for life as they undergo terminal differentiation. Moreover, the switch can have later consequences in diabetes, when the exposure of the heart to high glucose levels leads to the deposition of fat in the heart rather than metabolic consumption of glucose.

## The importance of energy balance

### Over-nutrition

Over-nutrition before and during pregnancy is common in developed countries, where there is an increasing prevalence of overweight and obesity and excessive weight gain among pregnant women [27, 28]. It is also becoming clear that obesity is rising rapidly and can coexist with under-nutrition in low- and middle-income countries undergoing nutritional transition [29]. Deposition of some fat in a woman during pregnancy is a natural process to provide energy stores to support lactation. This fat deposition results in part from the insulin resistance that develops in pregnancy in response to the secretion of placental hormones, as discussed above. However, excessive weight gain should be avoided, as over-nutrition leads to metabolic imbalances in both mother and fetus, with long-term adverse health consequences. For instance, over-weight women or those who gain too much weight during pregnancy have higher risks of developing GDM and possibly pre-eclampsia, and of their infants being large for gestational age (LGA) [30]. A positive association has been observed between excessive weight gain in pregnancy (>12.5 kg) and the risk of later childhood overweight, especially when the weight gain exceeds 20 kg [31]. Chapter 28 covers the impact of maternal body weight composition before and during pregnancy in more detail.

### Under-nutrition

Poor dietary intake during pregnancy remains a challenge in low- and mid-dle-income countries. Due in part to low socioeconomic status, low diet qual-ity, high intensity of agricultural labour, and frequent reproductive cycles, pregnant women in developing countries are particularly at risk for malnutri-tion. As with over-nutrition, inadequate nutrition during pregnancy has life-long health impacts on the offspring. During the Dutch Hunger Winter of 1944–1945, food supply to the western part of the Netherlands was cut dra-matically (with daily caloric intake restricted to 400–800 calories). Babies born to mothers who experienced this famine in late gestation were frequently of low birthweight and had decreased glucose tolerance at the age of 50 com-pared with individuals born the year before or after the famine [32]. Similarly, fetal and/or early postnatal life exposure to war-inflicted famine in Nigeria (1967–1970) or the Great Famine in China (1959–1961) was associated with an increased risk of adult hypertension [33, 34].

Lesser degrees of under-nutrition may also have effects. In the Gambia, where there is a marked seasonal variation in caloric intake, women who conceive during the 'hungry' season give birth to babies who are slightly preterm and weigh less on average than those conceived during the 'harvest' season [35, 36]. Those born during the hungry season have markedly shorter life expectancies, although this mortality difference, which is related primarily to infection, does not appear until adulthood [37, 38].

## The importance of physical activity

Adequate levels of physical activity are necessary for both cardiovascular fitness and for maintaining a healthy body composition. In non-pregnant adults 30 min-utes of vigorous exercise, five days a week, is recommended [39]. In chapter 29 we discuss the recommendations for pregnancy. Even lower levels of physical activity and reduction of sedentary lifestyle have beneficial effects on cardiovascular function and reduce the risk of cardiovascular disease [40]. In addition, exercise has beneficial effects on the skeletal muscle groups used, altering their metabolism and increasing the proportion of metabolically active fast twitch fibres [41]. Physical exercise is also recognized to act as a suppressor of appetite and hence can be a useful adjunct to dietary guidelines in weight loss programmes.

Individuals vary in their propensity to undertake vigorous physical exercise, and also in the extent to which it produces beneficial effects in them. In addition there is variation in metabolism not associated with exercise, sometimes termed non-exercising active thermogenesis [42]. Fidgeting and other minor body activities can be important sources of energy consumption, especially in children, and probably interact with other forms of energy consumption. The processes by which such interactions are regulated are unknown.

## Avoidance of risky exposures

One of the biggest concerns that potential parents have is about the safety of their food. Unpasteurized cheeses can contain the bacterium *Listeria* that can cross the placenta and cause fetal loss or preterm labour [43]. Other foods can contain potential toxins. The most well-known toxins in foodstuffs are those thought of as poisons (e.g. the atropine from deadly-nightshade berries, botulinum toxin from some types of poorly cooked meat, or mycotoxins associated with fungal contamination of poorly stored grains). Fungal mycotoxins are thought to be a significant source of stunting in some less developed countries [44]. Identification of safe and unsafe foods can be confusing for the mother-to-be, with the internet providing a very broad range of seemingly contradictory advice. In chapter 30 we provide a coherent set of information on such issues for health care professionals (HCPs) to provide to parents.

Components of modern diets can also be toxic if consumed in excessive quantities, the most well known being alcohol. However there is now considerable concern over other toxins in the environment that may find their way into foodstuffs even though they do not immediately exert obvious harmful effects on health. There are calls for the identification, measurement, and control of such substances in the environment although, with a few exceptions, there are at present no recommendations on their intake or exposure during development [45]. This is a very complex area of science where new measurement techniques allow extremely low concentrations to be measured, and yet there is no way to assess the significance of these concentrations.

While we would advocate the adoption of the precautionary principle, it is nevertheless easy to be alarmist without scientific justification—so a more balanced pragmatic approach is necessary [46–48]. For some exposures, however, there is no debate: attention to the toxic effects of smoking should not need reinforcing, although regrettably tobacco consumption is increasing in many low- and middle-income countries, especially in women and children. Smoking produces detrimental effects on the growth of many organs and systems in the fetal and neonatal body, including the brain, lungs, and cardiovascular system and produces long-term effects on health and the risk of disease in those individuals exposed to secondary smoke.

## Opportunities and challenges

Parents universally want the best for their children and hence the opportunities to reap the benefits of lifestyle and nutrition advice from HCPs are substantial. But while there is often no lack of motivation, finding a way of reinforcing the message about healthy diet and lifestyle over what may be a relatively sustained period in what can be a complex social milieu is not so easy. An important opportunity is linked to the health benefits for the parents themselves. Even relatively small changes in body mass index can produce beneficial effects on cardiovascular function. Positive messages derived from such measurements can help sustain the healthy lifestyle message.

Good maternal diet and body composition reduce the risk of pregnancy complications such as GDM, pre-eclampsia, or preterm birth. Associated problems such as fetal macrosomia, shoulder dystocia, and the adverse cerebral effects of neonatal hypoglycaemia are also important. Coupled with the effects of healthy early development on promoting healthy postnatal growth and development and reducing the later risk of non-communicable diseases in the offspring, there are clear and simple health messages to be transmitted to parents-to-be.

However, there are often barriers to changing diet and lifestyle in many at-risk groups of the population. Consumption of a healthy, balanced diet depends on access to retail outlets where healthy foods can be purchased, adequate resources to purchase the items, and knowledge of how to prepare and cook them. These three conditions are often not met and HCPs have to be aware that innovative solutions must sometimes be found to overcome these difficulties. Similar considerations can apply to exercise promotion, if it is perceived that this requires access and membership to a gym or other sporting facility that may be difficult, unacceptable, or unaffordable for some families.

The importance of cultural issues should not be underestimated. For example, in some cultures where exposure of the body is unacceptable among women, it is difficult to advocate some forms of sport or physical exercise, such as swimming. Brisk walking might be an alternative but this is sometimes challenging in hot climates and women are rightly concerned about safety issues. Another example is that covering the body and limited exposure to sunlight is responsible for the relatively high levels of vitamin D deficiency in women of reproductive age in some countries. There are also very distinct cultural attitudes to body shape.

As will be noted throughout this book, many of the benefits of diet and lifestyle result from healthy behaviours before pregnancy, and importantly this applies both to the mother and the father (see chapter 35 for information on paternal factors). However in many societies a substantial number of pregnancies are unplanned and, by the time that the couple knows that they have conceived and the women has seen a HCP, the opportunity for maximum effect of behaviour change has been lost. It is true that healthy diet and moderate exercise during pregnancy, coupled with appropriate weight gain especially during late gestation, confer benefits but sometimes these are too late for maximal effects on the health of the next generation.

A major focus in contemporary global health is therefore on adolescence, with a view to promoting healthy lifestyle before conception (see chapter 34 for specific consideration of adolescents). Adolescents have received less attention to their health in recent decades than have younger children, despite the fact that they form a substantial proportion of the world's population. Collectively, adolescents have a powerful capacity to instigate social change in their families or among their peer group. The challenge, however, is achieving a behaviour change in this group.

In many societies adolescents will not necessarily be attending school or other full-time education, and this is particularly true of girls after marriage or when they become pregnant. In addition, research has shown that health promotion initiatives in schools are relatively ineffective compared with learning outside the classroom activities. There is therefore a need to develop community-based health promotion activities outside the formal educational setting, where adolescents and young adults are more likely to engage more positively with the health promotion agenda.

The long-term goal is to promote what is termed health literacy, that is, the empowerment or self-efficacy needed to enable individuals to make choices about a healthy lifestyle for themselves, to influence their peers and their families, and to access health care and other services when appropriate. The wider issue is that even though adolescents and young parents may be currently healthy, their individual risks of later disease vary, because they lie on different trajectories of accumulating risk in their lives (see Fig. 1.2). Promoting health literacy in terms of nutrition and lifestyle is not only important for their future health but also so that they give their children the best start in life.

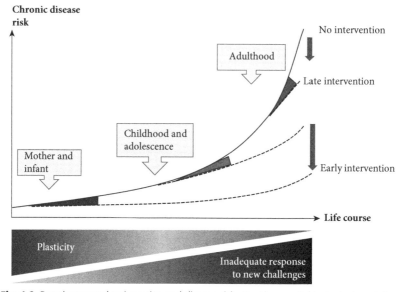

**Fig. 1.2** Developmental trajectories and disease risk. Developmental trajectories established in early life influence the response of the individual to later exposures, such as adult lifestyle. Risk increases throughout the life course as a result of declining plasticity and the resulting accumulative effects of inadequate responses to new challenges. The trajectory is influenced by factors such as the mother's diet and body composition before and during pregnancy, and fetal, infant and childhood nutrition and development. Early intervention can reduce later disease risk. Adapted from *Trends in Endocrinology and Metabolism*, Volume 21, Issue 4, Keith M. Godfrey et al., Developmental origins of metabolic disease: life course and intergenerational perspectives, pp.199–205, Copyright © 2010, with permission from Elsevier, <http://www.sciencedirect.com/science/journal/10432760>

Many current initiatives employ digitally based techniques to provide information, to engage adolescents and prospective parents, and to provide the interactive learning necessary to sustain change. Even in many low- and middle-income country settings, adolescents have access to smartphones or other tools for accessing the internet and are willing to engage with virtual communities and entertainment-based information provision services. There are therefore many positive ways in which HCPs can engage with young people to promote a healthy lifestyle.

Set against this, we have to recognize the role of the food and drinks industries, which not only produce a substantial proportion of the world's food but also sometimes target advertising and marketing techniques at young people. HCPs will have to play their part in addressing this problem. In some circumstances regulatory change may be needed, as well as better cooperation between public and private sectors so that desired goals can be achieved. There may therefore have to be hopefully more truces as well as battles, but in both situations it is hoped that the information provided in this book will assist the HCP in reaching better outcomes.

# Chapter 2

# Conceptual background to healthy growth and development

## Development is affected by early environment

### Growth

Growth of the body does not occur at a constant rate throughout development—there are spurts in the relative growth rate during both fetal life and adolescence, and not all tissues and organs develop to the same pattern (see Fig. 2.1). In utero, measures of fetal growth are obtained by ultrasound and necessarily only relate to body dimensions such as abdominal circumference, head circumference, head volume, crown-rump length or femoral length. These are useful because they give an indication of growth of the liver (abdominal circumference), brain (head circumference or head volume) and skeleton (crown-rump length or femoral length). Nutritional and other lifestyle factors such as smoking can affect these growth parameters.

Fetal growth is usually assessed by means of a growth chart. It is important to realize that the usefulness of such charts depends on a range of factors. First, as they are related to gestational age, knowing this age accurately is important. Frequently, however, the time of the women's last menstrual period is not known precisely. There can be a tendency to favour the ultrasound assessment of fetal age over the women's estimate of the date of conception, but this too can be problematic: it has been shown that first trimester fetal growth varies with maternal nutrition [49] and so this diminishes the accuracy of ultrasound dating measurements. Further the growth of male vs female fetuses differs from early gestation, and discordance in growth between dichorionic twins has been observed as early as 11–14 weeks gestation [50, 51]. In addition, there can be population differences in fetal growth, for genetic and other reasons. In this respect the derivation of standardized global fetal growth charts may need to be viewed with caution.

There are a number of circumstances that can affect fetal growth but are not necessarily associated with ill health. The most obvious example is multiple conception, where twins are each smaller than singleton babies at birth, and triplets smaller still. Male fetuses grow slightly faster than do female fetuses,

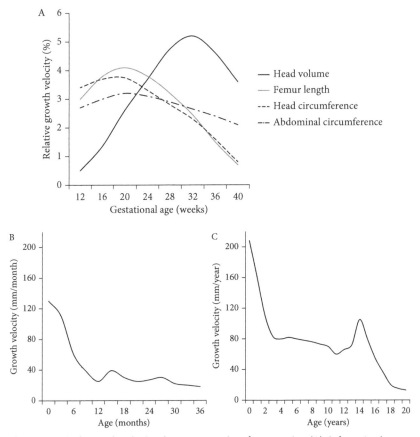

**Fig. 2.1** Typical growth velocity changes over time for gestation (A), infancy/early childhood (B), and childhood/adolescence (C). Panel A adapted from *Archives of Disease in Childhood Fetal Neonatal*, E. Bertino et al., Fetal growth velocity: kinetic, clinical, and biological aspects, Volume 74, Issue 1, pp. F10–F15, Copyright © 1996, with permission from BMJ Publishing Group Ltd.

and the fetus of a woman's first pregnancy grows slightly more slowly than subsequent siblings, especially in later gestation. This latter effect can be summarized as the operation of 'maternal constraint' processes [52], by which a woman down-regulates to a degree the growth of her fetus to ensure safe passage through the pelvic canal at birth. However, maternal constraint is overridden when maternal glucose levels are high: excessive glucose crosses to the fetus, as placental glucose transport is not saturable, and sets off a chain of hormonal changes that lead to increased fetal adiposity. Hence, offspring of women with gestational diabetes tend to be adipose.

In adopting a bipedal posture during our evolutionary past, and also evolving to have large brains, humans have a much tighter fit of the fetal head through the pelvis at delivery than our nearest cousins, the chimpanzees. For this reason the fetal head must turn during vertex delivery, and humans are the only mammalian species in which a birth attendant is usually present to assist the delivery. Even so, the risk of obstructed labour remains significant and, in the absence of advanced health care, is associated with a higher risk of maternal and fetal death and other complications such as fistulation of the genito-urinary tracts.

While these issues remain a major health problem in some low-income settings, they are also important to remember in other situations. Many women still fear the delivery process, with good reason. It remains associated with a high risk of haemorrhage, puerperal fever, and death of the woman in low- and middle-income countries. Some women attempt to reduce fetal growth by dieting (e.g. in some countries by avoiding milk as a source of calcium) or smoking in the hope of having an easier delivery. This is not only ineffective but can have longer-term detrimental effects on the health of the child.

Most parents are concerned about whether the postnatal growth of their infant is adequate. Usually this is thought of purely in terms of weight, but the weight-to-length ponderal index (weight/length$^3$) in the infant, and BMI (weight/height$^2$) in older children are more important. Infants lose weight (largely from water and some fat loss) in the first few days after birth and then gain weight subsequently. Patterns of body composition change in children in the first years of life, with an overall trend for fat mass to decline followed by its return—the so-called 'adiposity rebound'—by about age 4 to 6 years. There is much debate about the importance of these patterns to later adiposity and risk of non-communicable disease (NCD); for example, crossing two or more major growth centiles in the first six months is associated with a later risk of obesity [53]. The concept of the 'fat baby as a healthy baby' is now less appropriate for this reason, at least in developed countries, as it dates from the time when under-nutrition and infection were prevalent and the energetic stores present in fat were critical to survival.

## Body composition

Body composition is more important than simply a measure of size. Humans are the fattest mammals at birth—it is thought that this is to provide a metabolic buffer for the energetically expensive processes of thermoregulation and brain growth against the detrimental effects of malnutrition in infancy [54]. During prenatal life, inadequate nutrition or oxygen supply to the fetus can result from diseases such as pre-eclampsia, infections such as malaria, and poor placental function, and these problems are often interlinked.

In the face of such a challenge, the fetus reduces growth. In early gestation, this is usually manifest as a reduction in the growth of most organs but, in later gestation when the fetus is larger and its demands are correspondingly greater, the growth of specific organs including the brain, heart, and adrenal glands (the latter being important for cortisol production and organ maturation) is preserved at the expense of others. These changes in growth are usually preceded by changes in organ blood flow, measurable by ultrasound as a reduction in perfusion of muscle, kidneys, the lower body, and gut and either maintenance or an increase in flow to the head, neck, and heart. Placental blood flow is usually preserved under these conditions: in extreme conditions it may be reduced but this is likely to be an indication of a problem (i.e. placental dysfunction) rather than part of a coordinated response by the fetus. Unbalanced maternal nutrition leads to changes in the relative flow of blood to the fetal liver and blood which bypasses the liver through the ductus venosus, even at the expense of blood flow to the heart and brain [55]. This is thought to affect long-term metabolic physiology through effects on liver metabolism.

## Function

Cellular differentiation, tissue deposition, organ size, and higher-level neuroendocrine control systems are all affected by developmental factors, such as nutrition. Some organs show an ability to regenerate after damage or the effects of daily wear and tear. While this is a feature of the gut and skin, for example, it is not true of the heart and brain. Newer evidence suggests that these organs do possess stem cells that may under some conditions be induced to form new neurons or cardiomyocytes, respectively, although the extent of such repair appears to be limited.

Once a critical period for organ growth has occurred, or the set point of its control has been established, it is difficult or even impossible to change the outcome. For example, aspects of appetite are set very early in life, as are the levels of many neuroendocrine feedback loops such as that regulating cortisol production. These two concepts—that functional control systems are set early in response to cues received in early life, and that there is a critical period after which the setting can be difficult or impossible to change—are critical to the new approach to preventative developmental health, which is the context in which this book is written. This is not to say that opportunities for later preventative intervention do not exist, but these may be viewed as secondary interventions. Primary interventions to promote healthy early development have potentially greater impact.

## Developmental plasticity

Developmental plasticity refers to that set of changes in the development of an individual during early life in response to variation in the environment, especially the maternal state or conditions in infancy. Developmental plasticity can be considered normative and physiological, and evolved to allow the fetus and infant to tune its development to the environment in which it will live.

It is important to appreciate that these processes of developmental plasticity are ubiquitous. Evolved processes can only be adapted to the environment in which evolution occurred. Thus, because of the dramatic change in the way we now live our lives, our evolved biology is now almost inevitably mismatched to some extent to the world in which we now live [56]. But because this biology is also affected by the developmental experience affecting normative plasticity, the degree of mismatch can be enhanced, and this too can have consequences. Thus, how we start our lives can influence our relative risk of later developing various diseases (see Fig. 1.2). This is not to say that the disease process starts during development; rather, it is the developmental environment that sets the adequacy, or otherwise, of our responses to later challenges, and thus disease risk.

There are many developmental contexts which can affect the propensity for later disease risk, but which we would not normally view as 'abnormal'. For example, it appears that the later risk of obesity, diabetes, and heart disease is greater in first-born infants than in their subsequent siblings, in twins, in infants born slightly preterm or post-term, and in both infants of teenage mothers and older women. The increasing use of assisted reproductive technology is also revealing that children conceived by this method have a greater risk of these health problems either because of the technology itself or the associated context of greater maternal age and other factors. The effects may not be large, but it is important to be aware of them because it may influence the advice given to parents postnatally regarding the optimal growth patterns for their children.

Developmental plasticity can be understood from the perspective of evolutionary biology, which is driven by the need to reproduce so as to pass our genes to the next generation. However, what is best for survival to reproduce may not be best for health. It is clear from much theoretical and practical research that aspects of life-course biology set up during early development have important effects on the ability of the individual to respond to challenges in their adult life [57–59]. For example, the metabolic control processes established during development alter the amount of fat an adult individual will lay down in response to consuming a high glycaemic index diet, and thus their risk of obesity, diabetes, and the metabolic syndrome. Similar considerations apply to aspects of appetite control and perhaps even the propensity to exercise.

Experimental and clinical research has revealed some of the processes by which the environment of the embryo and fetus affects the characteristics of the individual. These characteristics are collectively called the *phenotype*. It is important to distinguish the phenotype from the *genotype*, which refers to the pattern of genes in the DNA inherited from the mother and father. There has been a tendency to view the role of genes and the environment as effectively independent. This is reflected in the rather trite but frequently used 'nature–nurture' dichotomy. What has become clear in recent years is that the concept of separating the genetic from the environmental, while a useful heuristic, is actually flawed. It turns out that the developmental environment can affect gene function in effectively fixed ways, and in ways that may cross generations [57, 60].

While we have tended to only think of two kinds of inheritance—that which is fixed in the genes through polymorphisms and other fixed genetic variation, and that which is culturally inherited (what we learn from our families and societies and pass on to the next generation; e.g. religion, language)—it is now clear that inheritance can occur in other ways. As we have already indicated, what the mother does can influence her offspring's biology, and because the oocyte formed when mother herself was a fetus, this environmental can affect her grandchildren. We term these phenomena *parental effects*. There are intriguing hints that this may even pass to more distant generations.

## Underlying mechanisms—the science of epigenetics

The term epigenetics refers to a number of biological mechanisms by which gene expression is altered in a stable manner without changing the underlying DNA sequence of the organism. This may involve methylation, acetylation, ubiquination, and other modifications at specific amino acid residues, or modifications to histones, around which the DNA is coiled. Epigenetics is central to understanding both developmental plasticity and why parental and intrauterine experience can have both short- and long-term effects.

Developmental plasticity allows the fetus and infant to take information from its mother and adjust its development in response to that information. Signals from the mother such as nutrients, hormones, and metabolites reach the developing embryo or fetus across the placenta, or the infant through the milk, and induce specific epigenetic changes which in turn drive developmental processes that are reflected in structure or function. Epigenetic processes allow one genotype to produce multiple phenotypes; thus, the physical and functional differences between identical (homozygous) twins can be explained by differences in their epigenetic profiles.

Genes are often thought of as discrete entities within the genome—particulate structures that are passed from parents to offspring. The definition of a gene has, however, become more complex. A gene can be considered as a functional segment of DNA, but whereas in the past genes were defined by their coding for messenger RNA (mRNA), which in turn was translated into proteins, we now know that many genes code for mRNAs that do not function as templates for protein production but as active molecules in their own right as regulators of gene action by interaction with DNA or other RNAs. These are called microRNAs or non-coding RNAs. Thus the simplistic model of gene to mRNA to protein has been replaced by an increasingly complex one involving molecular mechanisms by which gene expression is regulated (see Fig. 2.2). While 80 per cent of the human genome does not code for protein sequences, this is not 'junk DNA', as it was once termed, but contains many active DNA sequences that operate to regulate varied aspects of gene expression through the production of these microRNAs.

The most well-known epigenetic process is DNA methylation, in which a methyl group is attached by specific enzymes primarily to the cytosine of a cytosine–guanine dinucleotide (CpG) site. CpGs lie along the gene in particular patterns, and it is this patterning that provides multiple forms of epigenetic control. Some CpGs lie in clusters called CpG islands. Their function is important in determining whether a gene is turned on or off in a particular cell type. Other CpGs are more solitary and lie at a site where a transcription factor binds—these sites appear to be particularly important in developmental plasticity. Parental imprinting is a particular form of epigenetic change where a gene is silenced by methylation if it is derived from one parent but not if it comes from the other parent. Imprinted genes appear to be particularly important for placental function and some aspects of brain function. Loss of imprinting is

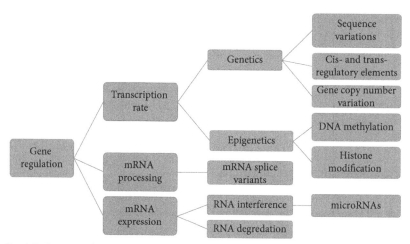

**Fig. 2.2** Gene regulatory mechanisms. Variations in gene expression occur via multiple mechanisms at the DNA level to control transcription rate, or at the RNA level to control mRNA expression, stability, or processing.

associated with some diseases such as Beckwith–Wiedemann syndrome. More recently it has been shown that DNA methylation has a higher level of complexity (e.g. some CpGs are hydroxy-methylated rather than simply methylated), and cytosines outside of CpGs may also be methylated.

DNA itself is coiled around protein cores which are termed histones, and the pattern of coiling makes the DNA either very tightly packed or more open. When it is more open, it is easier for transcriptional factors to bind and so for gene expression to occur. The pattern of coiling is very complex, and chemical modifications to histones affect the coiling and thus the function of DNA. This represents a second major type of epigenetic modification. DNA methylation and histone modifications are biochemically linked because they both have the effect of changing the conformation of the coiled DNA and thus its functionality. These complicated processes involve multiple enzymatic controls, and specificity appears to be conferred in part by the action of the small, non-coding RNAs. In turn, some of these can bind directly to DNA and thus affect coiling, giving another level of epigenetic control.

Epigenetic processes serve multiple functions, from X-chromosome inactivation in the female, to mediating cell differentiation and the induction of specific features of the cell. The specific details differ between these processes and those of plasticity. X-chromosome inactivation is clearly irreversible, and it has generally been assumed that this is also the case for epigenetic change associated with developmental plasticity. However, experimental studies suggest that this may not be completely correct [61].

The critical point to appreciate is that the developing organism is particularly sensitive to epigenetic modifications—indeed, some are essential for development because it is epigenetic change that allows the omnipotent zygote to differentiate into hundreds of distinct cell types as organogenesis proceeds. Moreover, epigenetic processes can be influenced by aspects of maternal lifestyle, such as diet and stress levels, and these more subtle maternally mediated epigenetic effects can have significant outcomes on offspring health and disease risk [62]. It is also clear that paternal lifestyle factors such as smoking can have epigenetic effects via the sperm.

## Critical periods and plasticity

The concept of critical periods is well known to the obstetrician and paediatrician—they are periods when the developing individual is particularly sensitive in some respect to external stimuli because a particular organ or system is developing at that time. It seems likely that epigenetic processes are central to mediating such plasticity. It may therefore be that, during such periods, the possibility exists of reversing undesirable changes, for example, if inappropriate epigenetic changes have occurred in some developing fetal tissues as a result of unbalanced maternal nutrition during pregnancy. Indeed in animals, proof-of-principle reversal of epigenetic changes in offspring has been produced by neonatal hormone treatment [63, 64]. We stress that this is purely experimental, and such studies should not be taken to provide evidence that such interventions should be tested in humans. However they do provide strong support for the concept that epigenetic changes can be measured at birth to indicate responses of the fetus to prenatal environment such as nutrition, and raise the possibility of appropriate interventions to reduce disease risk later.

Because a woman's oocytes are formed only during her fetal life, and only one generally matures per ovulatory cycle, it is possible for egg quality to be affected by what happens at any time during the mother's life from her conception to her offspring's conception. It seems probable that one way egg quality can be affected is via epigenetic modification. Similarly, the testis is formed when the father is also a fetus, and the germ cells from which sperm ultimately differentiate are sequestered in fetal life. Thus, it is possible that epigenetic changes can also occur in the father's sperm from his conception through to the production of mature sperm much later. As spermatogenesis is an ongoing process, with sperm production taking 2–3 months, then what the father does during the days and weeks before conception can affect his sperm and thus his offspring. There is growing evidence that obese fathers pass biological information to their offspring via the sperm that leads to a greater risk of obesity in the offspring [65].

These points are highlighted because there is growing evidence that parental behaviour prior to conception has influences on the embryo and fetus. This aspect will be discussed throughout the book. As every parent wishes the best for their offspring, it is important that health care professionals (HCPs) give information to prospective parents about what they can do, even prior to pregnancy as well as during pregnancy, to reduce the risk of a less than optimal pregnancy outcome.

Once conception has occurred, certain features of development are relatively consistent; for example, implantation occurs by about day 9, the fetal heart starts beating by the sixth week, fetal breathing movements start about week 10, etc. This does not, however, mean that every aspect of development is fixed; indeed, there is considerable variation. This developmental plasticity reflects the subtle changes in development as a result of variation in the information reaching the embryo and fetus from the mother and via the placenta. Many of these signals are hormonal, nutritional, or metabolic, and they can have both short-term consequences, such as altered fetal growth, and longer-term consequences, such as disease risk.

After birth, learning and experience are critical to brain development, leading to reinforcement of some pathways and pruning of excess neurons and synapses in others. Indeed, it may be that epigenetic mechanisms are involved in these neurodevelopmental processes. There is increasing evidence that brain development is subject to environmental influences, especially in the first years after birth, and this provides another stage when parental behaviour can have long-term consequences. For example, it is now clear that what a baby is weaned onto influences food preference for life through changes in neural pathways.

Much of this book will focus on the effects of maternal lifestyle on developmental plasticity. It is important to emphasize that developmental plasticity is a normative component of biology, and it is therefore inevitable that the fetus and infant will respond to changes in their environment. But there are situations that make a less than optimal outcome more likely. Similarly, plasticity for some organs, such as the brain, continues through life; but plasticity is obviously greatest in early life and, for many of the systems we are most interested in, remains apparent through infancy.

## Plasticity and mismatch

The major outcome of evolutionary processes is a life-course strategy that allows the lineage to pass its genes by reproduction successfully to the next generation in such a way that each generation is fit in turn to pass them to the next. Having the capacity to adjust the phenotype through environmentally sensitive plastic processes makes it more likely that the individual is better matched to its environment after birth and thus more likely to reproduce successfully [4, 56]. But plasticity is a complex process, and at some point for some systems it ceases— for example, once the kidney is fully formed, no more nephrons can be created. So, there may be an advantage in varying the number of nephrons that develop during the plastic phase, depending on environmental signals, to suit the phenotype of the individual. Indeed, there is considerable variation in nephron number between humans, being less in those who were born smaller [5, 66]. In animals, fetuses that were undernourished or exposed to elevated levels of glucocorticoids prenatally develop fewer nephrons [67, 68].

Such processes can be understood as an evolved mechanism to try and *match* the phenotype of the individual to the environment in which he or she lives. Developmental plasticity has the challenge, however, of predicting the environment in which the adult form of the organism will live during its reproductive phase. Thus, the risk of *developmental mismatch* is significant. If the embryo, fetus, or infant detects misleading signals about the world ahead, then it may adopt a less than optimal developmental plan. For example if a mother has placental dysfunction, her fetus will receive less nutrition, which could be interpreted as signalling a future environment of low nutrition; however, the baby may in fact be born into a world of nutritional excess, in which case it may have inappropriate settings of its metabolic physiology and be at greater risk of obesity and diabetes. There is now considerable evidence for the roles of these mismatch pathways in explaining much of metabolic and cardiovascular disease and aspects of human behavioural problems.

Striking examples of the health consequences of mismatch occur in developing countries that have gone through a socio-economic transition rapidly over one or two generations, and in the children of migrants from poor to richer conditions. Under these conditions the prevalence of obesity, diabetes, and heart disease is rising dramatically. That they are on a higher trajectory of risk is made clear by the fact that they are occurring in people whose lifestyles, by Western standards, are still not affluent; moreover, these diseases are becoming apparent at younger ages.

The mismatch phenomenon can however operate even in stable populations in a developed country. Many women and their partners consume an unbalanced or inadequate diet even though food is plentiful. Very often this is linked to low educational attainment, low socio-economic status, and a lack of empowerment, also termed low *health literacy*. Their children may benefit from social mobility, have a very different diet, and so a different risk trajectory.

## Other forms of developmental response

Sometimes the signals to the fetus are such that it must make immediately adaptive responses to survive. It must trade-off aspects of its development now in order to survive and cope with the consequences later. Fetal growth restriction may be the most appropriate response to under-nutrition even if it is associated with greater postnatal morbidity and mortality. Similarly, stunting as a result of prenatal or infant under-nutrition may be immediately adaptive even if it also carries later risks of ill health.

Both the plastic and immediate responses we have discussed represent physiologically appropriate adaptive responses of the developing individual in the attempt to preserve viability and reproductive potential. Sometimes, however, the normative programme of development is grossly disrupted by a teratogen, which can produce both immediate and later detrimental effects. Not all teratogens need involve novel agents—for example very high levels of maternal glucose associated with uncontrolled maternal diabetes can lead to cardiac malformations, and severe iodine deficiency can lead to thyroid agenesis.

## Taking a 'life-course' approach

These insights into our fundamental biology help to provide mechanistic explanations for the large body of epidemiological data that link measures of the developmental environment, such as birthweight, to the risk of diseases, such as diabetes, in adults. This is a major reason why there is a growing focus on a life-course approach to disease prevention, which must ideally start before conception. Indeed that is a major theme of this book. The key challenge is to take these conceptual ideas and reduce them to a practical guide for HCPs to use in advising parents.

Explaining the importance of these concepts to parents can be difficult. This is partly because many people do not really appreciate the concept of risk, especially the continuity of increasing risk that is associated with the life-course model of NCDs. It is often necessary to explain that the developmental processes that lead to such risk are inevitable and occur in every pregnancy, but to distinguish between this early origin of risk and a truly pathological disruption of development such as that resulting from exposure to a teratogen. The task of explaining why it is important to act to reduce risk of health problems such as NCDs in the next generation is made doubly difficult by the fact that pregnancy and early development are inherently very variable processes, which cannot be perfectly controlled or optimized and where the outcome is always uncertain to a degree. So, on the one hand the HCP has to explain to parents who have clearly an unhealthy lifestyle the greater risk of NCDs to which they are exposing their child as well as themselves, and on the other to manage the expectations of the parents who want a 'perfect' pregnancy outcome.

It is not possible to separate fully strands of advice that focus on the short term from those that address the longer-term issues. In general it is more helpful to provide advice by stage in the life course rather than by functional pathway. This is the purpose of section 4, which provides a checklist for HCPs and a guide for parents. However the following chapters of the book give the detailed information necessary to understand the basis for such nutritional and lifestyle guidance.

# Section 2

# Nutritional requirements of pregnancy and breastfeeding

Recommendations for nutrient intakes and the need for supplementation before and during pregnancy continues to be a source of confusion for parents. This section outlines our current knowledge of the effects of specific macro- and micronutrients on maternal and fetal health, and provides a reference manual to equip the health care professional (HCP) with sound advice on macronutrient balance and specific nutrient intakes for preconception, pregnancy, and lactation.

Chapter 3

# Practicalities: understanding nutrient recommendations

## Nutritional advice and caveats

There has been much research in recent years on the nutritional requirements of mothers during pregnancy, as well as an increasing focus on the nutrition of women before conception. Because there has been much confusion with regards to some nutrients such as vitamin D, iron, and polyunsaturated fatty acids, we provide here an in-depth assessment of the evidence. While this may give more detail than some HCPs require, as an increasing number of mothers turn to the internet for information of variable quality, we present sufficient evidence to give HCPs confidence in providing advice. This is particularly important, as there is much inconsistency in the rationale for supplementation with specific micronutrients. It is also important to note that the requirements for an individual woman may vary considerably depending on her context and/or health. We have also tried to provide sufficient guidance for HCPs to be able to adjust their advice to take account of such variation.

## Dietary reference intakes

There are a number of terms used by various agencies to describe nutrient requirements. The US Institute of Medicine (IOM), which sets these standards for the US, utilizes dietary reference intake (DRI) as a term encompassing the average, recommended, and upper limit reference intakes for various nutrients. The UK uses the term dietary reference value (DRV) for this purpose.

A key term is the RDA, or recommended dietary allowance, which is the daily intake amount of a nutrient that is expected to meet the needs of the majority (97.5%) of the population. The UK National Institute for Clinical Excellence and the WHO use the equivalent term RNI, or reference nutrient intake. The RDA (or RNI) is higher than the estimated average requirement (EAR) for the nutrient. The EAR is the intake level expected to meet the

**Table 3.1** Dietary reference intake terminology [69]

| Abbreviation | Term | Definition |
|---|---|---|
| **US/Canada** | | |
| RDA[a] | Recommended dietary allowance | Daily intake level to meet requirement for 97.5% of the population. |
| EAR | Estimated average requirement | Intake level expected to meet the needs of ~50% of the population. |
| AI | Adequate intake | Estimated average intake level—used when data are insufficient to set an RDA. |
| UL | Tolerable upper intake level | Highest level of daily intake at which no adverse effects have been observed. |
| LRNI[b] | Lower reference nutrient intake | Intake amount sufficient for a small proportion of the population with low needs. Intakes below this are likely to be inadequate. |

[a] Alternative term: RNI = reference nutrient intake. Used in the UK and by WHO; formerly used in Canada

[b] Used in the UK

Source: Institute of Medicine, *Dietary Reference Intakes: The Essential Guide to Nutrient Requirements*, The National Academies Press, Washington, D.C., US, Copyright © 2006.

needs of ~50 per cent of the population. In cases where data are insufficient to establish an RDA, the IOM sets a level considered to be an adequate intake (AI) for a specific group (by age or life stage). AI levels are generally used for infants and are based on an estimated average intake level of a specific nutrient in healthy breastfed infants.

The IOM also sets a tolerable upper intake level (UL) for most dietary nutrients. The UL is the highest level of daily consumption for which data indicate no adverse effects in humans when the nutrient is consumed indefinitely without medical supervision. In the UK, there is also a recommendation term for the lowest recommended nutrient intake (LRNI). For individuals, habitual intakes below the LRNI are likely to be inadequate, as the majority of people need more than the LRNI level. These terms are summarized in Table 3.1.

# Food labelling

Nutritional information provided on food labels is intended to guide the consumer in food selection. Standardized labelling formats, based on dietary recommendations, have been applied in different countries in order to assist consumers in comparing foods in terms of nutrients that are considered to be of nutritional importance. Nutrition labels are intended to help consumers make more healthful food choices, and to understand how a particular food product fits into their overall daily diet.

## Food labelling in the US and Canada

Food labels in the US and Canada (the 'Nutrition Facts' panel) show a per cent daily value (%DV) for each important nutrient [70]. The %DV is the proportion of the nutrient's recommended daily intake (based on a 2,000 kcal/day diet) that is provided in one serving of the food. This information is meant to enable consumers to determine the contribution a food would make to their total daily requirement or allowance. A %DV of 5 or less is considered low, and a %DV of 20 or more is high for all nutrients.

The Nutrition Facts panel includes information on serving size and servings per container, calories (kcal) per serving, and calories from fat. The labels first list nutrients that should be limited (e.g. total fat, cholesterol, and sodium), followed by nutrients that should be optimized (e.g., dietary fibre, vitamins, such as vitamin A and C, and minerals, such as calcium and iron). Other countries including the Philippines and Thailand have adopted strategies similar to those used in the US.

## Food labelling in the UK, Australia, and NZ

A 'nutrition information panel' (NIP) is used in the UK, Australia, and NZ. The labelling is based on typical values per serving, and per 100 g or 100 mL of the

**Table 3.2** UK guideline daily amounts (GDA) nutrition system advice on dietary components in food

| Dietary component | High vs low levels in foods |
|---|---|
| Total fat | High: more than 17.5 g of fat per 100 g |
| | Low: 3 g of fat or less per 100 g |
| Saturated fat | High: more than 5 g of saturated fat per 100 g |
| | Low: 1.5 g of saturated fat or less per 100 g |
| Sugars | High: more than 22.5 g of total sugars per 100 g |
| | Low: 5 g of total sugars or less per 100 g |
| Salt | High: more than 1.5 g of salt per 100 g (or 0.6 g sodium) |
| | Low: 0.3 g of salt or less per 100 g (or 0.1 g sodium) |

Note: ranges differ for drinks—all limits are half those for foods (e.g. 'high' for sugar in a drink is more than 11.25 g/100 mL).

Source: Reproduced from NHS Choices, *Nutrition labels on the back or side of packaging*, © Crown Copyright 2014, licenced under the Open Government Licence v.2.0, available from <http://www.nhs.uk/Livewell/Goodfood/Pages/food-labelling.aspx#Nutrition>.

food. The latter allows comparison of percentages between foods. Labels show a percentage of a reference intake, which is similar to %DV in the US.

The UK also uses a system based on 'guideline daily amounts' (GDA) to show food content percentages of the daily value for energy, macronutrients, fibre, and salt (sodium) [71]. The 'traffic light' system has been designed to indicate the content of food components that should be limited (e.g., fat, sugar, and salt), with ranges designated as high, medium, and low for each nutritional category. Other components of the GDA system are calories, protein, carbohydrates, and fibre. Guideline advice for high vs low levels of fats, sugars, and salt are shown in Table 3.2.

# Chapter 4

# Macronutrients and fibre requirements during pregnancy

## Macronutrient transfer to the fetus

Complex relationships exist between maternal macronutrient intake, energy expenditure, weight gain, and fetal growth and development [72, 73]. The placenta mediates the transfer of nutrients to the fetus and secretes hormone mediators of maternal and fetal physiology, maternal adaptation to pregnancy, and fetal maturation. The maternal metabolism adapts to the fetal requirements for nutrients as gestation progresses, transporting macronutrients by a number of mechanisms that can be affected by the maternal nutritional state.

Amino acids are actively and selectively transported from the maternal to fetal plasma, and impaired transport caused by poor maternal protein nutrition can result in intrauterine growth restriction [74]. Carbohydrates are transported to the fetus as glucose, which is taken up from the maternal plasma and transported in a concentration-dependent manner into the fetal plasma; thus, maternal plasma glucose levels directly affect those of the fetus [75]. Lipid transfer involves transport proteins, and the fetal supply is regulated by an interaction between maternal diet, which determines maternal lipid concentrations, and the placental capacity to produce, modify, and transport essential fatty acids and long-chain polyunsaturated fatty acids (PUFAs). This capacity is impaired in pregnancies affected by gestational diabetes mellitus (GDM) [76].

## Macronutrient balance during pregnancy

The maternal macronutrient profile can influence embryonic and fetal development. Energy balance was discussed in chapter 1. Here we consider the impact of varying intakes of protein, carbohydrates, and lipids, which are the key nutrients that contribute to calorie intake. Fibre is also an important food component that needs to be considered. Because these are always consumed as foods and not in the form of supplements, we do not take a biochemical perspective and consider them in isolation but focus on the issue of macronutrient balance as a proportion of energy intake. The exceptions are the long-chain PUFAs such as docosahexaenoic acid, which, while found in foods such as fish, have also been promoted as a specific supplement for pregnancy. PUFAs will be reviewed in more detail in chapter 5.

The proportions of macronutrients required for pregnancy are generally the same as for non-pregnant women, although macronutrient ratios in the diets of pregnant women can be quite variable. Daily dietary reference values for macronutrient intakes vary somewhat by geographical region. For the majority of women in developed countries, dietary intakes are not well aligned with country-specific recommendations [77]. Energy and fibre intakes tend to be lower than the recommendations, while the intakes of total fat and saturated fats are consistently above the recommendations. Mean energy intakes differ by socioeconomic status, with reported energy intakes increasing as status decreased [77].

A study in the UK found that maternal dietary intakes of protein, fat, and carbohydrates during pregnancy correlate with later child dietary intakes of the same nutrients. This association was stronger than the influence of either parent's postnatal diet, suggesting some effect of in utero programming on offspring dietary habits [78]. Getting the balance right in pregnancy may therefore be important not only for the immediate growth and development of the fetus, but also for its long-term health and well-being.

## Protein in the maternal diet

The ratio of protein to non-protein energy in the maternal diet has been shown to influence the offspring's body composition [79], and animal studies suggest it impacts the risk of metabolic disease in adult life [80, 81]. Both low and excessively high-protein intakes during pregnancy are associated with restricted growth [82–84], increased adiposity and elevated cholesterol, triglyceride, and leptin levels [82, 85], as well as impaired glucose tolerance and insulin resistance [81, 82, 85]. The percentage of protein in the maternal diet appears to be inversely associated with fetal abdominal subcutaneous fat, regardless of whether fats or carbohydrates are the diluents of the protein [79].

The source of protein may also matter to fetal growth. In a UK survey, differences in the both placental and fetal growth were observed between mothers consuming different balances of dairy protein and meat protein. In late pregnancy, low intakes of dairy protein were associated with low placental weight, and low intakes of meat protein were associated with lower birthweight. Overall, birthweight fell by 3.1 g for each gram decrease in meat protein intake in late pregnancy [86].

Studies have shown that early-pregnancy diets that are high in protein as a percentage of energy intake are associated with higher birthweight and placental weight [87], whereas high carbohydrate intakes in early pregnancy tend to produce lower placental and birthweights [86]. However, a follow-up study in Motherwell, Scotland, of adults whose mothers had been advised to consume a high-protein (red meat), low-carbohydrate diet in pregnancy exhibited higher blood pressure in adulthood than those whose mothers did not follow such dietary advice [88]. High-protein supplementation is not recommended for pregnant women; rather, balanced protein/energy supplementation (where proteins provide less than 25% of the total energy intake) appears to be beneficial, particularly for undernourished women [89].

## Fats in the maternal diet

Animal studies have shown that high-fat maternal diets can significantly increase susceptibility to diet-induced obesity and percentage total body fat in offspring [90]. Diets high in fat have been demonstrated to increase the risk for GDM recurrence in future pregnancies [91]. Early-pregnancy diets with increasingly higher fractional caloric intakes from carbohydrates relative to fats were found to decrease the risk of both glucose intolerance and GDM [92]. High intakes of saturated fat and trans-fat as a percentage of energy, and low intakes of vegetable and fruit fibre were individually associated with increased fasting glucose levels in the second trimester [93]. However, increased PUFA intake has been associated with a reduction in incidence of glucose intolerance during first pregnancies in Chinese women, highlighting the need to consider the type of fat ingested and to consider PUFAs separately from total fat [94]. Specific requirements for fatty acids are discussed in chapter 5.

## Carbohydrates in the maternal diet

### Glucose during pregnancy

Glucose is the main energy substrate for the fetus, and its concentration in the maternal bloodstream has a direct effect on the fetus. The type and content of carbohydrate (high- vs low-glycaemic sources) in the maternal diet influences blood glucose concentration [95]. Glycaemic index (GI) refers to the grouping of carbohydrate sources by the magnitude of their induced glucose response. Low-GI sources include whole grains, unprocessed rice, beans, most fruits, nontuberous vegetables, nuts, and dairy products; high-GI sources include processed grains (flour, bread, cereals), tuberous vegetables (potatoes, carrots), baked goods, soft drinks, snack foods, ripe bananas, and some tropical fruit. Recent data suggest that exposure to a high-GI diet in pregnancy is associated with markers of the metabolic syndrome (e.g. fasting glucose levels, triglycerides, cholesterol, blood pressure) in offspring at 20 years of age [96].

## Fructose during pregnancy

Fructose is one of the natural sugars found in fruits but until recently was a small component of diets. It has been widely used as a sweetener in canned foods, baked goods, processed foods, dairy products, and carbonated drinks, predominantly in North America and Japan [97, 98] and is thought to be contributing to the rapid rise in the prevalence of obesity and metabolic syndrome [99]. The main sources of fructose are table sugar (sucrose, a disaccharide composed of glucose and fructose), high-fructose corn syrup (a sweetener containing up to 55% fructose, the remainder being glucose), fruits, and honey. Fructose consumption in the US has increased to about 80 g/day [100], and its consumption accounts for 10–20 per cent of the daily caloric intake [99, 101].

Studies have demonstrated that dietary fructose disrupts lipid metabolism and decreases insulin sensitivity [102–105]. Evidence from both animal and human studies have also shown that excessive fructose consumption is associated with various adverse metabolic outcomes such as insulin resistance, increased adiposity, hypertriacylglycerolaemia, hyperleptinaemia, hyperglycaemia, hyperinsulinaemia, impaired glucose tolerance, and hepatic steatosis [106–110]. Epidemiological studies have also reported a correlation between fructose intake and cardiovascular disease, type 2 diabetes, and obesity [108, 109] A study of 13,475 women found a 22 per cent increased risk of GDM associated with consumption of 5 servings/week of sugar (fructose) sweetened beverages [111].

Gallbladder disease is a significant cause of maternal morbidity during pregnancy [112]. Studies have shown an association between high intake of carbohydrates and gallstone disease [113–117], and in a recent, large, prospective study [112], high intakes of fructose were associated with increased risk beyond the effect of total carbohydrate intake. Gallstones are associated with metabolic syndrome [118], and excessive fructose intake might also contribute to its development [119–122].

## Fibre in the maternal diet

Increased dietary intakes of fibre-rich fruits, vegetables, and whole grains are often recommended as part of a healthy dietary guideline. Fibre-rich ingredients such as wheat bran, beta-glucans from oats and barley, and soluble fibre from prebiotics are also recommended to ensure an adequate intake of dietary fibre [123]. High-fibre diets have been associated with reduced risks of cardiovascular disease, stroke, and diabetes [124–126]. Supplementary dietary fibre has also been shown to improve insulin sensitivity and plasma lipid profiles, and to reduce blood pressure [127–130].

Changes in physiological state during pregnancy may increase the risk of several gut disorders and metabolic diseases [123]. Thus, a pregnant mother's need for dietary fibre may be higher than that of the general population. Pregnant mothers have been recommended to consume between 25 and 30 g of total dietary fibre from various food sources such as fruits, vegetables, and whole grain cereals [131]. Consumption of dietary fibre during pregnancy has been reported to reduce the risk of GDM, pre-eclampsia, and postpartum weight retention [132–134].

The beneficial effects of dietary fibre on GDM seem to depend on foods such as whole grains, cereals, and fruits [135]. In the US Nurses' Health Study II cohort (>11,600 women), pre-pregnancy dietary fibre intake had a strong negative association with GDM risk, which decreased by 26 per cent with each 10 g/day increment in total fibre intake [134]. Lower intakes of vegetable and fruit fibre during the second trimester have been linked to increased fasting glucose, and in women with family histories of type 2 diabetes, a higher vegetable and fruit fibre intake has been associated with reduced insulin resistance and increased insulin sensitivity [93].

Higher dietary fibre intake during pregnancy has also been associated with reduced risks of pre-eclampsia [133, 136]. During pregnancy, maternal plasma lipids are significantly elevated, and pre-eclampsia exacerbates this situation [137, 138]. Pregnant women with higher intakes of dietary fibre tend to have lower levels of total triglycerides and higher levels of HDL cholesterol compared with those consuming diets low in fibre [133]. High-fibre diets have been associated with weight control and obesity prevention [139–141]. A daily intake of around 8.5 g fibre per day was found to have a protective effect against postpartum weight retention [132]; conversely, inadequate postpartum fibre intake has been reported to increase the risk of obesity [142].

## Recommended macronutrient and fibre intakes during pregnancy

The US Insitute of Medicine (IOM) recommends no increase in caloric intake during the first trimester, an additional 340 calories per day (1,423 kilojoules) during the second trimester, and an additional 452 calories per day during the third trimester. In general, it is recommended that pregnant women should consume 175 g/day of carbohydrates, 60–70 g/day of protein, 28 g/day of fibre, 10–13 g/day of omega-6 PUFAs, and 1–1.4 g/day of omega-3 PUFAs [131]. During pregnancy, a balanced protein–energy diet, where protein provides less

**Table 4.1** Australian National Health and Medical Research Council recommendations for macronutrient and fibre intakes for pregnant women [143]

| Nutrient class | Maternal age | | |
|---|---|---|---|
| | 14–18 yrs | 19–30 yrs | 31–50 yrs |
| Protein[a] | 58 g/day | 60 g/day | 60 g/day |
| Fat | | | |
| Linoleic acid (omega-6) | 10 g/day | 10 g/day | 10 g/day |
| Alpha-linolenic acid (omega-3) | 1.0 g/day | 1.0 g/day | 1.0 g/day |
| Carbohydrate[b] | No recommendation | | |
| Fibre | 25 g/day | 28 g/day | 28 g/day |

[a] As there is little additional weight gain during the first trimester, no additional protein is needed. The recommendations listed are for additional protein in the second and third trimesters

[b] Data were considered insufficient to make a recommendation.

Source: National Health and Medical Research Council, *Nutrient Reference Values for Australia and New Zealand, Including Recommended Dietary Intakes*, Department of Health and Ageing, Australian Government, Canberra, Australia, copyright © 2006.

than 25 per cent of the total energy content, has been recommended as an ideal dietary pattern that may help mothers to achieve appropriate weight gain, as well as to help reduce the risk of infants being small for gestational age. The recommended percentage of energy sources are 10–15 per cent from protein, 15–30 per cent from fat, and 55–75 per cent from carbohydrates. During the second and third trimesters, it is recommended that pregnant women should consume an additional ~25 g/day of protein, ~35 g/day of carbohydrates, and ~3 g/day of fibre [131]. The Australian National Health and Medical Research Council provides recommendations for pregnant women that are slightly lower than those of the IOM [143], as shown in Table 4.1.

## Our recommendations for macronutrient and fibre intake during pregnancy

The macronutrient profile of a woman's diet during pregnancy is clearly important to her own health and that of her fetus. The increased metabolic rate that occurs in pregnancy results in an increased fuel requirement in mid- and late pregnancy, as the energy and nutrient requirements of the fetus increase. By late pregnancy women require an extra ~35 g/day of dietary carbohydrates. This amount is supplied in portions of carbohydrate-rich foods such as one bagel, two slices of bread, a small baked potato, one average-sized tortilla, or four tablespoons of cooked rice. Refined sugars, in particular fructose, should be limited—low-GI carbohydrate sources should make up the majority of carbohydrate intake. With regard to protein, a single serving of meat (steak, hamburger, turkey, chicken) provides between 25 and 30 g of protein, which is sufficient for the daily needs of pregnant women. Good non-animal protein sources include legumes (e.g. 1 cup cooked chickpeas or lentils provides 12–18 g protein), tofu (9 g protein/4 oz serving), oats (7 g protein/cup), and soy milk (5 g protein/cup).

The requirement for fats in pregnancy can be met by typical Western diets, but the quality of the diet with respect to types of fats is a concern. Fats should represent 15–30 per cent of a woman's overall energy intake, although intake of saturated fats should be limited (reducing consumption of fried fast foods and processed snacks) and PUFA intake should be maintained or increased by consuming 1–2 meals/week of oily fish. However, women should be aware of fish species to limit or avoid because of possible contamination with industrial toxins (see chapter 5 and chapter 30). Fibre is important for pregnant women, and requirements for pregnancy should be achievable in a diet that includes a variety of whole grains, vegetables, fruit, and legumes. Overweight and obese women do not need to increase their energy intake during pregnancy but should focus on achieving a balanced diet in accordance with the above recommendations. Undernourished women require a balanced protein energy diet, which can be achieved via supplementation when the food components of a sufficient and balanced diet are not readily available.

# Chapter 5

# Polyunsaturated fatty acids in pregnancy and breastfeeding

## Polyunsaturated fatty acids are essential for fetal and infant development

There is increasing interest in the role of the omega-3 fatty acids in fetal and infant development and thus in the use of dietary supplements for pregnant women and/or infants, and in promoting intakes of oily fish as a source of omega-3 long-chain polyunsaturated fatty acids (PUFAs). The evidence for supplementation over and above promoting a healthy diet during pregnancy and breastfeeding is still uncertain, but this is a rapidly evolving area of nutritional research. Given the potential beneficial effects of greater omega-3 PUFA levels on fetal brain development and on reducing the risk of allergy and the likely detrimental effects on metabolic health of a high omega-6/omega-3 ratio, this is a subject in which objective evidence can be drowned by considerable pressure to act on anecdotal observations.

The omega-3 and omega-6 fatty acids represent the two major forms of PUFAs. [144]. The simplest omega-3 PUFA is alpha-linolenic acid (ALA), and the simplest omega-6 PUFA is linoleic acid (LA). ALA can be metabolized into the longer and more unsaturated fatty acids eicosapentaenoic acid (EPA) and docosahexaenoic acid (DHA), while LA can be synthesized into long-chain arachidonic acid (AA). However, the conversion rates from ALA to EPA and especially to DHA, and from LA to AA are usually low in humans, with estimates ranging from 1 to 10 per cent [145–147]. The conversion also varies depending on common single nucleotide polymorphisms in the fatty acid desaturase gene cluster, as these polymorphisms can result in different amounts of EPA, DHA, and AA being formed in different individuals [148, 149]. Conversion rates are lower in infants than adults, and insufficient conversion of ALA to EPA—and further to DHA—will have adverse effects on visual and neural development, particularly in premature infants [150, 151].

## Dietary sources of polyunsaturated fatty acids

Significant amounts of the omega-6 PUFA LA are found in vegetable oils such as corn, sunflower, soybean, and peanut oils as well as in products made from these oils, such as margarines; the omega-6 fatty acid AA is found in animal sources only (e.g. meat, eggs) [144, 152]. Sources for the omega-3 fatty acid ALA are green plant tissues, flaxseed, walnuts, beechnuts, butternuts, chia seeds, canola, and soy [144]. The omega-3 long-chain PUFAs EPA and DHA are found in cold-water fatty fish, such as salmon. In most Western diets, up to 98 per cent of dietary fatty acid intake is made up of LA and ALA, with LA intake being in excess of that of ALA. The intake of LA in the Western diet has increased markedly over the second half of the twentieth century, following the introduction and increased consumption of vegetable cooking oils and margarines, whereas ALA intake did not change much over this time [152].

The changed pattern of LA consumption has resulted in a marked increase in the ratio of omega-6 to omega-3 fatty acids in the diets of most Western populations [153]. For example, in men the LA:ALA ratio ranges from 5.5:1 in Denmark to 13.8:1 in France; a similar pattern is seen in women. However, the LA:ALA ratio for both Spanish men and women is 27:1. This ratio is important because high LA inhibits the synthesis of DHA as a result of competition for common converting enzymes. However, while increasing the intake of ALA provides more substrate for synthesis of EPA, the final step conversion to DHA (the desaturation of 24:5omega-3) is actually inhibited at high levels of dietary ALA. Therefore diets low in ALA may be preferred so long as the level of LA is also low [154].

## Polyunsaturated fatty acid status in pregnancy and lactation

Maternal transfer of long-chain PUFAs to the fetus is influenced by maternal fatty acid status, placental function, and the placental levels of fatty acid transporters and binding proteins that are involved in the selectivity of DHA for mobilization [155, 156]. Maternal PUFA status decreases progressively during pregnancy, especially in multiple pregnancies and in each subsequent pregnancy [157]. DHA status declines further after parturition, particularly in breastfeeding women, although other long-chain fatty acids increase [158].

Breast milk is sensitive to changes in fatty acid composition in the maternal diet. For a typical Western diet, the mean LA composition in breast milk has increased from 6 to 15 per cent of total fatty acids in the US from 1944 to 1990, and from 10 to 14 per cent in Australia from 1981 to 2000; while during the same period, the DHA content has decreased [159–161]. DHA levels in breast milk reflect dietary changes in the mother, although there is some selective transfer of DHA to breast milk at the expense of the maternal supply if the latter is low. The DHA levels in infant blood correlate significantly with the DHA levels in both maternal blood and milk [162]. Infants consuming human milk have higher levels of cerebral cortex DHA than do those fed with formula milk without DHA [163–165].

## Effects of polyunsaturated fatty acids on health

### Polyunsaturated fatty acids and maternal mental health

The prevalence rates for antenatal and post-partum depression range from 10 to 40 per cent worldwide [166]. Aside from genetic predisposition, environmental, social, and psychological factors, inadequate nutrition may also play a role in maternal depression. Intake of long-chain PUFAs, in particular the omega-3 fatty acids DHA and EPA, has been associated with mental health outcomes, and greater intake may improve maternal mental health. The omega-3 fatty acids play a role in serotonin functioning and thus may produce antidepressant effects [166].

PUFA status (especially omega-3 fatty acid status) declines during pregnancy and can be improved by supplementation [167]. The decline of maternal DHA status during pregnancy and/or lactation has been associated with post-partum depression, especially in women with a low intake of DHA. Analyses of data in published reports from 23 countries showed that higher concentrations of DHA in mothers' milk and greater seafood consumption predicted lower prevalence rates of post-partum depression [168, 169]. Nonetheless, intervention studies performed to evaluate the potential protective effects of omega-3 fatty acids in maternal depression have shown mixed, but generally negative, results [170–173].

### The effect of polyunsaturated fatty acids on offspring growth and development

Maternal intake of omega-3 fatty acids and AA during pregnancy has been shown to correlate positively with fetal growth and birthweight, whereas maternal LA intake correlated negatively with birth size [174–176]. In preterm infants, AA levels at birth are associated with both birth size and growth during the first year of life [177, 178]. A large cohort study in the US reported that higher omega-3 fatty acid concentrations in the maternal diet and umbilical cord plasma were associated with a lower obesity rate in 3-year-old children

[179]. However supplementation with 1.2 g omega-3 fatty acids daily, along with dietary counselling to reduce AA intake from mid-pregnancy through 4 months of lactation had no effect on adipose tissue development during early postnatal life, despite maternal fatty acids being positively correlated with infant weight, length, and lean body mass at birth [180].

Differentiation of pre-adipocytes is promoted by omega-6 fatty acids, and exposure to these PUFAs in utero and during early infancy promotes fat cell formation and excess fat deposition in early life [181]. Increasing consumption of omega-6 fatty acids relative to omega-3 fatty acids in the Western diet has been implicated as a contributing factor to the increased incidence of childhood obesity [159, 182]. It has been hypothesised that reduction of the omega-6 to omega-3 fatty acid ratio in the maternal diet may limit the offspring's early adipose tissue development, and this may be a novel strategy to prevent childhood obesity [183].

## The effect of polyunsaturated fats on cognitive/visual development

Long-chain PUFA supply during pregnancy is crucial for the optimal development of the brain and visual systems. Studies in non-human primates have reported impaired cognitive function and visual acuity in offspring of mothers who were deficient in omega-3 fatty acids, and this situation could not be salvaged by postnatal omega-3 fatty acid supplementation [184, 185]. In human observational studies, higher maternal DHA intake correlated with better motor functioning, attention, and sleep pattern development in infants and children [186–192]. The period of greatest accumulation of DHA in the developing brain is during the last trimester of pregnancy and the first year of life [162].

Observational studies suggest that consumption of oily fish (a source for omega-3 fatty acid) during pregnancy can improve the offspring's visual stereo-acuity, vocabulary comprehension, receptive vocabulary and verbal intelligence quotient from infancy to 9 years of age [189, 193–196]. Pregnant mothers who consume more than the recommended amount of fish are reported to have children who show higher cognitive performance [189, 192]. These results however, have not been validated in randomized, controlled trials. A recent meta-analysis of trials of maternal omega-3 fatty acid supplementation found no differences in cognitive, language, or motor development between offspring of supplemented vs non-supplemented mothers, despite some trials showing higher cognitive scores in young children [197]. Current evidence neither supports nor refutes the hypothesis that consumption of omega-3 fatty acid during pregnancy can improve cognitive or visual development in children.

## The effect of polyunsaturated fatty acids on the development of allergies and respiratory disease

The changing composition of long-chain PUFAs in human diets, with an increasing intake of omega-6 fatty acids relative to omega-3 fatty acids, has coincided with an increased prevalence of atopic diseases in children [198, 199]. This may be because the amount of omega-6 fatty acids in the diet influences the rate of formation of the inflammatory mediator prostaglandin E2 and thus the development of allergic sensitization [198]. These dietary changes are reflected in the fatty acid composition in breast milk, which has been shown to impact the susceptibility of breastfed infants to such disorders. Children who were breastfed by mothers with low levels of omega-3 fatty acids relative to omega-6 fatty acids in their milk (in particular, a high AA:EPA ratio) were found to be at increased risk of developing atopy by 18 months of age [200]. In non-atopic mothers, plasma long-chain fatty acid content was negatively correlated with the development of atopic eczema in their infants [201]. A report from the Southampton Women's Survey also provided some limited support that a low level of maternal omega-3 fatty acids relative to omega-6 fatty acids is linked to later wheeze and atopy in the offspring [202].

With the decline in the consumption of omega-3 fatty acids in favour of the more pro-inflammatory omega-6 fatty acids, numerous studies have suggested a potential protective role of omega-3 fatty acids in allergic diseases [203, 204]. Omega-3 long-chain PUFAs can be obtained from some fish and fish oils, and these fatty acids may oppose the actions of omega-6 fatty acids [203]. A study in Australia demonstrated that high-dose omega-3 long-chain fatty acid supplementation of 900 mg/day in pregnancy did not reduce the overall incidence of immunoglobulin E associated food allergy in the first 12 months of life, although it lowered the incidence of atopic eczema and egg sensitization [205].

Maternal fish intake during pregnancy has been consistently demonstrated to have protective effects on atopic or allergic diseases in infants and children, including eczema, asthma, and sensitization to dust mites or food [206–209]. However, this is not the case for fish intake during infancy or childhood, where the reported effects have been inconsistent. However, dietary supplementation of DHA and AA in infants and children is associated with delayed onset and reduced risk of upper respiratory infection and asthma, allergic rhinitis, allergic conjunctivitis, and atopic dermatitis up to 3 years of age [210], and a lower incidence of bronchiolitis in the first year [211], as well as fewer episodes and a lower incidence of respiratory illness [212].

## Agency guidelines on polyunsaturated fatty acid intake

Based on a joint expert consultation on fats and fatty acids in human nutrition, the FAO and WHO have formulated guidelines for dietary intakes of essential fatty acids for pregnant and lactating women [213]. These guidelines suggest that PUFAs should represent 6–11 per cent of total energy intake. The recommended minimum intake of omega-3 fatty acids for optimal maternal health and fetal and infant development is 0.3 g/day EPA + DHA, of which at least 0.2 g/day should be DHA. The European Food Safety Authority has also set an adequate intake (AI) value for ALA for all population groups, including pregnant and lactating women, as 0.5 per cent of the total energy intake. According to this set of recommendations, the AI value for total EPA + DHA is 250 mg/day for adults, which should be supplemented by 100–200 mg/day DHA during pregnancy and lactation [214].

## Our recommendations for polyunsaturated fatty acid intake during pregnancy and lactation

Transfer of long-chain PUFAs from a mother to her offspring during pregnancy and lactation relies on adequate maternal status, which correlates with her dietary intake and can be influenced by common genetic variants in fatty acid processing enzymes. There are large differences worldwide in dietary intake of long-chain PUFAs, particularly DHA. Although the main source is fish/fish oil and seafood, vegetable oils and cereals are other important sources of polyunsaturated fatty acids, especially for those who consume a mostly vegetarian diet.

It should also be noted that high consumption of oily fish carries an increased risk of exposure to lipophilic industrial contaminants such as polychlorinated biphenyls [215] and mercury (see chapter 30). However, the proportion of polychlorinated biphenyl exposure originating from fish is low (≤26%) compared with that from other foods of animal origin. Mercury contamination is an issue mainly with large predatory fish species such as swordfish, king mackerel, Chilean sea bass, Ahi tuna, shark, and tilefish [216]. Regional differences in environmental contaminants may be important, and health care professionals should be aware of any local or regional fish consumption advisories. Consumption of a variety of fish (not just oily fish) should be encouraged.

The LA: ALA ratio is important; diets low in ALA (from canola oil, flaxseed, walnuts, etc.) are acceptable so long as the level of LA (from other vegetable oils and meat) is also low. The FAO and WHO guidelines for dietary intakes for total fat and essential fatty acids should be followed in order to maintain adequate levels during pregnancy. At present the evidence is not sufficient to support specific additional supplementation for pregnant women, although intakes of DHA up to 1,000 mg per day and EPA up to 500 mg per day are safe and may have some beneficial effects. For children under 2 years of age, the key sources of omega-3 long-chain PUFAs are breast milk and fish. Therefore, continued breastfeeding and an increased intake of fish should be promoted.

# Chapter 6

# Vitamin A in pregnancy and breastfeeding

## Vitamin A functions

Vitamin A refers to a group of fat-soluble compounds (retinoids) that includes retinol, retinal (retinaldehyde), retinoic acid (RA), and retinyl esters. Retinoids are required for visual function and modulate the expression of many genes involved in embryonic development, tissue growth, epithelial tissue integrity, metabolism, reproduction, and immune function. The biologically active retinoid form is RA, except in the visual system, where retinal is also required. The pleiotropic effects of RA are mediated through two types of receptors: the RA receptors and the retinoid X receptors [217].

Retinol is known as 'preformed' vitamin A and is obtained from animal sources primarily in the form of retinyl esters stored in fats (see Fig. 6.1) The provitamin A carotenoids (beta-carotene, alpha-carotene, and beta-cryptoxanthin) are dietary precursors of retinol derived from plants and are converted in the body by the retinaldehyde dehydrogenase enzymes to retinol and then to two active retinoids, all-*trans*-RA and 9-*cis*-RA. All-*trans*-RA binds to RA receptors, and 9-*cis*-RA binds to retinoid X receptors, forming heterodimers that regulate gene transcription by binding chromosomal RA response elements. RA receptors and retinoid X receptors also form heterodimers with thyroid hormone receptors and vitamin D receptors, mediating the interaction between vitamin D and thyroid hormones with their receptors [218].

Retinol is absorbed in the small intestine via a carrier-mediated and saturable process, with high absorption efficiency (70–90%). Carotenoids are absorbed passively in the small intestine; the efficiency of absorption is 9–22 per cent, decreasing with increasing carotenoid intake. Most vitamin A reserves are stored in the liver as retinyl esters, but carotenoids are also deposited throughout the body in fatty tissues [219]. The release of vitamin A from the liver and vitamin A transport in plasma is dependent on retinol binding protein. Carotenoids are fat soluble and are transported in plasma via lipoproteins [217, 220]. The maintenance of RA levels in cells and tissues is regulated by positive and negative feedback controlled by the cytochrome P450 enzymes CYP26A1, CYP26B1, and CYP26C1, which are expressed in different tissues [221].

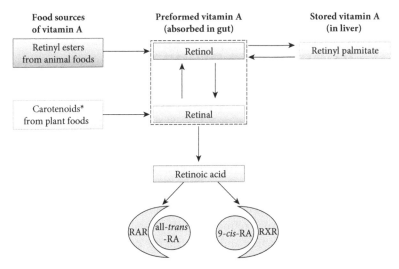

*beta-carotene, alpha-carotene, beta-cryptoxanthin

**Fig. 6.1** Vitamin A precursor forms, sources, and conversion pathways; 9-*cis*-RA, 9-*cis*-retinoic acid; all-*trans*-RA, all-*trans*-retinoic acid; RAR, retinoic acid receptors; RXR, retinoid X receptors.

## Vitamin A deficiency

The WHO classifies individuals as being at risk for biochemical vitamin A deficiency (VAD) at a serum retinol threshold of <0.7 µmol/L [222]. However, serum retinol is not well correlated with vitamin A intake or signs of deficiency, as its levels are homeostatically controlled unless liver vitamin A stores are either very low or very high. The effect of vitamin A on the visual system is reflected in early signs of deficiency or excess. The most specific evidence of VAD is xerophthalmia (dry eyes and night blindness). Other eye symptoms include keratomalacia (ulceration of the cornea), keratin debris in the conjunctiva (Bitot spots), and photophobia [223]. The visual pigment rhodopsin, which is critical for dim-light vision, is formed from the binding of 11-*cis*-retinal (derived from isomerization of retinal) to the membrane receptor opsin in photoreceptor cells of the retina [224]. Night blindness is a precursor sign of hypovitaminosis A, whereas double vision is a sign of hypervitaminosis A.

Vitamin A is essential for proper functioning of both male and female reproductive systems; deficiency causes infertility [225]. In addition, vitamin A supports several functions that are key to resistance to infection. VAD disrupts neutrophil development [226] and reduces Th2-mediated antibody responses as well as natural killer cell activity and number, thereby impairing both innate and adaptive immune responses to infection [227]. Vitamin A is also involved in mucosal epithelial barrier function, and deficiency compromises the ability of such barriers in eye conjunctiva and the respiratory, gastrointestinal, and urogenital tracts to resist penetration by pathogenic microorganisms [228]. Infection itself can impair vitamin A status and exacerbate deficiency in several ways primarily related to malabsorption. VAD is associated with an increased risk of death from common infections in pregnant women, infants, and young children [222]. As signalling molecules in embryogenesis, in part via their effects on hormone receptor activation, retinoids are required for development and maintenance of multiple organ systems, including the heart, lungs, kidneys, and skeleton. Both excess and deficiency of vitamin A in pregnancy are associated with birth defects, most typically malformations of the eye, skull, lungs, and heart [229].

## Vitamin A in pregnancy

Vitamin A homeostasis in pregnancy is altered to meet fetal demands, dependent on the mother's vitamin A status. Maternal serum retinol levels decrease prior to depletion of hepatic stores, particularly in the third trimester, because accelerated fetal growth during this period is dependent on vitamin A acquired from the maternal circulation [230]. Under conditions of moderate deficiency, accumulation of sufficient vitamin A in the fetus occurs at the expense of maternal vitamin A stores. Pregnant women are therefore most susceptible to deficiency in the third trimester, and night blindness most commonly occurs at this time in women with relative deficiency [222].

It is estimated that the growing fetus requires ~100 μg of vitamin A per day during the third trimester of pregnancy. In non-vitamin A deficient populations, maternal liver stores of vitamin A are thought to be sufficient to cover this increased requirement. The active transfer of vitamin A to the fetus from the placenta during pregnancy compensates for a wide range of maternal intakes. Nonetheless, women with low vitamin A intake or reduced liver stores should increase their intake throughout pregnancy to ensure adequate stores are available for rapid fetal growth in late gestation [231]. It is assumed that an insufficient supply of vitamin A to the fetus restricts growth, and there is some evidence for a positive association of vitamin A status in pregnancy with infant birthweight and length [232]. Low birthweight was significantly more prevalent among infants whose mothers were vitamin A deficient (affected by night blindness) in a study in rural south India [233]. However, controlled trials have tested the effect of maternal vitamin A supplementation on birth/infant size and thus far have not shown a clear benefit [234, 235].

VAD in pregnant women is highly prevalent in developing countries. In such areas of high VAD risk, an estimated 7.8 per cent of pregnant women have xerophthalmia (night blindness), and >15 per cent have low serum retinol concentrations. Over 19 million women are globally affected annually [222]. A UN/WHO report estimated that 160 million preschool children in developing countries were affected by VAD (prevalence 30%) [236]. In these countries, VAD is associated with growth failure, depressed immunity, and increased morbidity and mortality due to infectious disease.

On the other hand, a high intake of vitamin A in pregnancy also presents adverse health risks, particularly to the developing fetus. Vitamin A (as retinol) is considered to be teratogenic if present in excess in early pregnancy. Fetuses exposed to high-dose retinol between the fifth and seventh week after the last menstrual period (third to fifth week postconception) are most at risk of serious birth defects [229].

## Vitamin A supplementation in pregnancy

Because of the potential teratogenic effects from exposure to excess preformed vitamin A in the first trimester of pregnancy, vitamin A supplementation in pregnant women who are not deficient is not recommended. In areas of high VAD prevalence, however, vitamin A supplementation of pregnant women has been found to reduce the risks of night blindness, anaemia, and infection [237]. On the basis of the observed association between vitamin A and infectious disease resistance, supplementation has been specifically studied in HIV-positive women living in areas of high VAD risk, as well as those in areas where malaria is endemic. Vitamin A supplementation in pregnancy enhanced maternal immunity to malaria [238] but did not did not affect perinatal HIV transmission or improve birthweight and neonatal growth [239]. Supplementation of pregnant women in Bangladesh with weekly doses of vitamin A or beta-carotene had no effect on birth size [235] or neonatal mortality [240] A lack of effect of vitamin A supplementation on stillbirth or neonatal/perinatal mortality was also reported in two large randomized trials [238, 241] and a recent meta-analysis, which concluded that data do not currently support a role for antenatal vitamin A supplementation to reduce maternal or perinatal mortality.

Increasing maternal vitamin A late in gestation may reduce complications of neonatal respiratory insufficiency, particularly if preterm delivery is anticipated [242]. Preterm infants have low vitamin A stores at birth and are at increased risk of retinopathy, lung disease, and respiratory infections. Maternal supplementation appears to reduce mortality and oxygen requirements in preterm infants, but no evidence of either benefit or harm with regard to neurodevelopmental status at 18–22 months has been observed [242].

VAD is linked to impaired iron mobilization from body stores. VAD often coexists with iron deficiency in developing countries. Vitamin A supplementation was found to improve anaemia in pregnant women when added to an iron supplementation regimen in some studies [243], but others did not observe a benefit [244, 245] Data are currently insufficient to recommend vitamin A supplementation to improve anaemia in pregnancy.

## Vitamin A in lactation and infancy

Newborn infants have low liver vitamin A stores and require an intake of around 100 µg retinol daily to meet their needs for growth. The sources of vitamin A at this stage are colostrum and breast milk, which serve to increase infant stores during the first few months of life unless the breast milk vitamin A content is inadequate. Breast milk from well-nourished mothers is rich in vitamin A. Not surprisingly, the mean retinol concentration in breast milk from women in developing countries is lower than that from women in developed countries [246].

In contrast to placental vitamin A transfer during pregnancy, breast milk is more sensitive to maternal intake [247]. The amount of vitamin A transferred from mother to infant in the first 6 months of lactation is 60 times that which the fetus accumulates throughout gestation. Breastfed infants are generally protected from clinical VAD, although improving vitamin A stores during infancy is important to protect against symptoms of deficiency after weaning [248]. High-dose supplementation of breastfeeding women at risk of VAD has been suggested as a possible intervention for improving both child and maternal health [249]. However, limited benefits of vitamin A supplementation (mainly single dose) were seen in post-partum women in populations with high VAD prevalence. Although supplementation enhanced serum and breast milk retinol concentrations, this effect was not sustained [250].

In a study of very low birthweight infants, poor vitamin A status (low plasma vitamin A) in the first week of life was associated with the development of chronic lung disease and increased the risk of infant death [251]. Supplementing low birthweight infants with vitamin A reduced the incidence of death in the first month and reduced chronic lung disease. It has been suggested that vitamin A supplementation may also reduce incidence of retinopathy of prematurity [242]. In middle- and low-income countries, vitamin A supplementation in infants and children under 5 years of age is associated with significant reductions in all-cause mortality, including a 27 per cent reduction in deaths from diarrhoea [252] Infections were also reduced in supplemented infants (15% decrease in diarrhoea incidence; 50% decrease in measles).

## Sources and metabolism of vitamin A

In the diet, vitamin A can be found as provitamin A carotenoids (found in darkly colored fruits and vegetables, oily fruits, and red palm oil), or preformed as retinol or retinyl esters (found in fatty acids from animal products). Retinols are found in the highest concentration in the livers and liver oils of marine animals. The potency of vitamin A activity differs markedly depending on the dietary source. Beta-carotene is less easily absorbed than retinol, and food sources have poorer absorption than beta-carotene from supplements (2 µg of beta-carotene as a supplement supplies the equivalent of 1 µg retinol, but 12 µg beta-carotene from food is required to provide 1 µg retinol). Other provitamin A carotenoids are even less easily absorbed. The different retinoid potencies can be expressed as retinol activity equivalents (RAEs), as follows: 1 µg RAE = 1 µg retinol, 12 µg beta-carotene, and 24 µg alpha-carotene or beta-cryptoxanthin.

Supplemental beta-carotene is more efficiently converted to vitamin A than dietary beta-carotene, because the food matrix affects the release of carotenoids from food for conversion. Products of fat digestion are required for solubilization of retinol and carotenoids, and this process occurs more efficiently with animal sources than with vegetable sources. Absorption of vitamin A depends on the amount of lipids in the diet. Diets very low in fat result in low absorption of retinol and carotenoids [253].

Vegetarian diets do not include preformed vitamin A, which is derived only from animal sources. Therefore the intake of deeply colored (red and yellow) vegetables should be increased, or fortified foods (e.g. some margarines, cereals) should be consumed during pregnancy. Consuming the recommended 5 servings of fruits and vegetables a day should contribute between 5 and 6 mg of provitamin A carotenoids, which equates to over 400 µg RAEs, or over half of the pregnancy recommended dietary allowance (RDA) [71].

Intestinal infections and diarrhoea can cause malabsorption of vitamin A; this is a common problem in developing countries. Because of an overlap in metabolic pathways, alcohol (ethanol) can compete with retinol for metabolism and also competitively inhibits the conversion of retinol to RA. Alcohol consumption thereby potentiates the effects of VAD by further depleting liver vitamin A stores [254]. Inhibition of RA synthesis by ethanol has been suggested as a potential mechanism for defects observed in fetal alcohol syndrome [255].

## Risks of excess vitamin A during pregnancy

Vitamin A has a relatively narrow range of safe intake. Excess vitamin A is hepatotoxic, and the effect on liver function is the basis for setting the upper intake limit in non-pregnant adults. Hypervitaminosis A is caused by overconsumption of preformed vitamin A, not carotenoids. In addition to liver damage, severe cases can result in haemorrhage, coma, and death. Signs of toxicity are associated with consumption around 10 times the RDA (8,000–10,000 μg/day or 25,000–33,000 IU/day). The upper intake level (UL) for adults has been set at 3,000 μg (10,000 IU)/day of preformed vitamin A.

Excess vitamin A in pregnancy is known to cause birth defects. Pregnant women should avoid multivitamin or prenatal supplements that contain more than 1,500 μg (5,000 IU) preformed vitamin A. Synthetic derivatives of vitamin A (e.g. etretinate and isotretinoin) can cause serious birth defects and should be avoided in pregnancy or if there is a possibility of becoming pregnant [256, 257]. In populations at low nutritional risk for VAD, intake of prenatal multivitamins containing vitamin A may result in excess, and potentially dangerous, levels of serum retinol [258]. These synthetic derivatives have teratogenic effects on structures derived from the cranial neural crest, resulting in abnormal external ear (e.g. microtia and anotia), small mandible, cleft palate, and conotruncal and aortic arch defects as well as brain defects (e.g. hydrocephaly and microcephaly) and a small or absent thymus. Neuro-functional deficits are reported in children without major malformations [259].

Taken as supplements in pregnancy, vitamin A (but not beta-carotene) can have teratogenic effects at levels not far above the recommended intake levels [229]. The threshold vitamin A intake above which the risk of teratogenicity increases is still debated. Most of the human data on teratogenicity of vitamin A involve doses ≥7,800 μg/day [260]. Individuals with high alcohol intakes, liver disease, hyperlipidemia, or protein malnutrition may be particularly susceptible to adverse effects of high vitamin A intake [71].

## Agency guidelines for vitamin A intake

Recommendations for vitamin A intakes are now based on RAEs. A microgram quantity of RAE is based on the activity of 1 μg of all-*trans*-retinol. Previously, the unit 'retinol equivalent' was used, which expressed vitamin A activity based on retinol equivalent weights, but this measure has since been found to overestimate the activity of the carotenoids [261]. A further complication for vitamin A nutrition is the fact that food and supplement labels usually state vitamin A levels in IUs. Vitamin A measurements expressed as IUs tend to overstate the contribution of activity provided by provitamin A carotenoids. Because the conversion of IUs to RAEs is different for retinol and carotenoids, IUs cannot be directly converted to RAEs (or vice versa) for total vitamin A unless the proportion of retinol to carotenoids in the sample is known (Box 6.1).

## Box 6.1 Vitamin A conversions

One IU of retinol is equivalent to 0.3 µg of retinol (1 µg = 3.33 IU) or 0.3 µg retinol activity equivalent (RAE).

One IU of beta-carotene in supplements is equivalent to 0.5 IU of retinol or 0.15 µg RAE (0.3 × 0.5).

One IU of dietary beta-carotene is equivalent to 0.165 IU retinol or 0.05 µg RAE (0.3 × 0.165).

One IU of other dietary provitamin A carotenoids is equivalent to 0.025 µg RAE.

Source: Institute of Medicine, *Dietary Reference Intakes: The Essential Guide to Nutrient Requirements*, The National Academies Press, Washington, DC, copyright © 2006. [71]

For some food groups the conversion to RAEs is simple. If vitamin A activity is being contributed by only provitamin A carotenoids, the IU value can be divided by 20 or the retinol equivalent value divided by 2 to get the RAE value. These food groups include plant foods such as fruits, vegetables, spices, nuts, seeds, and legumes. For food groups such as meats, where all of the vitamin A is being contributed by retinol, the IU value can be divided by 3.33, and the retinol equivalent value and RAE value are the same. Dietary intake recommendations for vitamin A are based on intake levels needed to ensure adequate vitamin A stores in the liver. The tolerable UL for the general population is based on the lowest intake level reported to be associated with liver abnormalities; for pregnancy (or women of childbearing age), the UL is based on the lowest level reported to induce teratogenicity [71].

According to the US Institute of Medicine, pregnant women have an estimated average requirement of 550 µg RAE per day (530 µg/day for women 18 years and younger), with a maximum dose (tolerable upper limit; UL) of 3,000 µg/day (2,800 for ≤18 years; Box 6.2). The RDA is 770 µg/day (750 µg/day for ≤ 18 years) [71, 260]. The RDA represents an increase of 50 µg/day for pregnant adolescents, and 70 µg/day for adult females, above their pre-pregnancy requirements (RDA = 700 µg RAE/day). The recommended intake for lactation is substantially higher, to account for infant requirements and losses in breast milk. The estimated average requirement for adult lactating women is 900 µg RAE/day (885 µg/day for women ≤ 18 years), and the RDA is 1,300 µg RAE/day (1,200 µg/day for ≤ 18 years). The UL for pregnancy and lactation is 2,800–3,000 µg RAE/day. The UL for vitamin A applies only to preformed vitamin A (e.g. retinol—the form of vitamin A found in animal foods, most fortified foods, and supplements). It does not apply to vitamin A derived from carotenoids.

## Box 6.2  US Institute of Medicine recommended dietary allowances for vitamin A

Infants 0–6 months (adequate intake (AI)) = 400 µg retinol activity equivalent (RAE)/day

Infants 7–12 months (AI) = 500 µg RAE/day

Children 1–3 years = 300 µg RAE/day

Females 14+ years = 700 µg RAE/day

Pregnancy 14–18 years = 750 µg RAE/day

Pregnancy 19+ years = 770 µg RAE/day

Lactation 14–18 years = 1,200 µg RAE/day

Lactation 19+ years = 1,300 µg RAE/day

Tolerable upper intake level (pregnancy) = 3,000 µg RAE/day (10,000 IU/day)

Source: Institute of Medicine, Food and Nutrition Board, *Dietary Reference Intakes for Vitamin A, Vitamin K, Arsenic, Boron, Chromium, Copper, Iodine, Iron, Manganese, Molybdenum, Nickel, Silicon, Vanadium, and Zinc*, The National Academies Press, Washington, DC, copyright © 2001. [260]

In light of new knowledge about the potency of provitamin A carotenoids in foods, WHO/FAO guidelines have suggested that previously recommended number of servings of green leafy vegetables needed to meet vitamin A requirements should be at least doubled, particularly during the third trimester of pregnancy [231]. The most recent WHO guidelines (2011) do not recommend routine vitamin A supplementation during pregnancy or lactation for the prevention of maternal and infant morbidity and mortality, and state that high-dose vitamin A should be avoided in pregnancy, particularly between day 15 and day 60 after conception [262, 263]. However, the WHO recommends supplementation for at least 12 weeks in late pregnancy and during lactation in areas with endemic VAD, for the prevention of night blindness (populations at risk are those where the prevalence of night blindness is ≥5% in pregnant women or ≥5% in children 24–59 months of age). Specifically, pregnant women should receive up to 10,000 IU vitamin A daily or up to 25,000 IU vitamin A weekly as an oral, liquid, oil-based preparation of retinyl palmitate or retinyl acetate, beginning after day 60 of gestation. Supplementation should be continued for a minimum of 12 weeks during pregnancy until delivery [262]. The WHO previously issued guidelines on safe supplementation in light of the potential adverse effects of excess vitamin A exposure in early pregnancy [264].

UK and Australian guidelines acknowledge that there is little evidence to support routine supplementation with vitamin A and that excessive quantities of fat-soluble vitamins may be harmful. Pregnant women should be informed to avoid supplement intake above 10,000 IU of retinol (>700 μg), as this level of intake may cause birth defects [265, 266]. These guidelines recommend that pregnant women avoid consuming liver and liver products, which contain high levels of vitamin A. There is wide variation in recommendations for vitamin A throughout Europe. The individual European recommendations range from 700 to 1,100 μg and from 850 to 1,500 μg for pregnant and lactating females, respectively [267]. The government of India recommends that children should be given vitamin A supplements every 6 months from the age of 9 months until the age of 3 [268].

## Our recommendations for vitamin A intake during pregnancy and lactation

Clinical deficiency for vitamin A still affects significant numbers of pregnant women in developing countries. Low intake during the nutritionally demanding periods of pregnancy, lactation, infancy, and childhood increases the risk of serious health problems in both mothers and children. These risks include growth failure, depressed immunity, and increased morbidity and mortality due to infectious disease.

Most women who are at low nutritional risk can meet their early pregnancy vitamin A requirement from food sources. An increased intake from food sources is recommended during the third trimester and throughout lactation. Although supplementation in pregnancy may be warranted in a subset of the population, both pregnant and lactating women should be encouraged to receive adequate vitamin A nutrition by consuming at least five servings a day of darkly colored fruits and vegetables (e.g. carrots, pumpkin, sweet potato, butternut squash, dried apricots, cantaloupe, red pepper, and spinach), and animal sources of retinol, although liver products should be avoided during pregnancy. In deficient areas, the WHO recommendation of vitamin A supplementation (10,000 IU/day or 25,000 IU/week) for 12 or more weeks prior to delivery should be followed.

## Chapter 7

# Vitamin B₁ (thiamine) in pregnancy and breastfeeding

## Thiamine functions

Vitamin B₁ (thiamine) is a water-soluble vitamin involved in nervous system and muscle function, acting by multiple enzymatic processes via the enzyme cofactor thiamine pyrophosphate. Thiamine pyrophosphate catalyses the production of acetyl coenzyme A, which provides a link between carbohydrate, fat, and protein metabolism. Thiamine is essential for carbohydrate metabolism, via the enzyme transketolase, and for intermediary metabolism [269]. Thiamine at low concentrations is mainly transported from the gastrointestinal tract by a saturable, energy-dependent mechanism [270]. At higher concentrations thiamine appears to be absorbed by passive diffusion. Blood and tissue concentrations of thiamine are not subject to physiological regulation but are dependent on dietary intake. The total body thiamine content in an adult is approximately 30 mg, and the biological half-life is in the range of 9–18 days [271].

## Indicators of thiamine status

Biochemical alterations reflecting poor thiamine status occur before overt signs of deficiency. The urinary excretion rate of thiamine reflects its intake and is used to assess intake. Urinary thiamine excretion of <40 µg/day is indicative of thiamine deficiency, and excretion of <100 µg/day reflects marginal deficiency [269]. A widely used measure to detect thiamine deficiency is the indirect, functional measurement of thiamine diphosphate in erythrocytes with either the transketolase activation test or the transketolase activity assay. This assay is not particularly sensitive to recent thiamine intake [272], and there are inter-individual and genetic factors that can affect transketolase activity. The measurement of thiamine pyrophosphate effect is an assay for transketolase that is performed in the absence and presence of added thiamine, expressed as an activity coefficient. The normal range is 0–14 per cent; 15–24 per cent reflects marginal thiamine deficiency, and ≥25 per cent signifies clinical deficiency.

**Table 7.1** Thiamine status indicators [269]

| Indicator | Marginal deficiency | Deficiency |
|---|---|---|
| Erythrocyte transketolase activity[a] | 1.2–1.25 | >1.25 |
| Erythrocyte thiamine (nmol/L) | 70–90 | <70 |
| Thiamine pyrophosphate effect (%)[a] | 15–24 | ≥25 |
| Urinary thiamine | | |
| (nmol [μg]/g creatinine) | 90–220 [27–66] | <27 μg/day |
| (nmol [μg]/day) | 133–333 [40–100] | <40 μg/day |

[a] Activity coefficient representing fold-stimulation above baseline following addition of thiamine pyrophosphate

Reproduced with permission from Institute of Medicine, Food and Nutrition Board, *Dietary Reference Intakes: Thiamin, Riboflavin, Niacin, Vitamin B₆, Folate, Vitamin B₁₂, Pantothenic Acid, Biotin, and Choline*, Dietary Reference Intakes, National Academy Press, Washington, DC, copyright © 1998. Courtesy of the National Academies Press, Washington, DC.

Erythrocyte thiamine pyrophosphate level has also been used to provide an indication of thiamine status [273]. The direct measurement of erythrocyte thiamine by high-performance liquid chromatography has also been used to assess thiamine status, with comparable results [274]. Indicators of thiamine status are summarized in Table 7.1.

## Thiamine deficiency

Thiamine deficiency can be caused by inadequate intake, typically in populations that consume diets that are high in milled or polished rice and low in other food sources of thiamine. Severe thiamine deficiency causes beriberi, which is still endemic in Asia and occurs frequently in refugee and displaced populations [275]. Symptoms include severe lethargy/fatigue, weight loss, impaired sensory perception, emotional disturbances, and irregular heart rate. Beriberi is also seen in alcoholics, who often have poor nutrition and low intakes of thiamine-containing foods. In addition to poor dietary intake in alcoholics, thiamine deficiency is exacerbated by the interference of alcohol with thiamine absorption [276]. Thiamine deficiency associated with alcoholism is known as Wernicke–Korsakoff syndrome (or Wernicke's encephalopathy) [277]. Deficiency for thiamine is associated with HIV infection and AIDS and may result from low intake, increased metabolic rate (catabolic state characteristic of AIDS), and gastrointestinal disturbances [278]. Thiamine deficiency impairs cardiac function and can lead to congestive heart failure. Low thiamine intakes are associated with increased risks of cataracts [279] and age-related lens opacification [280].

## Thiamine in pregnancy

In pregnancy, thiamine is important for fetal growth and development, and production of ATP from glucose in the brain. Deficiency in pregnancy can lead to widespread metabolic disturbances affecting the placenta and fetus. Pregnancy imposes an increasing requirement for thiamine over the course of gestation, and the increased utilization of thiamine is reflected in decreased thiamine excretion or by the erythrocyte transketolase activation test [281, 282]. Women with marginal thiamine status are at risk for developing symptomatic thiamine deficiency in pregnancy, which is associated with anorexia, maternal weight loss, neurological symptoms, muscle degeneration, and intrauterine growth restriction. Women of low socioeconomic status may be particularly vulnerable because of poor pre-conception nutritional status and an inadequate diet in pregnancy [281].

Prolonged vomiting in pregnancy results in thiamine depletion. Thiamine deficiency is thus evident in approximately 60 per cent of women with hyperemesis gravidarum [283] and can result in ketonuria. Thiamine replacement therapy has been shown to prevent or reverse maternal neurological complications of hyperemesis gravidarum [284, 285].

Free thiamine crosses the placenta, and its concentration is higher in cord blood than in maternal blood [281]. It appears that the fetus is able to sequester thiamine at the expense of the mother and has an enhanced metabolism which further stimulates the extraction of thiamine from the maternal circulation There is no evidence that thiamine deficiency causes fetal malformations, even in cases of overt maternal beriberi [282]. Nonetheless, prenatal supplementation may protect newborns from deficiency.

## Thiamine in lactation and infancy

Thiamine deficiency in infants is very rare in developed countries. However, if a breastfeeding mother has low thiamine status, her infant will be vulnerable to developing symptoms of deficiency (infantile beriberi). The thiamine concentration is low in colostrum, at around 0.01 µg/L. Mature milk contains around 0.21 µg/L. Lactating women secrete approximately 0.16 mg thiamine into breast milk each day and therefore require an increase in intake to compensate for this loss. Thiamine concentrations in blood decrease over the first 12–18 months of life [286].

The essentiality of thiamine in infant nutrition was made very clear in 2003, when a number of infants in Israel developed life-threatening thiamine deficiency after being fed a defective infant formula lacking thiamine [287]. Symptoms included cardiac failure, and seizures that progressed to epilepsy in some children [288]. At 8 years of age, all of the children displayed developmental delay, and varying degrees of speech impairment [289]. Overall, the thiamine deficient formula resulted in the deaths of four children [290]. The European Community has since established specific standard requirements for infant formulae [291].

## Thiamine sources

Thiamine is found in a wide variety of foods, including meats, legumes (beans, lentils), milk, nuts, oats, oranges, rice, seeds, wheat, and wholegrain cereals. The outer layer of seeds and grains are rich in thiamine, and excessive refining and polishing of cereal grains depletes them of the vitamin. Yeast and yeast extract are particularly high in thiamine.

## Effects of excess thiamine

Thiamine is rapidly cleared by the kidneys, and excess intake is not associated with known adverse effects. The US Institute of Medicine (IOM) has not set a tolerable upper intake level because of a lack of data on which to base such a recommendation. Supplements containing up to 50 mg/day of thiamine are available in the US without a prescription, but the possible adverse effects of chronic high intake have not been extensively studied [269]. Thiamine is administered intravenously to treat malnourished patients with suspected Wernicke's encephalopathy.

## Agency guidelines for thiamine intake

The amount of thiamine needed in the body is proportional to caloric intake (~0.5 mg thiamine required per 1,000 kcal). Larger body builds appear to require more thiamine than smaller individuals, as signs of deficiency during starvation occur earlier in larger people [292]. The IOM and the WHO recommendations for thiamine are in agreement for infants in the first year of life (see Box 7.1 for IOM recommendations). The WHO recommended nutrient intake [231] and the IOM adequate intake (AI) recommendation [269] for babies from birth to 6 months of age is 0.2 mg/day, which is approximately 0.03 mg/kg bodyweight. For infants between 1 and 3 years of age, the reference nutrient intake is 0.5 mg/day and the IOM AI is 0.4 mg/day. Similarly, the WHO recommendation is slightly higher for adolescents, at 1.1 mg/day for girls from the age of 10 years, whereas the IOM recommended dietary allowance (RDA) is 0.9 mg/day for 9–13-year-old adolescents (girls and boys). For girls aged 14–18 years, the RDA is 1.0 mg/day [269].

## Box 7.1 US Institute of Medicine recommended dietary allowances for thiamine

Infants 0–6 months (adequate intake (AI)) = 0.2 mg/day
Infants 7–12 months (AI) = 0.3 mg/day
Children 1–3 years = 0.3 mg/day
Females 14–18 years = 1.0 mg/day
Females 19+ = 1.1 mg/day
Pregnancy = 1.4 mg/day
Lactation = 1.4 mg/day

Source: Institute of Medicine, Food and Nutrition Board, *Dietary Reference Intakes: Thiamin, Riboflavin, Niacin, Vitamin B$_6$, Folate, Vitamin B$_{12}$, Pantothenic Acid, Biotin, and Choline*, Dietary Reference Intakes, National Academy Press, Washington, DC, copyright © 1998. [269]

The WHO recommended nutrient intake and the IOM RDA recommendations for adults are 1.1 mg/day for women and 1.2 mg/day for men. Both agencies recommend an increase in thiamine intake of at least 10 per cent to cover increased energy utilization in pregnancy. This is reflected in a reference nutrient intake/RDA for pregnancy of 1.4 mg/day. The WHO recommends a further increase to 1.5 mg/day during lactation to account for the energy cost of milk production [231]. The RDA for lactation remains at the pregnancy level of 1.4 mg/day of thiamine [269].

## Our recommendations for thiamine intake during pregnancy and lactation

Nutritional deficiency for thiamine and other B vitamins rarely occurs in people consuming a moderately varied diet. However, the body does not store thiamine, so a continuous supply is needed. The consequences of thiamine deficiency are potentially severe, and insufficient maternal and/or infant thiamine intake may have long-lasting negative effects on child development. We recommend a varied diet during pregnancy and lactation, preferably substituting wholegrain (unpolished) rice for the more highly refined varieties, if rice is a staple of the diet. Supplementation with thiamine and other B vitamins as found in typical antenatal vitamin supplements may be beneficial for women who experience excessive vomiting in pregnancy or who otherwise find it difficult to consume a varied diet containing thiamine-rich foods.

Chapter 8

# Vitamin B$_2$ (riboflavin) in pregnancy and breastfeeding

## Riboflavin functions

Riboflavin is a water-soluble B vitamin (also known as vitamin B$_2$) that acts as a cofactor for an array of flavocoenzymes involved in energy-producing, biosynthetic, detoxifying, and electron-scavenging pathways. Riboflavin exerts minimal intrinsic enzymatic activity until it is converted to flavin mononucleotide (FMN) by riboflavin kinase, and from FMN to flavin adenine dinucleotide (FAD) by FAD synthetase. These active flavins form complexes with flavoprotein dehydrogenases and oxidases that participate in oxidation–reduction reactions in metabolic pathways [293]. FAD and FMN act as electron acceptors in oxidative metabolism of proteins, fatty acids, and carbohydrates. They also donate electrons to the electron transport chain and are critical for mitochondrial function and energy generation in aerobic cells.

Several human disorders are caused by mutations in flavoprotein genes. Many are mitochondrial disorders, as most flavoproteins are localized to mitochondria (e.g. Leigh syndrome) [293]. Flavocoenzymes also catalyse reactions in biosynthetic pathways of cell-signalling molecules, including steroid hormones [294].

Riboflavin is involved in the metabolism of other B vitamins. For example, synthesis of niacin (vitamin B$_3$) from tryptophan requires FAD as a cofactor of kynurenine mono-oxygenase. Conversion of naturally occurring vitamin B$_6$ (pyridoxine) to its active form, pyridoxal 5′-phosphate, requires the FMN-dependent enzyme pyridoxine 5′-phosphate oxidase. The interconversion of the folate metabolites tetrahydrofolate (THF) and 5-methyl-THF requires the action of the FAD-dependent enzyme methylenetetrahydrofolate reductase (MTHFR) [295].

The active folate and vitamin B$_6$ metabolites generated by flavocoenzymes link riboflavin to both the trans-sulphuration and remethylation pathways in homocysteine metabolism, and the methyl cycle. FMN-dependent generation of pyridoxal 5′-phosphate is necessary for trans-sulphuration of homocysteine to cysteine, and FAD-dependent MTHFR is required for remethylation of homocysteine to produce methionine.

Riboflavin is involved in heme biosynthesis via the FAD-dependent enzyme protoporphyrinogen IX oxidase (PPOX). Reduction in PPOX activity leads to porphyria. Deficiency for riboflavin also alters iron metabolism; correction of the deficiency improves the response to iron therapy in people with iron-deficiency anaemia [296,297].

Riboflavin is present in all tissues, although tissue depletion and repletion can occur rapidly, as very little excess riboflavin is stored. Tissue riboflavin is mainly in the liver as FAD, although it is also present in spleen, kidney, and cardiac muscle, and these organs are initially spared from riboflavin deficiency. Circulating plasma contains riboflavin in three forms: free riboflavin (50%), FAD (40%), FMN (10%) [298].

## Indicators of riboflavin status

Assessment of the activity of the FAD-dependent enzyme erythrocyte glutathione reductase provides an indicator of functional riboflavin status using an activity coefficient expressing the ratio of activities in the presence and absence of added FAD. An erythrocyte glutathione reductase activity coefficient of less than 1.2 indicates adequate activity; 1.2–1.4 indicates low riboflavin status, and above 1.4 indicates deficiency [231,299].

Urinary riboflavin excretion reflects intake in excess of tissue requirements but is not considered an accurate measure of riboflavin status. Erythrocyte flavin level is primarily a measure of FMN. Values greater than 40 nmol/L are considered adequate [231,299].

## Riboflavin deficiency

Riboflavin deficiency is rare in developed countries; it is encountered almost invariably in combination with deficit of other water-soluble (B) vitamins in areas of poor overall nutrition. Deficiency is endemic in populations whose staple diet consists of rice and wheat, with low or no consumption of meat and dairy products [231]. Disorders causing abnormal digestion, such as lactose intolerance or celiac disease, may result in decreased assimilation of riboflavin. The high prevalence of lactose intolerance in Asian and African populations coincides with a lower intake of milk, and poor riboflavin absorption. Hypothyroidism may be a predisposing factor in riboflavin deficiency, because thyroid hormones are involved in riboflavin metabolism [300].

Because of its interactions with other B vitamins, a severe deficiency of riboflavin affects a large number of enzyme systems, and symptoms of deficiency overlap with those associated with other B vitamin deficiencies. Signs of riboflavin deficiency are sore throat, pharyngeal and oral oedema, cracks/splits at corners of mouth (cheilosis), inflammation of the tongue (glossitis), dermatitis, and normochromic–normocytic anaemia [269]. When faced with an inadequate intake of riboflavin, the activity of flavin-dependent enzymes is hierarchically reduced. Enzymes involved in the core electron transfer chain required for ATP synthesis are preserved, while those required for the first step of fatty acid beta-oxidation are decreased. Most flavocoenzymes are FAD dependent; therefore concentrations of FAD are maintained at the expense of FMN [301].

Riboflavin deficiency ultimately leads to the depression of mitochondrial beta-oxidation, and an altered fatty acid profile of triacylglycerols and phospholipids. Diets high in lipids increase the requirement for riboflavin for growth. Deleterious effects of high-fat intake have been reported in riboflavin-deficient animals, including the development of fatty liver [302,303].

## Riboflavin in pregnancy

Placental transfer of riboflavin involves binding proteins that are specific to pregnancy [304,305]. Free riboflavin accumulates in the fetal circulation, ultimately resulting in a concentration that is fourfold higher than that in maternal plasma [306]. Flavin-binding proteins are also present in the fetus at higher levels than in the mother [307]. Preterm birth is a risk for riboflavin deficiency, as most transport and fetal accumulation occurs in late pregnancy.

Infants of riboflavin-deficient mothers tend to be deficient themselves at birth and remain deficient through breastfeeding and weaning. This was noted in a study in Gambia, where the local diet was deficient in riboflavin, consisting of very little meat or dairy products [308]. Yet in two separate small studies, no correlation was found between the riboflavin status of the mother and the outcome of pregnancy, even when riboflavin deficiency was present [309,310]. This may be because riboflavin status improves transiently in the neonatal period, even when maternal status is poor, but declines again at weaning if the diet is nutritionally lacking [308].

## Riboflavin in lactation

During lactation, the maternal requirement for riboflavin is almost 50 per cent higher than prior to pregnancy. Riboflavin is secreted in breast milk, and the concentration in milk is somewhat sensitive to increased maternal intake if the mother's status is low [311]. However, supplementation of well-nourished mothers does not significantly alter the amount of riboflavin present in milk [312]. A small increase in intake of dairy products may be sufficient to meet the riboflavin need in lactating women consuming a varied diet.

Women in some regions may require different interventions or dietary changes. A recent study found that, prior to vitamin fortification of foods, >80 per cent of lactating women in South Africa did not meet the estimated average requirement for most B vitamins, including riboflavin, as well as vitamins A, C, and D, folate, zinc, iodine, and calcium. After fortification for these nutrients, >70 per cent still did not meet the estimated average requirement for riboflavin, in addition to zinc, vitamin A, and vitamin $B_6$ [313]. Even in developed countries, a substantial proportion of pregnant and lactating women may be lacking in riboflavin and will have breast milk concentrations below the level considered adequate (800 nmol/L) [314]. Infants receiving phototherapy for neonatal jaundice are at risk for riboflavin deficiency, because riboflavin is photosensitive and is degraded by this treatment [231,315].

## Riboflavin sources

A balanced diet with a variety of foods should contain ample amounts of riboflavin, which is obtained from the diet as free riboflavin or as FAD or FMN. Dairy products and milk are the most significant sources of riboflavin in Western diets, although meats (particularly organ meats) eggs, dark/leafy green vegetables (spinach, asparagus, and broccoli), legumes, and nuts are also sources. Nutritional yeast is a good source of riboflavin for vegetarians and vegans. Breads and cereals are often fortified with riboflavin and other B vitamins [269].

Absorption is better from animal sources than from vegetable sources; vegetarians and vegans are therefore at higher risk for deficiency. Because riboflavin degrades in light, foods containing riboflavin should be stored in lightproof containers. The riboflavin content of grains and vegetables can be leached away by boiling/cooking, unless the liquid is reused as soup or in sauces [269].

## Risks of excess riboflavin

Toxicity from excessive intake of riboflavin has not been observed in humans. This is assumed to be because riboflavin exhibits low solubility, which limits its absorption from the gastrointestinal tract and prevents exposure to amounts sufficient to produce toxic effects. Because of a lack of evidence on adverse effects, a tolerable upper intake level has not been set for riboflavin.

## Agency guidelines for riboflavin intake

According to the US Institute of Medicine (IOM), the daily requirement for riboflavin is 1.1 mg for adult females (1.3 mg/day for males), increasing to 1.4 mg/day during pregnancy, and to 1.6 mg/day during breastfeeding (Box 8.1) Intake requirements vary somewhat depending on metabolic challenges and

## Box 8.1   US Institute of Medicine recommended dietary allowances for riboflavin

Infants 0–6 months (adequate intake) = 0.3 mg/day; 7–12 months = 0.4 mg/day

    Children 1–3 years 0.5 mg/day

    Females 14–18y = 1.0 mg/day

    Females 19+ years = 1.1 mg/day

    Pregnancy = 1.4 mg/day

    Lactation = 1.6 mg/day

Source: Institute of Medicine, Food and Nutrition Board, *Dietary Reference Intakes: Thiamin, Riboflavin, Niacin, Vitamin B$_6$, Folate, Vitamin B$_{12}$, Pantothenic Acid, Biotin, and Choline*, Dietary Reference Intakes, National Academy Press, Washington, DC, copyright © 1998. [269]

the efficiency of uptake. In the US, the normal intake for an adult is slightly above the recommended dietary allowance (RDA), at an estimated 1.6–2.6 mg/day [269]. There is evidence of tissue saturation with intakes above 1.1 mg/day [316,317]. The IOM AI level for infants aged 0–6 months is 0.3 mg/day, and from 7–12 months it is 0.4 mg/day [269].

The American Association of Pediatrics advises that maternal riboflavin supplementation poses minimal risk in pregnancy and lactation [318].

## Our recommendations for riboflavin intake during pregnancy and lactation

A varied diet including dairy products and meat is the best way to achieve a sufficient riboflavin status in pregnant and lactating women and ensure adequate riboflavin supplies in both mother and infant. An increase in dairy products and/or meat consumption, particularly during lactation, may be necessary in some women. Vegans and vegetarians should consider nutritional yeast in addition to legumes, nuts, and dark green vegetables as a source of this nutrient.

Riboflavin deficiency rarely occurs in isolation in human populations but is seen in conjunction with other nutritional deficiencies in those whose intake of dairy products and meat is limited. An increase in consumption of milk/dairy products is recommended in areas where lactose intolerance is not an issue. In such cases, supplementation at least to the level of the RDA is recommended. Supplementation with riboflavin is generally unnecessary in individuals with a varied diet and healthy lifestyle.

Chapter 9

# Vitamin B$_3$ (niacin) in pregnancy and breastfeeding

## Niacin functions

Niacin, a term encompassing nicotinamide and nicotinic acid (and their biologically active derivatives), is one of the water-soluble B-complex vitamins and is also known as vitamin B$_3$. Nicotinamide is a component of the pyridine nucleotide coenzymes nicotinamide adenine dinucleotide (NAD) and NAD phosphate and acts as an electron donor or acceptor in redox reactions. NAD is involved in the oxidative degradation of fuel molecules (carbohydrates, proteins, fats, and alcohol), and NAD phosphate functions in the reductive biosynthesis of fatty acids and steroids, including cholesterol. Niacin is an accepted treatment for the correction of low levels of HDL cholesterol and high levels of LDL cholesterol and triglycerides. Doses of 1–3 g/day of nicotinic acid are used for this purpose.

NAD is also involved in DNA repair and replication as the substrate for poly-ADP–ribose polymerase enzymes. These enzymes catalyse the transfer of ADP–ribose pairs from NAD to arginine, lysine, or asparagine residues of proteins that are involved in these processes [319]. Niacin deficiency can therefore lead to DNA instability. NAD is also the substrate for mono-ADP-ribosyltransferases, which play a role in G protein-mediated cell signalling [320].

Niacin is rapidly absorbed from the stomach and small intestine, and supplemental niacin absorption does not appear to be significantly inhibited by food [321]. Doses of up to 3–4 g niacin can be almost completely absorbed [269]. Excess niacin is excreted in urine. All body tissues synthesize NAD and NAD phosphate from nicotinic acid and nicotinamide, and nicotinamide can also be synthesized from tryptophan, so proteins containing tryptophan are an important dietary source. The conversion of tryptophan to niacin requires riboflavin (vitamin B$_2$) and pyridoxine (vitamin B$_6$).

## Indicators of niacin status

The most reliable and sensitive measures of niacin status are urinary excretion of the two major methylated metabolites, $N$1-methyl-nicotinamide and its

2-pyridone derivative (N1-methyl-2-pyridone-5-carboxamide) [322]. Excretion rates of less than 5.8 μmol/day indicate deficient niacin status, and those of 5.8 to 17.5 μmol/day indicate low niacin status. Erythrocyte NAD concentration is sensitive to changes in niacin intake and is therefore a reasonable functional blood measure of niacin status [323].

## Niacin deficiency

Niacin deficiency is uncommon in developed countries, although it is still present in developing countries and during famines, and marginal deficiency can occur with low dietary protein intakes. Deficiency has been observed in populations for whom the chief dietary staple is corn or sorghum (including poor communities in the southern US in the early 1900s) [324]. The late stage of severe niacin deficiency is known as pellagra, a chronic wasting disease characterized by erythematous dermatitis, diarrhoea, and dementia. If untreated, pellagra can be fatal. Some sequelae of niacin deficiency reflect roles played by riboflavin or pyridoxine (vitamin B$_6$), as both are essential for conversion of tryptophan to niacin. Alcoholism is a significant cause of niacin deficiency [269]. Malabsorption disorders such as Crohn's disease, hepatic dysfunction, and diabetes [269], as well as the use of oral contraceptives, also affect niacin status [325].

## Niacin in pregnancy and lactation

There is an increased conversion of tryptophan to niacin during pregnancy [326], possibly controlled by the altered hormonal environment [327, 328]. This increased capacity for tryptophan metabolism is reflected in an increased urinary output of N1-methyl-nicotinamide in pregnancy [325]. Nicotinamide is actively transported across the placenta such that fetal plasma levels are higher than maternal plasma levels. Additional energy and growth requirements in pregnancy and lactation are reflected in an increase in niacin requirement of 2–4 mg/day above the pre-pregnancy recommendation [269].

Lactating women secrete approximately 1.4 mg of niacin per day into breast milk, and an additional 3 mg/day above pre-pregnancy requirements is recommended. Breast milk provides approximately 1.5 mg (12.3 μmol) of niacin per litre [231], or the equivalent of 9.9 mg niacin per 1,000 kcal (derived from tryptophan at ratio of 60:1) [329]. Infants who are exclusively breast fed would consume twice the level necessary to prevent deficiency.

## Niacin sources

The daily requirement for niacin can be met by food sources, and also via synthesis from tryptophan, which is present in dietary proteins. Niacin equivalents from tryptophan are based on the ratio of 60:1; i.e. 60 mg of tryptophan provides 1 mg of niacin, or 1 mg of niacin equivalents [329]. Food sources of niacin include dairy products, eggs, fish, lean meats, liver, poultry, legumes (peanuts), brewer's yeast, beets, nuts, and seeds. Bread and cereals are usually fortified with niacin. Grains naturally contain niacin, but in complexed forms with low bioavailability [330]. As mentioned, the prevalence of niacin deficiency is higher in populations consuming mainly corn or sorghum as a dietary staple. Corn contains niacin, but only in a bound form that is nutritionally unavailable. Heating or soaking corn in an alkaline solution (e.g. lime (calcium oxide)) releases bound niacin and improves its bioavailability [331]. Infant formulas are usually fortified with niacin and other B vitamins.

## Risks of excess niacin

Long-term administration of high-dose nicotinic acid (as a therapy for lowering serum cholesterol) can lead to dermatological manifestations and hepatotoxicity. There is no evidence of adverse effects from the consumption of niacin as it occurs naturally in foods. The advised upper limit for niacin intake is 35 mg/day, which applies to synthetic forms obtained from supplements and/or fortified foods [269].

## Agency guidelines for niacin intake

The US Institute of Medicine recommends 2 mg/day as an adequate intake of niacin for infants aged 0–6 months, increasing to 4 mg/day between 7 and 12 months, and 5 mg/day up to the age of 3 years (Box 9.1) [269]. For females aged 14 and older, the recommended dietary allowance (RDA) is 14 mg/day [269],

---

### Box 9.1 US Institute of Medicine recommended dietary allowances for niacin

Infants 0–6 months (adequate intake) = 2 mg/day; 7–12 months = 4 mg/day
  Children 1–3 years = 5 mg/day
  Females 14+ years = 14 mg/day
  Pregnancy = 18 mg/day
  Lactation = 17 mg/day

Source: Institute of Medicine, Food and Nutrition Board, *Dietary Reference Intakes: Thiamin, Riboflavin, Niacin, Vitamin $B_6$, Folate, Vitamin $B_{12}$, Pantothenic Acid, Biotin, and Choline*, Dietary Reference Intakes, National Academy Press, Washington, DC, copyright © 1998. [269]

although the WHO recommended nutrient intake is 16 mg/day for adolescents up to 18 years of age [231]. The RDA for pregnant women is 18 mg/day, and 17 mg/day for lactation. In the US and Canada, intakes of niacin often exceed the RDA [269]. Although there are no reports of adverse effects of niacin or nicotinamide on the human fetus, niacin supplementation in doses above the RDA for the treatment of high cholesterol is not recommended in pregnancy (FDA category C).

## Our recommendations for niacin intake during pregnancy and lactation

Diets deficient in niacin are likely to be deficient in other B vitamins. Consumption of a balanced, mixed diet is generally sufficient to meet niacin requirements. The additional needs for niacin during pregnancy are mirrored by the increased energy intake needs, and dietary supplementation is only necessary in cases of overall poor nutritional intake.

# Chapter 10

# Vitamin B$_6$ (pyridoxine) in pregnancy and breastfeeding

## Vitamin B$_6$ functions

Vitamin B$_6$ is a water-soluble vitamin required for the activity of around 100 enzymes, with key roles in amino acid and carbohydrate metabolism, lipid bio-synthesis, hormone function, synthesis of neurotransmitters and nucleic acids, red blood cell formation, and immune system function. The term vitamin B$_6$ refers to six related compounds: pyridoxal (PL), pyridoxine, pyridoxamine, and their respective active forms, pyridoxal-5′-phosphate (PLP), pyridoxine-5′-phosphate, and pyridoxamine-5′-phosphate. The main forms in animal tissues (and animal-derived foods) are PL and PLP, while pyridoxine and pyridoxine-5′-phosphate predominate in plants. All forms of vitamin B$_6$ can be converted to the key coenzymatic form, PLP [332].

Although they display catalytic diversity, most PLP-dependent enzymes, including oxidoreductases, transferases, hydrolases, lyases, and isomerases, act on amino acids. PLP covalently binds its substrate, acting as an electrophilic catalyst that stabilizes reaction intermediates [333–335]. In this way, vitamin B$_6$ is involved in basic metabolic pathways rather than in specialized regulatory functions.

Enzymes involved in the metabolism (trans-sulphuration) of homocysteine to cysteine depend on vitamin B$_6$ (PLP) as a cofactor. Disruption of this reaction leads to elevated blood homocysteine, which is associated with cardiovascular disease, neuropsychiatric problems, and other adverse effects. Adequate levels of vitamin B$_6$, along with vitamin B$_{12}$ and folate, are required to keep homocysteine levels low [336].

Vitamin B$_6$ is also involved in synthesis and metabolism of neurotransmitters, which are formed by PLP-dependent decarboxylation of amino acids, and production of polyamines necessary for cell growth [337]. Lipid metabolism depends on vitamin B$_6$ as a cofactor in decarboxylation of phosphatidylserine. Because of its role in the synthesis of sphingosine [338], vitamin B$_6$ also affects the development of brain lipids and myelination. PLP and PL accumulate in erythrocytes, where they modulate the oxygen-binding affinity of haemoglobin [339,340].

## Indicators of vitamin B$_6$ status

Plasma PLP is used as an indicator of vitamin B$_6$ status, also reflecting the status of liver stores [341]. Plasma levels change slowly in response to vitamin B$_6$ intake, plateauing around 7–10 days after a change in intake. The suggested value for adequate vitamin B$_6$ status is PLP >30 nmol/L, although this varies somewhat with age, sex, and protein intake [342]. The US Institute of Medicine (IOM) recommendations are based on achieving a PLP level of ≥20 nmol/L [269].

## Vitamin B$_6$ deficiency

Although vitamin B$_6$ is widely available in foods, mild to moderate deficiency is still common, even in developed countries such as the US [343]. In addition to poor dietary intake, various conditions including malabsorptive disorders, inflammatory bowel disease, and diabetes, can decrease plasma vitamin B$_6$ levels. Classic symptoms relate to vitamin B$_6$ functions in neurotransmitter and haemoglobin biosynthesis, and include epileptic convulsions, depression and confusion, microcytic anaemia, and dermatitis.

Low levels of vitamin B$_6$ (PLP) have been linked to inflammatory disorders such as rheumatoid arthritis [344] and inflammatory bowel disease [345]. Plasma PLP concentrations are inversely correlated with cardiovascular disease risk, independent of major atherosclerotic risk factors including high homocysteine [346]. Drugs such as isoniazid (for tuberculosis) and L-DOPA interfere with vitamin B$_6$, reducing its plasma concentration and increasing the risk for deficiency [269].

## Vitamin B$_6$ in pregnancy

PLP levels decline during pregnancy, beyond the effects of haemodilution. In fact, the most significant drop occurs in the third trimester, when blood volume plateaus. The fetus sequesters vitamin B$_6$ throughout pregnancy, and after the first trimester, the fetal concentration is higher than the maternal concentration. Low maternal intakes during pregnancy can lead to compromised vitamin B$_6$ status in the infant, as the vitamin B$_6$ status of cord blood correlates with maternal B$_6$ status [347].

As noted previously, vitamin B$_6$ deficiency can lead to hyper-homocysteinaemia, which in pregnancy is associated with pre-eclampsia, preterm birth, low birthweight, and small-for-gestational-age infants [348–350]. However, currently there is no evidence that vitamin B$_6$ supplementation in pregnancy reduces the risk of these adverse pregnancy outcomes. Specific other effects of vitamin B$_6$ in pregnancy are noted below.

## Vitamin B$_6$ in conception

Vitamin B$_6$ has been implicated in regulating the length of the luteal phase in the menstrual cycle, and deficiency for the nutrient has been shown to reduce the likelihood of conception [351]. A pre-conception 'Mediterranean diet' (high in vegetables and vegetable oils, legumes, and fish, and low in saturated fats, meats, and refined carbohydrates), was shown to produce healthy levels of vitamin B$_6$ both in blood and follicular fluid. Couples undergoing in vitro fertilization who were following such a diet were more likely to achieve pregnancy than those following a diet that was higher in whole grains, meat, fruits, fatty dressings (e.g. mayonnaise), and snacks, despite the latter diet being low in processed foods and considered 'health conscious'. Both diets increased folate concentrations, but the Mediterranean diet led to an additional rise in vitamin B$_6$ [352].

## The effect of vitamin B$_6$ supplementation on nausea and vomiting in pregnancy

Vitamin B$_6$ supplementation has long been considered as a remedy for morning sickness. Doses between 10 and 40 mg/day were shown to reduce the severity of symptoms of nausea and vomiting in pregnancy in two small randomized trials [353,354]. However, a recent systematic review found no strong evidence that vitamin B$_6$ supplementation reduces vomiting more than placebo or other interventions, including ginger and acupressure [355]. Nonetheless, the American Congress of Obstetricians and Gynecologists continues to recommend taking vitamin B$_6$ supplements for nausea and vomiting in pregnancy [356].

## Vitamin B$_6$ and anaemia

Vitamin B$_6$ deficiency can contribute to anaemia in pregnancy. Some pregnant women with anaemia are nonresponsive to iron, but anaemia improves with administration of vitamin B$_6$ [357]. Deficiency for vitamin B$_6$ should be considered in cases of anaemia that do not respond to supplemental iron.

## Vitamin B$_6$ and fetal brain development

Vitamin B$_6$ deficiency during pregnancy alters the concentrations of the neuro-active amino acids glutamate and glycine, which are endogenous ligands of the N-methyl-D-aspartate (NMDA) receptor. NMDA receptors are involved in synaptic plasticity during development and are important for learning and memory. Abnormalities in brain NMDA receptor function have been observed in rats postnatally following vitamin B$_6$ restriction during gestation [358].

In addition to glutamate and glycine, synthesis of the neurotransmitters gamma-aminobutyric acid (GABA), serotonin, epinephrine, norepinephrine, histamine, and dopamine requires PLP-dependent enzymes. Seizures can occur in utero, when GABA neurotransmission is disrupted by mutations in genes involved in vitamin B$_6$ metabolism [359], and in infants, when vitamin B$_6$ intake is deficient.

## Vitamin B$_6$ in lactation and infancy

Gestationally accumulated stores of vitamin B$_6$ are important to maintain adequate levels for the breastfed neonate in the first weeks of life [360,361]. Weight gain and linear growth in early infancy have been correlated with infant vitamin B$_6$ intake [362]. Breast milk vitamin B$_6$ concentrations are influenced by maternal vitamin B$_6$ status and respond rapidly to changes in dietary intake. Milk from mothers receiving 2.5 mg/day of vitamin B$_6$ as a supplement had average vitamin B$_6$ concentrations that ranged from 0.15 to 0.21 mg/L [360]. However, there is significant inter-individual variation in breast milk levels despite similar intakes. Some women receiving supplements of 2.5 mg/day had breast milk vitamin B$_6$ concentrations well below the goal of 0.13 mg/L in milk [360], the concentration deemed adequate for infant needs [269]. A more recent study found that only infants of mothers supplemented with 10 mg/day met or exceeded the vitamin B$_6$ recommended dietary allowance (RDA) of 0.3 mg/day [363].

Seizures have been observed in infants consuming milk formula with low vitamin B$_6$ content. The seizures respond to vitamin B$_6$ supplementation [364,365]. Breast milk vitamin B$_6$ concentrations of <0.1 mg/L are thought to place infants at risk for the development of seizures [365].

Maternal vitamin B$_6$ nutritional status may influence infant behaviour. A study of a cohort of Egyptian mothers and their breastfed infants found that aspects of infant behaviour (mother–infant interactions, consolability, and irritability) were better in infants whose mothers had the highest vitamin B$_6$ status. In addition, in these mothers, vitamin B$_6$ was the only nutrient present in insufficient levels in breast milk (compared with breast milk from a group of well-nourished Western women). There was also a significant positive association between maternal vitamin B$_6$ and birthweight in this cohort [366].

## Vitamin B$_6$ sources and metabolism

Plants, fungi, and single-celled organisms can synthesize vitamin B$_6$, but animals must ingest it from external sources. Vitamin B$_6$ is widely distributed in foods, particularly poultry, fish (especially tuna), and meats, legumes (e.g. chickpeas), potatoes and other starchy vegetables, non-citrus fruits, and nuts and seeds (e.g. pistachios, sunflower seeds, and sesame seeds). Fortified cereals and fortified soy-based meat substitutes also provide vitamin B$_6$ and may be important food sources for individuals consuming vegan diets [269].

The availability of vitamin B$_6$ from foods is approximately 75 per cent. Food of plant origin contains mostly pyridoxine and pyridoxine-5′-phosphate, which have lower bioavailability than PL and PLP from animal-source foods. Non-phosphorylated vitamin B$_6$ absorbed from the diet is stored in the liver. At high intakes, the capacity for protein binding of PLP limits its accumulation in tissues [367]. However, the high PLP-binding capacity of proteins in muscle and plasma, and haemoglobin in erythrocytes allows high accumulation when other tissues are saturated.

## Risks of excess vitamin B$_6$

There are no reported adverse effects of vitamin B$_6$ derived from food sources. The tolerable upper level of intake from supplements is based on sensory neuropathy as the critical adverse event. Levels below 100 mg/day are considered not to be associated with adverse effects, so this amount is set as the tolerable upper intake level [269].

## Agency guidelines for vitamin B$_6$ intake

Both the IOM and the WHO guidelines advise intakes of 1.3 mg/day for females aged 19–50 years (1.5 for over 50 years), with reference nutrient intakes/RDAs for pregnancy and lactation of 1.9 and 2.0 mg/day, respectively [231,269]. Most people in the US and other developed countries have access to foods that offer adequate amounts of vitamin B$_6$ in their diets. Diets lacking B$_6$ would be nutritionally poor overall and would lack other B vitamins, so primary deficiency of vitamin B$_6$ is rarely encountered [269]. However, vitamin B$_6$ levels were found to be low in ~11 per cent of people who take supplements, and in ~24 per cent of people who do not take supplements, in a 2008 report of the National Health and Nutrition Examination Survey [368]. The findings suggested that the current vitamin B$_6$ RDAs did not guarantee adequate nutritional status for the whole population and that intakes between 3 and 4.9 mg/day would still leave some subgroups (the elderly, people of African descent, smokers, and current and former users of oral contraceptives) with inadequate vitamin B$_6$ status.

The CDC also considers vitamin B$_6$ deficiency to be a fairly common occurrence in the US [343]. Nonetheless, a study of middle–high income pregnant women in the US found that the usual intake of vitamin B$_6$ exceeded the estimated average requirement of 1.6 mg/day, and generally met the RDA (1.9 mg/day). The probability of intake less than the estimated average requirement was 21 per cent [369].

## Box 10.1  US Institute of Medicine recommended dietary allowances for vitamin B$_6$

Infants 0–6 months (adequate intake (AI)) = 0.1 mg/day (≈0.014 mg/kg)
  Infants 7–12 months (AI) = 0.3 mg/day (≈0.033 mg/kg)
  Children 1–3 years = 0.5 mg/day
  Females 14–18 years = 1.2 mg/day
  Females 19–50 years = 1.3 mg/day
  Pregnancy = 1.9 mg/day
  Lactation = 2.0 mg/day

Source: Institute of Medicine, Food and Nutrition Board, *Dietary Reference Intakes: Thiamin, Riboflavin, Niacin, Vitamin B$_6$, Folate, Vitamin B$_{12}$, Pantothenic Acid, Biotin, and Choline*, Dietary Reference Intakes, National Academy Press, Washington, DC, copyright © 1998. [269]

There is an additional requirement of 0.6–0.7 mg/day during pregnancy and lactation. Some degree of deficiency may be present in infants whose sole source of nutrition is breast milk, and whose mothers have marginal vitamin B$_6$ intake and/or are not supplemented (Box 10.1).

According to European Commission recommendations, supplements of 2.5–4 mg/day are required to maintain the plasma concentration of vitamin B$_6$ at pre-pregnancy levels [370]. This is to account for the drop in plasma concentrations during pregnancy that are a consequence of preferential uptake by the fetus. The view of this board is that there is no evidence that vitamin B$_6$ metabolism changes during lactation, so unlike the IOM RDA, the recommendation is the same as for non-lactating women (15 µg/g dietary protein or 1.1 mg vitamin B$_6$/day) [370].

## Our recommendations for vitamin B$_6$ intake during pregnancy and lactation

Although increased amounts of vitamin B$_6$ are recommended for pregnant and breastfeeding women, supplementation is usually not required if the diet is adequate and nutritionally balanced. A diet similar to the Mediterranean diet is recommended during pregnancy and lactation to provide a variety of sources for vitamin B$_6$ and other B complex vitamins. Most prenatal vitamins contain vitamin B$_6$ in adequate daily amounts. Additional vitamin B$_6$ supplements for alleviating nausea and vomiting in pregnancy should only be taken under the advice of a physician and should not be combined with prenatal vitamins that also contain vitamin B$_6$.

# Chapter 11

# Vitamin B₇ (biotin) in pregnancy and breastfeeding

## Biotin functions

Biotin is a water-soluble B vitamin (vitamin $B_7$) that acts as a coenzyme for carboxylases, with roles in gluconeogenesis, fatty acid synthesis, and amino acid catabolism. Reduced activity of biotin-dependent enzymes (acetyl-CoA carboxylase I and II, and propionyl-CoA carboxylase) alters lipid metabolism and may impair synthesis of polyunsaturated fatty acids and prostaglandins [371]. Impaired hepatic gluconeogenesis results in fatty liver and kidney syndrome in animals (chickens) and is responsive to biotin supplementation [372]. Biotin has effects on gene expression by binding covalently to histones [373].

## Indicators of biotin status

Biotin is a cofactor for beta-methylcrotonyl-CoA carboxylase, which is required for the degradation of leucine. Biotin deficiency causes inactivation of this enzyme and accumulation of the leucine metabolite 3-hydroxyisovalerate, which is formed via an alternate pathway. Urinary excretion of biotin and/or 3-hydroxyisovalerate, assessed via an avidin-based immunoassay, is used to determine biotin status [374]. Overt cases of biotin deficiency show decreased excretion of biotin and/or abnormally increased excretion of 3-hydroxyisovalerate (>195 µg/day) [375]. The normal range for biotin excretion is 19–62 nmol/day. Excretion decreases rapidly during biotin depletion. Low plasma biotin is not a sensitive indicator of biotin deficiency or inadequate intake [374].

## Biotin deficiency

Prolonged consumption of egg whites can lead to biotin deficiency, as egg whites contain the biotin-binding protein avidin. Otherwise, dietary deficiency is rare. Clinical signs of deficiency include erythematous or seborrhoeic dermatitis, conjunctivitis, hair loss, and CNS abnormalities including lethargy, hypotonia, hallucinations, depression, paraesthesia, and developmental delay in infants [269]. Biotin deficiency has adverse effects on immune function, including reduced antibody synthesis and a lower percentage of B lymphocytes in spleen [376]. Animal studies suggest biotin deficiency can cause birth defects, primarily manifesting as cleft lip and palate, and impaired skeletal long bone growth [377]. Even marginally deficient biotin status that does not confer symptoms in the mother appears to increase the risk of these defects in various animal species. Smoking accelerates the degradation of biotin, resulting in marginal biotin deficiency [378].

## Biotin in pregnancy

Placental transport of biotin is not rapid and does not generate a substantial fetal-to-maternal gradient, despite the presence of a biotin transporter in the trophoblastic villus membrane. As in other tissues, carrier-mediated biotin transport in the placenta is saturable and sodium dependent [379]. Pregnancy increases biotin breakdown and may impair absorption of biotin, resulting in maternal biotin depletion. In a small study, biotin status was abnormally low in ~75 per cent of women in late pregnancy [380]. This may reduce fetal histone biotinylation, causing altered gene expression with the potential for teratogenesis. The effects of biotin deficiency on lipid metabolism are also potentially teratogenic [381]. Yet, despite evidence that marginal biotin deficiency in human pregnancy is common, there is currently no direct evidence of teratogenicity in humans.

## Biotin in lactation

The biotin content of human milk is estimated to be approximately 6 μg (24 nmol)/L [382,383]. Based on this, the estimated intake for breastfed infants is 5 μg/day (assuming consumption of ~0.75 L/day). Symptomatic biotin deficiency has not been reported in breastfed infants.

## Biotin sources

Biotin is synthesized by intestinal bacteria and is present in a wide variety of foods at low concentrations. In some foods, such as wheat bran, biotin is present in reasonable quantities but is not bioavailable. Liver and egg yolks are the most significant natural sources of biotin. Egg whites contain avidin, which binds and sequesters biotin. Raw egg whites should be avoided, and cooked egg whites should be consumed in moderation to prevent biotin depletion. Other sources include legumes (particularly soybeans and lentils), sunflower seeds, milk, cheese, chicken, pork, beef, and some fruits and vegetables. The availability of biotin from cereals is low.

## Risks of excess biotin

The intestinal absorption of biotin is limited, so the risk of excess is considered minimal. Biotin has been shown to be relatively non-toxic at high doses in mice (>60 mg/day) [384]. Although some individuals taking biotin supplements may experience mild nausea, stomach cramps, or diarrhoea, these effects are relatively rare. Toxicity from food sources is considered unlikely.

## Agency guidelines for biotin intake

The WHO reference nutrient intakes [231] and the US Institute of Medicine (IOM) recommended dietary allowances (RDAs) [269] are in agreement with regard to biotin requirements (see Box 11.1 for the IOM recommendations). The adequate intake recommendation for infants 0–6 months is 5 µg/day and then increasing to 6 µg/day until the age of 1. Children 1–3 years of age require 8 µg/day. The RDA/reference nutrient intake for adolescents aged 13–18 years is 25 µg/day. For females 19+ years (including pregnancy), the RDA/reference nutrient intake is 30 µg/day (123 nmol/day), rising to 35 µg/day (143 nmol/day) during lactation. Despite some questions about the potential teratogenicity of biotin deficiency, and the impact of pregnancy on reducing biotin levels, the IOM does not consider the evidence strong enough to warrant an increase in the RDA for pregnancy, except in pregnant adolescents, for whom the RDA increases to 30 µg/day from 25 µg/day pre-pregnancy. However, an additional 5 µg/day is recommended during lactation to account for losses due to excretion into breast milk (Box 11.1) [269].

---

### Box 11.1 US Institute of Medicine recommended dietary allowances for biotin

Infants 0–6 months (adequate intake (AI)) = 5 µg/day
  Infants 7–12 months (AI) = 6 µg/day
  Children 1–3 years = 8 µg/day
  Females 14–18 years = 25 µg/day
  Females 19+ = 30 µg/day
  Pregnancy = 30 µg/day
  Lactation = 35 µg/day

Source: Institute of Medicine, Food and Nutrition Board, *Dietary Reference Intakes: Thiamin, Riboflavin, Niacin, Vitamin $B_6$, Folate, Vitamin $B_{12}$, Pantothenic Acid, Biotin, and Choline*, Dietary Reference Intakes, National Academy Press, Washington, DC, copyright © 1998. [269]

## Our recommendations for biotin intake during pregnancy and lactation

Deficiency is unlikely unless a biotin antagonist (e.g. avidin) is present in the diet. Currently available evidence suggests that supplemental biotin is generally not required in pregnancy, although high consumption of egg whites should be avoided. Women who smoke have a greater risk of biotin deficiency resulting from accelerated biotin metabolism.

# Chapter 12

# Vitamin B$_9$ (folate) in pregnancy and breastfeeding

## Folate functions

Folate is an essential B-group vitamin (sometimes called vitamin B$_9$) that is synthesized by microorganisms and higher plants but not by mammals. It is a coenzyme in multiple biochemical pathways involving one-carbon metabolism, including amino acid metabolism, purine and pyrimidine nucleotide biosynthesis, the methylation cycle, and homocysteine–methionine metabolism.

Homocysteine, an amino acid that is not found in proteins, serves as an intermediate in methionine metabolism. It is formed by removal of a methyl group from methionine and can be remethylated back to methionine or converted to cysteine via the action of folate, vitamin B$_{12}$, and vitamin B$_6$ (see Fig. 12.1). Folate serves as a methyl donor, and homocysteine status is therefore influenced by the supply of folate [385]. Low folate intake results in elevated serum homocysteine, which has been implicated as a risk factor for vascular disease, especially stroke [386]. Folate supplementation has been shown to decrease homocysteine levels, improve endothelial function, and reduce the risk of stroke [387, 388].

Folate also serves as the principal source of the one-carbon group used for DNA methylation, which is central to epigenetic processes. Methylation patterns can be transmitted through mitosis, perpetuating the epigenetic pattern through subsequent cell generations. Folate deficiency may influence the ability to maintain DNA methylation patterns in replicating cells and thus may induce lasting phenotypic changes [389, 390]. Altered methylation has been associated with some cancers [391].

The key role of folate in nucleotide biosynthesis, and thus in DNA and RNA synthesis, means that folate requirements increase during periods of rapid cell division. The most overt consequence of folate deficiency is megaloblastic (pernicious) anaemia, which is caused by the inhibition of DNA synthesis in red blood cell (RBC) production [392, 393]. Embryogenesis and fetal growth also require higher levels of folate.

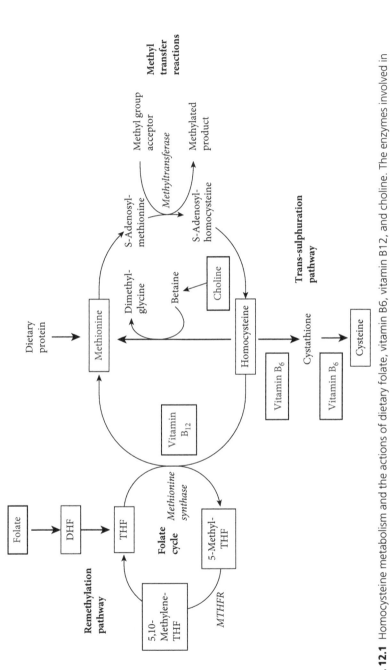

**Fig. 12.1** Homocysteine metabolism and the actions of dietary folate, vitamin B6, vitamin B12, and choline. The enzymes involved in the conversions are shown in italics. DHF, dihydrofolate; MTHFR, methylenetetrahydrofolate reductase; THF, tetrahydrofolate

Fetal requirements for folate must be supplied maternally during pregnancy. A link between low maternal folate levels and the occurrence of neural tube defects (NTDs, e.g. spina bifida, anencephaly, and encephalocele), has long been recognized [394, 395]. Low folate may induce NTDs by either inhibiting DNA synthesis or through the disruption of DNA methylation [396]. Maternal folate requirements increase by 50 per cent during pregnancy, and even if the daily diet consists of food rich in folates, the high requirement usually cannot be met through the consumption of unfortified foods alone. It is for this reason that peri-conceptional supplementation with folic acid is recommended internationally for the prevention of NTDs. 'Folic acid' specifically refers to the fully oxidized monoglutamate form that is used in supplements and fortified foods, and rarely occurs in nature. Randomized clinical trials have shown that folic acid taken in very early pregnancy can markedly reduce the risk that an infant will be born with a NTD [397–399].

## Indicators of folate status

Clinical folate deficiency is usually defined as a serum folate concentration <7 nmol/L (~3 ng/mL) or an RBC folate concentration that is <315 nmol/L (~140 ng/mL) [269]. Low serum folate is inversely correlated with serum homocysteine. Although plasma homocysteine is very sensitive to changes in folate level, the concentration of homocysteine in plasma can also be influenced by vitamin $B_{12}$ status [400] and is therefore not a specific indicator.

## Folate deficiency

Irrespective of the clinical definition of folate deficiency, NTD-affected pregnancies may yet occur among women who are not classified as deficient. A dose–response study which aimed to determine if supplementation to increase folic acid levels beyond the threshold of 'deficient' status would further reduce NTD risk found that maximal risk reduction occurred at RBC folate levels >906 nmol/L [401]. Earlier studies showed that peri-conceptional supplementation of 800 μg folic acid/day together with multivitamins achieved a near 100 per cent reduction of NTDs as well as marked reductions of congenital heart defects [398, 399]. Folate deficiency can also occur as a result of alcohol abuse, malabsorption, liver disease, certain anaemias, and because of concomitant intake of medications that interfere with folate utilization (e.g. anticonvulsants, metformin, sulfasalazine, triamterene (a diuretic), methotrexate, and barbiturates) [402].

Obese women have a significantly higher risk of having a NTD-affected pregnancy than do normal-weight women [403, 404]. This increased risk is independent of their use of supplements containing folic acid [405], or consumption of flour fortified with folic acid [406]. Adequate folate intake thus appears to protect against NTDs in lean but not overweight women [407].

Folate levels are not specifically modified by BMI, although obesity may affect body distribution, resulting in a lower plasma folate level and a higher RBC folate level. It is not yet clear whether obese women require higher doses of folate supplements [408]. A recent pharmacokinetic study has provided evidence that obesity affects the pharmacokinetic response to supplemental folic acid and its tissue distribution, resulting in lower circulating levels of folate [409]. However other data suggest that folate deficiency may not be the primary cause of the elevated NTD risk in this population [410].

Achieving effective folate concentrations (≥906 nmol/L) is challenging. A Canadian study found that in 2006, 40 per cent of women of childbearing age and 36 per cent of pregnant women had RBC folate below the recommended level, despite nationwide flour fortification [411]. In Canada, a high (5 mg/day) dosage is recommended for pregnant women with a family history of NTDs and those trying to conceive. The relationship between folic acid intake and RBC concentration is non-linear; a study of 1.1 mg vs 5 mg folic acid per day for 30 days observed a twofold increase in RBC folate concentration from a fivefold increase in folic acid intake [412].

## Folate in pregnancy

### Folate in pre-eclampsia, placental vascular disorders, and gestational hypertension

Maternal folate deficiency and elevated homocysteine may increase the risk of placental vascular disorders. Folate deficiency was observed as a prominent risk factor for placental abruption/infarction in a systematic review of four early studies [413]. A study using data from the Medical Birth Registry of Norway found that women who used folic acid and/or multivitamin supplements containing folic acid had a significantly lower risk of placental abruption, particularly preterm abruption, than did women who did not use supplements [414]. The recent Generation R Study in the Netherlands, using a prospective cohort of >5,800 women, reported an association between low maternal folate concentrations and vascular-related pregnancy complications [349]. Homocysteine concentrations are higher in pre-eclamptic pregnancies than in normal pregnancies [415, 416], and levels may associate with the severity of pre-eclampsia [417]. Folic acid supplement use was reported to be associated with a lower risk of gestational hypertension in a retrospective study [418].

## The effect of folate on preterm birth

A study of >34,000 low-risk singleton pregnancies found that pre-conceptional folic acid supplementation for one year or longer, compared with no supplementation, was associated with a 70 per cent decrease in the risk of spontaneous preterm delivery between 20 and 28 weeks, and a 50 per cent decrease between 28 and 32 weeks. The risk of early spontaneous preterm birth was inversely proportional to the duration of pre-conceptional folate supplementation. Pre-conceptional folate supplementation was specifically related to early spontaneous preterm birth and not associated with other complications of pregnancy [419]. Low folate levels were also associated with preterm birth in the Generation R Study [349].

## The effect of folate on birthweight

Maternal folate status is thought to have a role in promoting normal fetal growth and placental function. Folate requirements peak in the third trimester to account for rapid fetal growth and fetal accumulation of folate stores. Low folate (and high homocysteine) concentrations were associated with lower birthweight and a higher risk of having a small-for-gestational-age infant in the Generation R Study [349]. Other studies report a positive association between birthweight and maternal RBC folate status or intake [420, 421].

## Folate in the prevention of birth defects

### Supplemental folic acid and NTD prevention

Multiple case–control and epidemiological studies have demonstrated a positive effect of folic acid supplementation or dietary intake of folate on reducing the risk of NTD-affected pregnancies [394, 422–424]. Epidemiological findings were strengthened by the results of a non-randomized intervention study in China that included 130,142 women who took folic acid before pregnancy, and 117,689 who did not. The study concluded that pre-conceptional intake of 400 µg/day folic acid could reduce risk of NTDs in areas with both high and low rates of defects [425].

The first randomized controlled trial of pre-conceptional folic acid treatment involved 112 women with a prior NTD pregnancy and showed a statistically significant effect [426]. The UK's Medical Research Council Vitamin Study was an international, multicentre, double-blind randomized controlled trial in women with a previous NTD pregnancy (from the UK, Hungary, Israel, Australia, Canada, the USSR, and France). The study found that folic acid alone can reduce NTD recurrence by 71 per cent [397]. To determine if folic acid could prevent the first occurrence of NTDs, a randomized trial was conducted using what was considered a physiological folic acid dose (800 µg/day), along with minerals and trace elements (copper, manganese, zinc, low-dose vitamin C), and compared with results obtained from supplementation with the trace elements alone [398]. The study included >4,800 women and observed no NTDs in the folic acid group, as compared with six NTDs in the group that received trace elements alone (p = 0.01). A meta-analysis of five trials in >6,100 women has confirmed that folic acid supplementation helps prevent both first occurrence and reoccurrences of NTD [427].

## Folic acid and orofacial clefts

In a large prospective cohort study of over 240,000 pregnancies, daily maternal consumption of 400 µg of folic acid without other vitamins, started before the mother's last menstrual period, was associated with a reduced risk of cleft lip (with or without cleft palate) in babies born in a high-prevalence region of China [428]. However, an earlier Hungarian study suggested that higher doses (6 mg/day) were required in the critical period of primary and secondary palate development to reduce the incidence of isolated orofacial clefts [429]. A 2010 meta-analysis found insufficient evidence to support folic acid use for the prevention of orofacial clefts [427], but a more recent population-based cohort study of >11,000 infants in Ireland indicated that folic acid use (generally 400 µg/day) by mothers during the first trimester of pregnancy was associated with a more than fourfold lower incidence of cleft lip (with or without cleft palate) in their infants [430].

## Folic acid and neurodevelopment

An increase in folic acid intake resulting from fortification and/or supplementation may increase folate levels sufficiently to avoid NTDs but not to eliminate more subtle neurodevelopmental effects of marginal folate status on the offspring. Low folate concentrations in the brain have been proposed to be a causative factor in some forms of developmental delay and autism [431, 432]. Higher peri-conceptional maternal folic acid intake was shown to correlate with a decreased risk of autism in the developing child when the mother and/or child possessed the *MTHFR* 677 C>T variant (see 'Folic acid genetics') [433]. A recent population-based analysis within the Generation R Study found that low maternal folate status in early pregnancy was associated with an increased risk of emotional and behavioural problems in offspring at 18 months (n = 4,214 children) [434] and 3 years of age (n = 3,209 children) [435]. The data suggest that folic acid supplementation in early pregnancy can help reduce the risk of later behavioural problems in children.

## Folic acid genetics

There appears to be a genetic component to the causation of NTDs, as suggested by results of twin and family studies, and the higher prevalence in some ethnic groups such as Celts [436], Sikhs [437], and Northern Chinese [438]. Folate status is modified by activity of the enzyme methylenetetrahydrofolate reductase (MTHFR), which controls a rate-limiting step in the methylation cycle (remethylation of homocysteine to methionine—see Fig. 12.1). MTHFR diverts one-carbon units towards methylation reactions at the expense of nucleotide synthesis [439]. Inactivating mutations in the *MTHFR* gene, which encodes this enzyme, and particularly the 677C>T polymorphism, result in lower plasma folate, and elevated plasma homocysteine levels. The TT genotype renders individuals more susceptible to epigenetic alterations in response to low folate status; the combination of such *MTHFR* mutations in the presence of low folate intake can increase the risk of NTDs [440]. An examination of international variation in the distribution of the TT genotype in ~7,000 newborns from 16 geographic regions found that trends in frequencies of NTDs follow the genotype distribution to some extent [441, 442].

## Folate interactions with vitamin B$_{12}$ and choline

Folate and vitamin B$_{12}$ interact in common biochemical reactions (see Chapter 11 on vitamin B$_{12}$), and when either is in deficit, a very similar picture of megaloblastic anaemia emerges, reflecting a derangement of DNA synthesis in erythropoietic cells [443]. Supplementation with folic acid in the presence of low vitamin B$_{12}$ can correct the anaemia but allows the neurological pathologies associated with vitamin B$_{12}$ deficiency to progress. These manifestations result from inactivation of vitamin B$_{12}$-dependent methylmalonyl-CoA mutase, correction of which cannot be addressed by increasing folate [443].

Low levels of either vitamin B$_{12}$ or folate leads to an elevation in plasma homocysteine, and its associated adverse effects. The vitamin B$_{12}$-dependent enzyme methionine synthase is inactive when this nutrient is in deficit, causing folate to be trapped in the form of 5-methyl-tetrahydrofolate, compounding folate deficiency [444]. Supplementation with folate can lower homocysteine levels in the presence of vitamin B$_{12}$ deficiency, although other consequences of this nutritional imbalance are becoming evident. Children born to women with high erythrocyte folate but low vitamin B$_{12}$ status appear to be at high risk for developing insulin resistance [445].

There is also an intersection of the pathways of choline and folate in the formation of methionine from homocysteine. Betaine, the primary oxidative product of choline, can act as an alternate methyl donor to 5-methyl-tetrahydrofolate in this conversion. Choline becomes a limiting nutrient during folate deficiency [446].

## Food folate sources

The most concentrated food sources of folates are liver (320 µg/100 g), yeast extract, green leafy vegetables, legumes, citrus fruits, and fortified breakfast cereals. Natural food folates are heat labile and may be destroyed by storage, processing, and cooking [269]. They are also less easily absorbed than synthetic folic acid, which is the most bioavailable form. The bioavailability of food folate is likely to be less than 50 per cent [447]. A strong correlation exists between serum folate concentration and daily use of a supplement containing folic acid.

## Food fortification with folic acid

Despite strong confirmation of the protective effective of folic acid supplementation, and the recommendations of many agencies that women take folic acid in supplement prior to and during pregnancy, this approach alone has not translated into population-wide declines in NTD prevalence. There are reports that consumption of enriched cereal grain products (e.g. bread, pasta, etc.), produced from flour fortified with folic acid to a level of 140 µg/100g, does not appear to significantly increase serum folate to levels that are considered protective against NTDs [448, 449].

A recent survey in the US found that 77 per cent of pregnant women were taking supplements, mostly daily prenatal vitamins containing an average of 817 µg folic acid and 48 mg iron, but fewer were taking supplements in the first trimester (55%) [450]. Evaluations of NTD trends in countries that have folic acid dietary intake and supplementation recommendations, but not mandatory food fortification programmes, found that the incidence of NTDs has not fallen significantly [451, 452]. For example, an epidemiological study in France of 202,670 births did not observe a decrease in incidence of NTDs before and after recommendations were publicized in 1991–1992 [453].

Therefore, combined strategies of fortification and supplementation are likely to be required to meet population recommendations for folic acid intake [454]. Globally, around 75 countries have initiated nationwide policies of mandatory flour fortification with folic acid and other nutrients. This is meant to ensure that the entire population receives at least a small additional amount of folic acid, regardless of access to supplements (see *Flour Fortification Initiative* (<http://www.ffinetwork.org/regional_activity/index.php>) for country and regional data). A randomized trial of several doses of folic acid (100, 200, or 400 µg/day) concluded that a fortification programme that delivered 100 µg folic acid daily to women would produce an important decrease in NTD prevalence, without the expense of unnecessarily high exposure for the general population [455]. Following the introduction of folic acid fortification of enriched cereal grain products in the US, a 19 per cent reduction in NTD birth prevalence was observed [456]. In Nova Scotia, Canada, the incidence of NTDs decreased by more than 50 per cent after mandatory fortification was implemented [457]. These reduction figures are substantially different because the US data was based only on live births and, unlike the Canadian study, did not include prenatally diagnosed cases that resulted in early termination of the pregnancy [458].

## Risks of excess folate

No adverse effects have been associated with the consumption of excess folate from foods. Adverse effects are exclusively reported from use of the synthetic compound folic acid [459]. The European Scientific Committee considers the risk of progression of the neurological symptoms in vitamin $B_{12}$-deficient patients (as a result of masking the signs of pernicious anaemia) as the most serious potential adverse effect of folic acid supplementation. This generally occurs with folic acid dosages >5 mg/day, whereas dosages up to 1 mg of folic acid are unlikely to cause this masking effect. Therefore the tolerable upper intake level in the EC is set at 1 mg of folic acid [460]. The same tolerable upper intake level of 1 mg/day is used in the US by the Institute of Medicine (IOM) and is the same for both pregnant and lactating women [269]. The recommendation of 4 mg/day for the prevention of NTD recurrence is well above the tolerable upper intake level and should be monitored by a physician.

It has been suggested that high folic acid intake could overwhelm the liver's metabolic capacity, leading to exposure to unmetabolized folic acid. Although no adverse effects have been observed at high doses (5 mg) [461], another study found that excess unmetabolized folic acid correlated with decreased activity of natural killer cells, which are important for antiviral and anticancer immunity [462]. There has been some debate over whether folic acid supplementation and/or fortification is responsible for an increasing incidence of colorectal cancer in areas where this has been implemented [463]. However, a recent meta-analysis of studies involving 50,000 individuals on the effect of folic acid supplementation on cancer incidence suggested that consuming supplements for five years has no substantial effect on this outcome [464]. As food fortification generally involves much lower doses than supplementation trials, it seems unlikely that cancer risk would be affected by the consumption of fortified foods in moderate quantities.

There is evidence from animal studies (in mice) that a maternal diet supplemented with methyl donors (folic acid, vitamin $B_{12}$, choline, L-methionine, zinc, and betaine) leads to decreased transcriptional activity and increased severity of allergic airway disease in offspring (via excessive methylation of the *RUNX3* transcription factor gene, a negative regulator of allergic airway disease) [465]. A few human studies have supported this idea, reporting that folic acid supplementation in early pregnancy was associated with a small increase in risk of infant wheezing (up to 18 months) [466], or with an increased risk of asthma at 3 years of age [467]. High maternal folate levels (>17.84 nmol/L) in the second trimester were also associated with an increased risk of asthma at 3 years [468]. However, results from the recent KOALA Birth Cohort Study (n = 2,834) in the Netherlands found no association between either maternal folic acid supplement use in pregnancy, or maternal intracellular folic acid levels, and impaired lung function or the development of atopic manifestations in offspring at 6 to 7 years of age. On the contrary, there was a dose-dependent correlation between high maternal folic acid levels in late pregnancy and decreased childhood asthma risk [469]. This is in agreement with a study in adults and children ≥2 years of age, in whom serum folate levels were inversely correlated with IgE levels and the presence of atopy and wheeze [470]. A recent systematic review and meta-analysis did not support a causal link between the use of antenatal folic acid supplements and increased risk of asthma in children [471]. However, to date no randomized controlled trials have been performed to assess allergic outcomes of folic acid supplementation.

Excess folate during late pregnancy may affect other aspects of the developmental course in the offspring. Recent animal studies suggest that the trajectory to peak bone mass may be sensitive to nutritional folate exposure in utero. High folate diets (equivalent to 10× recommended levels) fed to pregnant rats resulted in lower weight and reduced bone mass in female offspring [472]. If this holds true in humans, it may be of concern in light of the number of pregnant women who take folic acid well above the generally recommended amounts.

## Agency guidelines for folate intake

The general recommendation prior to conception and throughout pregnancy is for supplementation with 400 μg of folic acid in tablet form, in addition to dietary sources, which can reduce the risk of NTD by approximately 50 per cent [473, 474]. Fortification of flour in some countries (providing ~25–100 μg/serving of breads or cereals) has also contributed to a marked reduction in the incidence of NTDs, as has been seen, for example, in Canada [475] and South Africa [476]. Whether fortification of flour is independently correlated with

## Box 12.1 Conversions for dietary folate equivalents

1 dietary folate equivalent = 1 µg food folate = 0.6 µg folic acid from supplements and fortified food

Source: Institute of Medicine, Food and Nutrition Board, *Dietary Reference Intakes: Thiamin, Riboflavin, Niacin, Vitamin B$_6$, Folate, Vitamin B$_{12}$, Pantothenic Acid, Biotin, and Choline*, Dietary Reference Intakes, National Academy Press, Washington, DC, copyright © 1998. [269]

decreasing incidence of NTDs is not clear [477], and supplementation is still recommended even for women consuming diets including fortified grain products in order to further reduce the risk of NTDs [478].

The recommendations for folate intake set by the IOM express the units of intake as dietary folate equivalents (DFEs) in order to account for differences in absorption of food folate (<50% absorbed) compared with synthetic folic acid (85% absorbed) [269]. DFE conversions are shown in Box 12.1

The IOM advises an intake of 400 µg DFE/day as the recommended dietary allowance (RDA) for individuals (both male and female) above the age of 14 years (estimated average requirement = 330 µg/day). Prior to and during pregnancy, the RDA increases to 600 µg DFE/day; it is recommended that 400 µg/day is taken as a folic acid supplement, in addition to a varied diet providing natural food folate. The RDA drops to 500 µg DFE/day during lactation (Box 12.2). Women with a prior NTD-affected pregnancy are advised to take 4 mg

## Box 12.2 US Institute of Medicine recommended dietary allowances for folate

Infants 0–6 months (adequate intake (AI)) = 65 µg dietary folate equivalents (DFE)/day

Infants 7–12 months (AI) = 80 µg DFE/day

Children 1–3 years = 150 µg DFE/day

Females 14+ years = 400 µg DFE/day

Pregnancy = 600 µg DFE/day

Lactation = 500 µg DFE/day

Source: Institute of Medicine, Food and Nutrition Board, *Dietary Reference Intakes: Thiamin, Riboflavin, Niacin, Vitamin B$_6$, Folate, Vitamin B$_{12}$, Pantothenic Acid, Biotin, and Choline*, Dietary Reference Intakes, National Academy Press, Washington, DC, copyright © 1998. [269]

DFE/day at least 1 month before conception and throughout the first trimester [269]. The adequate intake level for infants is 65 µg DFE/day up to 6 months of age, and 80 µg DFE/day from 7 to 12 months. These intakes are based on amount consumed by healthy breastfed infants [269].

In agreement with the IOM, CDC guidance states that all women of child-bearing age should consume 400 µg of folic acid daily in supplement form [479, 480]. For prevention of recurrence in women who previously had an NTD-affected pregnancy, supplementation with 4 mg/day is suggested, beginning 1 month before trying to conceive and continuing through the first 3 months of pregnancy. This higher dosage should be supervised by a health care professional.

The US Preventive Services Task Force recommends that all women capable of becoming pregnant take folic acid supplements of 400–800 µg/day. Their most recent review of potential harms of this preventive measure found no evidence of significant drug interactions, allergic reactions, or carcinogenic effects associated with intake of the recommended dosages [481]. Canadian Clinical Practice Guidelines [482] advise that women who have not had a prior NTD-affected pregnancy should consume a multivitamin supplement delivering 0.4–1 mg folic acid/day from at least 2 months before conception and continuing through to the end of lactation. For women with a family history of NTDs, as well as for those in high-risk ethnic groups (e.g. Sikh) or who take anticonvulsant medications, a daily dose of 5 mg folic for 3 months both before and throughout the first 12 weeks of pregnancy is recommended as the standard of care. From 12 weeks until the end of gestation and throughout breastfeeding, these women should take a daily multivitamin supplement containing between 0.4 and 1 mg folic acid. Although the peri-conceptional use of 5 mg folic acid/day is uncommon outside this specific group of women, the Society of Obstetricians and Gynae-cologists of Canada also recommends 5 mg folic acid under a broader list of indications, including for women with histories of poor medication compliance, poor or variable diets, or inconsistent/non-use of birth control.

The UK National Institute for Clincal Excellence guidelines recommend that pregnant women supplement with 400 µg folic acid/day from pre-conception through the first 12 weeks of pregnancy [266]. Regarding folic acid supplementation in obese women, the UK Centre for Maternal and Child Enquiries and the Royal College of Obstetricians and Gynaecologists have issued a joint guideline which advises women with a BMI ≥30 who are contemplating pregnancy to supplement with 5 mg folic acid daily, starting at least 1 month before conception and continuing during the first trimester of pregnancy [483]. However, there is some debate about this recommendation, as peri-conceptional hyperglycaemia may be an independent risk factor, not modifiable by folic acid intake, which contributes to the higher prevalence of NTDs in offspring of obese women [484]. The European Scientific Committee on Food advises women who are contemplating pregnancy to use a daily supplement containing 400–500 µg folic acid from 4 weeks before conception to 8 weeks postconception to reduce NTD risk [370, 460].

## Our recommendations for folate intake during pregnancy and lactation

Most data are consistent with the recommendation that women who are contemplating pregnancy should consume a multivitamin supplement containing 400 µg folic acid/day, from 2 months prior to conception and through the first 12 weeks of pregnancy. This advice is in addition to consuming a varied diet containing natural food folate. Although liver is a rich source of folate, it is not recommended during pregnancy because of its high content of preformed vitamin A. A diet rich in fruits and vegetables, including legumes, is recommended, along, where available, with moderate amounts of foods fortified with folic acid. We recognize that women who have had a previous NTD-affected pregnancy require higher-dose folic acid supplementation prior to and throughout the first part of pregnancy. A dosage of 4 mg/day should be considered, under the guidance of a physician.

Translating the known protective effect of folic acid into population-wide reductions in NTD prevalence has not been straightforward. Maternal lifestyle factors such as smoking, alcohol consumption, bodyweight/BMI, and folic acid supplement use can be viewed as a proxy of nutrition and lifestyle, all of which can affect a woman's folate and homocysteine status and have important repercussions for her pregnancy. Recent data support the idea that BMI has a significant impact on folate metabolism, and recommendations based on BMI may be warranted. The current recommendations were based largely on data from several decades ago, when obesity was not as prevalent and the average BMI was in the normal range [485, 486]. It may be prudent to suggest higher folic acid supplementation for overweight or obese women.

# Chapter 13

# Vitamin B$_{12}$ (cobalamin) in pregnancy and breastfeeding

## Vitamin B$_{12}$ functions

Vitamin B$_{12}$ (cobalamin) has multiple functions in human physiology. It is required for the synthesis of fatty acids and myelin, and so is crucial for normal neurological function and maintenance of the CNS. In conjunction with folate, vitamin B$_{12}$ is involved in red blood cell formation and DNA synthesis. In embryogenesis, vitamin B$_{12}$, like folate, is important for proper neural tube formation and brain development.

The terms cobalamin and vitamin B$_{12}$ refer to a group of cobalt-containing compounds composed of ribose, phosphate, and a base attached to a corrin ring structure. Vitamin B$_{12}$ can be converted to either of two metabolically active cobalamin enzyme cofactors. One of these, methylcobalamin, is a cofactor for methionine synthase, which catalyses the conversion of homocysteine to methionine. The second cofactor is 5-deoxyadenosylcobalamin, which is required by methylmalonyl coenzyme A mutase for the metabolism of odd-chain-length fatty acids and some branched-chain amino acids [487]. Methylcobalamin may serve as a direct methyl donor in the DNA methylase reaction [488]. Because of its role in one-carbon metabolism, vitamin B$_{12}$ interacts metabolically with folate, and these micronutrients are nutritionally interdependent (see 'Interaction with folate').

Three soluble vitamin B$_{12}$-binding proteins are known to be involved in the uptake and transport of cobalamins in humans: intrinsic factor, transcobalamin, and haptocorrin. Following ingestion, dietary vitamin B$_{12}$ enters the stomach bound to proteins and is released by pepsin and hydrochloric acid to bind to haptocorrin. In the small intestine, haptocorrin is degraded by pancreatic enzymes, and the released vitamin B$_{12}$ is taken up by intrinsic factor. Absorption of vitamin B$_{12}$ occurs via an active process whereby the complexes of B$_{12}$ and intrinsic factor attach to receptors in the ileal mucosa and are internalized. Vitamin B$_{12}$ later enters the circulation bound to transcobalamin I, II, or III. Lack of intrinsic factor results in vitamin B$_{12}$ malabsorption [489].

## Indicators of vitamin B$_{12}$ status

Serum cobalamin concentration has limited specificity as a marker of vitamin B$_{12}$ deficiency, as there are other causes of abnormal levels, including pregnancy, folate deficiency, transcobalamin deficiency, and some diseases such as HIV infection and myeloma [490]. Nonetheless, measurement of vitamin B$_{12}$ in blood is the current routine procedure for determining deficiency [491]. The WHO suggests a plasma vitamin B$_{12}$ concentration of <150 pmol/L (203 pg/mL) for defining vitamin B$_{12}$ deficiency [492].

Methylmalonic acid and homocysteine are metabolites that accumulate in serum when vitamin B$_{12}$-dependent reactions are impaired. Serum levels of methylmalonic acid and homocysteine have been used to establish diagnosis of vitamin B$_{12}$ deficiency. However, these tests are more expensive than ones that rely on the measurement of serum B$_{12}$, and the results can be affected by poor renal function [493]. Holotranscobalamin is considered the active form of vitamin B$_{12}$; it is a complex of vitamin B$_{12}$ bound to transcobalamin that is available to cells. Measurement of holotranscobalamin may be more suitable than serum vitamin B$_{12}$ measurement for the diagnosis of vitamin B$_{12}$ deficiency in populations, but to date this test has not achieved wide clinical acceptance [494, 495]. The US National Health and Nutrition Examination Survey reviewed biomarkers for vitamin B$_{12}$ deficiency and concluded that at least one biomarker of circulating concentrations of vitamin B$_{12}$ (vitamin B$_{12}$ itself or holotranscobalamin) and one biomarker of functional vitamin B$_{12}$ status (methylmalonic acid or homocysteine) should be measured to determine subclinical vitamin B$_{12}$ deficiency, as these have shown associations with anaemia and cognitive decline in various studies [496, 497].

## Vitamin B$_{12}$ deficiency

Under normal circumstances, dietary vitamin B$_{12}$ is accumulated and stored in the liver. Relative to daily needs, the body stores large amounts of vitamin B$_{12}$; therefore signs of deficiency appear only after 2–5 years of insufficient intake [498]. Some gastric dysfunctions, such as hypochlorhydria or atrophic gastritis, can cause malabsorption of food-bound vitamin B$_{12}$, lowering serum levels and eventually resulting in deficiency [499]. Long-term use of drugs that affect gastric acid production (e.g. proton pump inhibitors) can worsen deficiency because gastric acid is needed to release vitamin B$_{12}$ bound to proteins in food. However, such drugs have not been shown to cause deficiency [500]. Vitamin B$_{12}$ levels are reduced among alcoholics [501] and in smokers due to increased excretion [502]. Dietary deficiency is common in vegans and those who have very low meat intakes. This is a particular issue in Asia, where vitamin B$_{12}$ deficiency has a high prevalence.

## Interaction with folate

Deficiency for either vitamin B$_{12}$ or folate impairs the production of tetrahydrofolate, preventing DNA synthesis and cell division in blood cells. This disruption of cell division produces the enlarged erythrocytes characteristic of megaloblastic or pernicious anaemia. The megaloblastic process affects all rapidly dividing bone marrow cells and so can also lead to neutropenia and thrombocytopenia [503]. Pernicious anaemia can be caused by a lack of intrinsic factor, triggered by an autoimmune response whereby antibodies attack intrinsic factor-producing parietal cells in the gut. This results in impaired absorption of vitamin B$_{12}$, and subsequent signs of deficiency.

The haematological consequence of vitamin B$_{12}$ deficiency is indistinguishable from folate deficiency, and the effects can be reversed by treatment with either vitamin B$_{12}$ or folic acid [495]. However, folic acid treatment does not correct the neurological complications of vitamin B$_{12}$ deficiency, which include sensory disturbances in the extremities (tingling and numbness), motor disturbances, and demyelinating degeneration of the spinal cord and peripheral nerves. Cognitive impairment (loss of concentration, memory loss, disorientation, mood changes, and dementia), visual disturbances, insomnia, and impotency, and impaired bladder and bowel control may also occur. Thus, large amounts of folic acid can temporarily mask vitamin B$_{12}$ deficiency by correcting the megaloblastic anaemia, while allowing the neurological disease to progress [504, 505]. This is considered to be the biggest risk associated with high-dose folic acid supplementation (see 'Interaction with folate').

The interdependence of these two nutrients means that both are ultimately required for proper homocysteine metabolism (see Fig. 12.1 in chapter 12). Even in the presence of adequate folate, a functional folate deficiency can develop if vitamin B$_{12}$ is lacking. This is because once 5,10-methylene-tetrahydrofolate is reduced by methylenetetrahydrofolate reductase to form 5-methyltetrahydrofolate, it requires the vitamin B$_{12}$-dependent enzyme methionine synthase in order to be recycled to tetrahydrofolate and therefore to participate in DNA biosynthesis and cell division. Thus, in vitamin B$_{12}$ deficiency, cellular folate becomes trapped as 5-methyl-tetrahydrofolate, and the availability of other folate coenzymes is ultimately reduced.

Women with low vitamin B$_{12}$ status in a background of high folate are also at risk for intrauterine growth restriction and having small-for-gestational-age infants, as seen in a study in South India, where many women are supplemented with 5 mg/day of folic acid but are deficient in vitamin B$_{12}$ [506]. Thus, high plasma folate resulting from the enthusiastic promotion of pre- and early pregnancy folic acid supplementation may, in some women, exacerbate the effects of existing vitamin B$_{12}$ deficiency.

# Vitamin B$_{12}$ in pregnancy and lactation

Vitamin B$_{12}$ crosses the placenta and is present in breast milk. There is some evidence, mainly from animal studies, that the absorption of vitamin B$_{12}$ may increase during pregnancy, coincident with a lactogen-dependent recruitment of intrinsic factor receptors that allows increased intestinal uptake [507, 508]. Nonetheless, serum total vitamin B$_{12}$ concentrations begin to decline early in the first trimester, to about half of non-pregnancy concentrations by the sixth month of gestation [509]. The decrease is greater than could be accounted for by haemodilution. The decrease does not reflect a tissue depletion of vitamin B$_{12}$ [510].

Fetal and maternal vitamin B$_{12}$ serum concentrations are correlated, in that lower maternal levels are associated with lower fetal levels [511]. Maternal intake during pregnancy is important, as only newly absorbed vitamin B$_{12}$, and not that acquired from maternal liver stores, is concentrated in the placenta. Vitamin B$_{12}$ is transferred from the placenta to the fetus by active transport against a concentration gradient. During the last two trimesters of pregnancy, it is estimated that 0.1–0.2 µg/day of vitamin B$_{12}$ is transferred to the fetus if the mother's diet is adequate [512, 513]. By the end of pregnancy, the serum vitamin B$_{12}$ concentration of the newborn is approximately twice that of the mother [514].

## Deficiency in pregnancy

Vitamin B$_{12}$ status has been considered as a modifiable risk factor for neural tube defects (NTDs) and other adverse pregnancy outcomes, given the close metabolic association between vitamin B$_{12}$ and folate and the importance of vitamin B$_{12}$ status as a determinant of plasma homocysteine. Elevated homocysteine, which can arise from a suboptimal intake of vitamin B$_{12}$, is associated with pre-eclampsia, preterm birth, low birthweight, and small-for-gestational-age infants [348–350]. Early observations on the relationship between maternal vitamin status and birth defects suggested that the primary cause of some cases of anencephaly (a severe NTD) could be a deficiency of vitamin B$_{12}$, with accompanying depletion of folate [515]. Low maternal vitamin B$_{12}$ was later reported as an NTD risk factor that is independent of maternal folate status [516].

Low vitamin B$_{12}$ levels, but high vitamin B$_{12}$-carrier protein levels, were detected in amniotic fluid from pregnancies affected by either NTDs or the abdominal-wall birth defect omphalocele, suggesting abnormal vitamin B$_{12}$ production, transport, or metabolism was associated with these defects [517]. Mothers of infants with spina bifida had vitamin B$_{12}$ levels that were 20 per cent lower than controls in a small case–control study wherein a vitamin B$_{12}$ serum concentration of $\leq$185 pmol/L (~250 ng/L) conferred a 3.5-fold increased risk of this NTD [518]. Similarly, a population-based case–control study in Canada reported a nearly threefold increase in NTD risk in women with low vitamin B$_{12}$ status, despite folic acid fortification of flour [519]. A study in a population at high risk for NTDs prior to folic acid fortification found a highly significant, dose-dependent correlation between increasing vitamin B$_{12}$ level and decreasing NTD risk [520]. The addition of vitamin B$_{12}$ to prenatal folic acid tablets and to foods fortified with folic acid has been suggested.

## Vitamin B$_{12}$ in the neonate

Despite the active transfer during pregnancy, the vitamin B$_{12}$ content in the newborn is low, and the infant is dependent on breast milk for ongoing needs. Lactating women with adequate vitamin B$_{12}$ status are estimated to secrete 0.4 µg/day of vitamin B$_{12}$ in breast milk and therefore require an extra intake of 0.4 µg vitamin B$_{12}$ per day while they are breastfeeding. This is in addition to the recommended dietary allowances (RDAs) for adults of 2.4 µg/day, giving a total RDA of 2.8 µg/day during lactation [269]. Breast milk can have insufficient concentrations of vitamin B$_{12}$ if the mother consumes a strict vegetarian or vegan diet, or in developing countries where the usual consumption of animal products is low. Signs of vitamin B$_{12}$ deficiency develop by 4 to 6 months of age in breastfed infants of mothers consuming strict vegetarian diets [521].

Infants who are exclusively breastfed by women who consume no animal products may have very limited reserves of vitamin B$_{12}$ and can develop vitamin B$_{12}$ deficiency within months of birth. Undetected and untreated vitamin B$_{12}$ deficiency in infants can result in severe and permanent neurological damage [522]. Clinical, biochemical, and metabolic monitoring is required for infants within strict vegetarian families. Vitamin B$_{12}$ deficiency after birth manifests in anaemia, failure to thrive, recurrent infections, and later psychiatric and neurological symptoms [523].

## Vitamin B$_{12}$ sources

Most microorganisms (including bacteria and algae) synthesize vitamin B$_{12}$, which enters the human food chain through animal ingestion. In herbivorous animals, gastric fermentation supports growth of microorganisms that synthesize B$_{12}$, which is subsequently absorbed and incorporated into animal-origin foods. Animal products including milk/dairy products, meat (especially liver), poultry, fish, and eggs are therefore the primary sources of vitamin B$_{12}$ in the human diet. The vitamin B$_{12}$ intake of individuals consuming strict vegetarian or vegan diets is thus very low, unless fortified foods or supplements are added to the diet.

Foods that are fortified with vitamin B$_{12}$ in some areas include breakfast cereals, soy-based beverages, and vegetarian burgers [269]. Vitamin B$_{12}$ from algae preparations (e.g. spirulina) does not appear to be bioavailable in humans, and should not be considered as a vegan/vegetarian source of the vitamin [524]. Some foods of animal origin, particularly beef and some types of fish, contain amounts of vitamin B$_{12}$ that exceed the RDA in a single serving (see <http://www.dietitians.ca/Nutrition-Resources-A-Z/Factsheets/Vitamins/Food-Sources-of-Vitamin-B12.aspx>). Areas of cobalt deficiency produce animal products that are low in vitamin B$_{12}$ [231]. The most commonly available synthetic form of vitamin B$_{12}$ in supplements is cyanocobalamin.

## Risks of excess vitamin B$_{12}$

According to the US Institute of Medicine (IOM), there is insufficient evidence on which to base the tolerable upper intake level for vitamin B$_{12}$. Absorption is limited by the binding capacity of intrinsic factor (1.2–2.0 µg vitamin B$_{12}$ per meal), with an additional 1–3 per cent absorbed by passive diffusion. There are no reports of adverse effects from intake of supplements of 1 mg/day. However, there are no established benefits associated with high doses, so these should be avoided in individuals who do not have conditions conferring vitamin B$_{12}$ malabsorption [269].

## Agency guidelines for vitamin B$_{12}$ intake

The IOM RDA for vitamin B$_{12}$ is based on the amount needed for the maintenance of haematological status and normal serum vitamin B$_{12}$ values. An assumed absorption of 50 per cent is included in the recommended intake. The RDA for adolescents and adults (≥14 years) is 2.4 µg/day of vitamin B$_{12}$, which does not change with age (Box 13.1). The estimated average requirement is 2.0 µg/day. The increased demands of the fetus during gestation, and the infant during breastfeeding, mean that an additional 0.2µg/day of vitamin B$_{12}$ is required during pregnancy, and an additional 0.4 µg/day is needed during lactation, such that the RDA for pregnancy is 2.6 µg/day (estimated average requirement, 2.2 µg/day), and the RDA for lactation is 2.8 µg/day (estimated average requirement, 2.4 µg/day) [269].

## Box 13.1  US Institute of Medicine recommended dietary allowances for vitamin B$_{12}$

Infants 0–6 months (adequate intake (AI)) = 0.4 µg/day
Infants 7–12 months (AI) = 0.5 µg/day
Children 1–3 years = 0.9 µg/day
Females 14+ years = 2.4 µg/day
Pregnancy = 2.6 µg/day
Lactation = 2.8 µg/day

Source: Institute of Medicine, Food and Nutrition Board, *Dietary Reference Intakes: Thiamin, Riboflavin, Niacin, Vitamin B$_6$, Folate, Vitamin B$_{12}$, Pantothenic Acid, Biotin, and Choline*, Dietary Reference Intakes, National Academy Press, Washington, DC, copyright © 1998. [269]

The recommendation for infants in the first 6 months of life is 0.4 µg/day (~0.05 µg/kg/day), which is based on the adequate intake level (AI) that is obtained from breast milk of well-nourished mothers. For infants aged 7–12 months, AI is 0.5 µg/day (~0.05 µg/kg/day). Children 1–3 years of age have an RDA of 0.9 µg/day (estimated average requirement, 0.7 µg/day). The IOM recommends that infants of vegan mothers be supplemented with vitamin B$_{12}$ at 0.4 µg/day from birth [269].

Vitamin B$_{12}$ deficiency is not common in industrialized countries, except in individuals who do not consume animal-derived foods (particularly vegans) or in those who have conditions affecting vitamin B$_{12}$ absorption. Women and children in developing countries who have limited access to animal food products are considered to be at risk for deficiency [231, 492] and supplementation should be considered, to the level of the RDA for women and the AI for infants. There is little variation from these recommendations across other agencies [143, 492].

## Our recommendations for vitamin B$_{12}$ intake during pregnancy and lactation

Maternal intake and absorption of vitamin B$_{12}$ during pregnancy have a more important influence on the vitamin B$_{12}$ status of the infant than do maternal vitamin B$_{12}$ stores. As the vitamin B$_{12}$ concentration in breast milk is also correlated with maternal intake, it is important for pregnant and lactating women to ensure that their diet contains sufficient sources of the vitamin, or supplements should be taken such that intake is 2.4 μg/day during pregnancy, and 2.8 μg/day during lactation. Pregnant women consuming vegan or strict vegetarian diets should either take vitamin B$_{12}$ supplements of this dosage, or seek foods that have been fortified with vitamin B$_{12}$. Given the interplay of folate and vitamin B$_{12}$, the status of both should be assessed in parallel, particularly if high doses of folate are considered.

Chapter 14

# Choline in pregnancy and breastfeeding

## Choline functions

Choline is an essential nutrient, sometimes classified with the B-group vitamins, that is required for the structural integrity of cell membranes and is involved in methyl-group metabolism, neurotransmission, transmembrane signalling, and lipid and cholesterol transport and metabolism. It is a component of the phospholipids phosphatidylcholine and sphingomyelin, which are key building blocks of cell membranes and the myelin sheath, and precursors for the intracellular signalling molecules diacylglycerol and ceramide. Platelet activating factor and shingophosphorylcholine are choline metabolites that also act as cell-signalling molecules. The provision of choline is critical during fetal and neonatal life to ensure optimal brain and cognitive development [525].

Pathways involving choline, folate, and vitamin $B_{12}$ intersect in the formation of methionine from homocysteine (see Fig. 12.1 in chapter 12). Betaine, the primary oxidative product of choline, can act as an alternate methyl donor to 5-methyl-tetrahydofolate in this conversion. Choline becomes a limiting nutrient during folate deficiency [446], and conversely, when choline supply is low, the demand for folate is increased. Folate metabolism is disturbed during choline deficiency, and vice versa [526].

Choline is mainly provided in the diet, although it is also synthesized in the liver in small amounts via the enzyme phosphatidylethanolamine $N$-methyltransferase. The rate of de novo synthesis is not adequate to meet the demands for choline, especially under circumstances of increased need, such as pregnancy and lactation. All tissues accumulate choline by diffusion or by mediated transport, and choline is actively transported across the blood–brain barrier.

## Indicators of choline status

Plasma choline concentration is sensitive to changes in dietary choline intake; it can increase twofold after a meal containing high amounts of choline, and three- to fourfold after a supplemental choline dose [269]. Choline concentrations average around 10 μmol/L. Plasma phosphotidylcholine also declines in choline deficiency but is influenced by other factors that affect plasma lipoproteins [527].

## Choline deficiency

Food sources of choline are plentiful, and deficiency is unlikely in individuals who consume a variety of foods including eggs, meat, legumes, and cruciferous vegetables [528,529]. However, certain population groups are at risk for choline deficiency, including pregnant and lactating women and infants. Liver damage and fatty infiltration of the liver can result from choline deficiency in an otherwise adequate diet [527,530]. This occurs because a lack of phosphatidylcholine limits the export of excess triglyceride from the liver.

## Choline in pregnancy

Choline, as a precursor of membrane phosphatides, is needed for the growth and development of the fetus and is particularly important for the developing brain. The placenta transports choline to the fetus, resulting in a choline concentration in amniotic fluid that is ten times higher than in maternal blood. Plasma concentrations in neonates at birth are much higher than those in adults [525,531]. The placental transport depletes maternal stores, so mothers must consume substantial amounts of choline during pregnancy to ensure an adequate supply to the fetus. Recent studies suggest that choline intake above the current agency recommendations (see 'Agency guidelines for choline intake') may be beneficial to improve placental function [532] and lower circulating cortisol levels in cord blood [533]. Because of altered choline metabolism in pregnancy, intake of 930 mg choline/day was found to elevate plasma betaine concentrations to levels closer to those of non-pregnant women, compared with intakes in the recommended range (480 mg/day) [534].

### Choline–folate–homocysteine interactions in pregnancy

There is a positive association between maternal choline and homocysteine levels during pregnancy. Homocysteine is an indirect product of the phosphatidylethanolamine *N*-methyltransferase enzymatic pathway, which synthesizes choline in the liver. The high fetal demand for choline appears to stimulate the de novo synthesis pathway, and this reaction also causes a rise in homocysteine concentrations [535]. Thus, it may be appropriate to advise intake of choline supplements during pregnancy to prevent activation of the de novo pathway and the resulting elevation of homocysteine, which is detrimental to cardiovascular health and has other adverse effects in pregnancy, including increased risks of pre-eclampsia, preterm birth, and low birthweight [536,537].

## Choline and neural development

Maternal peri-conceptional deficiency for choline, like folate, is associated with an increased risk of neural tube defects in the offspring [538]. A linear relationship between increasing serum choline concentration and decreasing risk of neural tube defects was found in a recent large prospective study using data from over 180,000 pregnant women [539]. In animal studies, maternal choline supplementation could reverse some but not all of the effects of folate deficiency on brain development [540].

Choline is a precursor of the neurotransmitter acetylcholine and is needed for the formation of cholinergic neurons. Choline availability from 8 weeks gestation through 3 months postpartum modulates the development of the hippocampal cholinergic system over this period [541]. The formation of synapses between these neurons also requires choline; this process occurs at a high rate from fetal life through the fourth year of life [542]. Although in animal studies maternal choline supplementation during pregnancy has been shown to be neuroprotective to the fetus [543], supplementation of pregnant women with 750 mg choline/day in the form of phosphatidylcholine (in addition to dietary choline intake) did not enhance the cognitive development in the offspring (assessed at 10–12 months of age), compared with women who received a placebo [544].

## Choline in lactation

During lactation, choline is secreted in relatively large amounts and is concentrated in breast milk. Choline and choline esters in human milk can be derived from the maternal circulation or by de novo synthesis within the mammary gland [545]. The concentration of phosphocholine in human milk is significantly higher than in cow's milk and in infant formulas, but other choline forms, including glycerophosphocholine, phosphotidylcholine, and sphingomyelin, are similar in human milk and cow's milk-derived formulas [546]. The average choline content of human milk is around 116 μmol/L.

Common polymorphisms in the *MTHFR* gene appear to attenuate the response to dietary choline intake and the concentration of choline in breast milk and may explain some of the variation in choline concentrations observed between women with similar dietary intakes [547]. These gene variants also affect folate and vitamin B$_{12}$ status. Further study is required in order to incorporate genotype information into individualized recommendations for intake of these nutrients.

## Choline and epigenetic mechanisms

As a methyl donor, choline affects DNA and histone methylation and is therefore involved in epigenetic regulation of gene expression. High choline intake during gestation in animals has been shown to influence the expression of cortical and hippocampal genes involved in learning and memory [548]. Other body systems will also be affected by appropriate maintenance or inappropriate epigenetic modification induced by the presence or absence of dietary methyl donors such as choline [549].

## Choline sources

Choline is available in many foods as free choline or in a number of esterified forms including sphingomyelin and phosphatidylcholine. A phosphatidylcholine-enriched fraction produced through commercial purification, termed lecithin, is often added to foods as an emulsifying agent. Free choline is found in highest quantities in beef liver, eggs, peanuts, soybeans, and some vegetables (iceberg lettuce, cauliflower, broccoli). In some countries, eggs enriched with choline through feeding of hens are available. Beef liver and eggs also have a very high content of phosphatidylcholine [528]. The dietary intake of phosphatidylcholine is approximately 6–10 g/day [527].

## Agency guidelines for choline intake

Few countries include choline in their nutrient intake recommendations, because the information on intake requirements in humans in sparse. In the US and Canada, the US Institute of Medicine recommends a choline intake (adequate intake (AI)) of 450 mg/day for pregnant women and 550 mg/day for lactating women [269] (Box 14.1). The pregnancy AI represents an increase over the non-pregnant AI (425 mg/day) to cover the needs of both the fetus and the placenta, based on body organ weight estimates. The main criteria for setting the AI is the level necessary to avoid liver damage from choline deficit. The AI for infants aged 0–6 months is 125 mg/day of choline, or approximately 18 mg/kg. For infants aged 7–12 months, the AI is 150 mg/day or ~17 mg/kg. This intake level should be obtainable from breast milk, which is rich in choline in well-nourished mothers.

---

**Box 14.1  US Institute of Medicine recommended adequate intakes for choline**

Infants 0–6 months = 125 mg/day
Infants 7–12 months = 150 mg/day
Children 1–3 years = 200 mg/day
Females 14–18 years = 400 mg/day
Females 19+ years = 425 mg/day
Pregnancy = 450 mg/day
Lactation = 550 mg/day
Tolerable upper intake level for 14–18 years = 3.0 g/day; 19+ years = 3.5 g/day

Source: Institute of Medicine, Food and Nutrition Board, *Dietary Reference Intakes: Thiamin, Riboflavin, Niacin, Vitamin B$_6$, Folate, Vitamin B$_{12}$, Pantothenic Acid, Biotin, and Choline*, Dietary Reference Intakes, National Academy Press, Washington, DC, copyright © 1998. [269]

---

# Our recommendations for choline intake during pregnancy and lactation

We recommend that pregnant women eat a variety of foods and do not restrict fat severely from their diets, as choline is derived from the lipid content of food. Eggs are a good source of choline and should not be restricted. Although liver is also a rich choline source, we do not recommend its excessive consumption during pregnancy because of the potential risk of excess vitamin A intake. Strict vegetarian or vegan diets may be low in choline. The high secretion rate of choline into breast milk means that lactating women have a high demand for this nutrient. Multivitamins containing choline at around the AI levels (450 mg/day) may be helpful for maintaining adequate choline levels in pregnant and lactating women.

# Chapter 15

# Vitamin D in pregnancy and breastfeeding

## Vitamin D functions

Of all the micronutrients considered essential in pregnancy, recommendations regarding vitamin D have been arguably the most controversial, and the requirement for and dosage of vitamin D in pregnancy has undergone substantial recent reconsideration and redefinition. That vitamin D is essential to health is undisputed, but how much is needed, and how it should be acquired (not only for pregnant women, but for the general population), is the subject of both intensive research and some difference of opinion. Vitamin D is a fat-soluble steroid best known for its key role in maintaining bone integrity via the regulation of calcium and phosphorus homeostasis. However, vitamin D influences a number of other extra-skeletal processes, including immune function and blood glucose homeostasis. Additionally, it has been suggested to have anti-proliferative and pro-differentiation actions that may explain its reported beneficial effects on cancer risk [550].

There are two major forms of vitamin D (vitamins $D_2$ and $D_3$); the term calciferol refers to both of these forms. Vitamin $D_2$ (or ergocalciferol) is synthesized by plants, while vitamin $D_3$ (or cholecalciferol) is produced in humans from an endogenously synthesized cholesterol metabolite (7-dehydrocholesterol) upon exposure of skin to UVB radiation. Vitamins $D_2$ and $D_3$ are hydroxylated in the liver to the primary inactive vitamin D storage form, 25-hydroxyvitamin D (25(OH)D; also known as calcidiol) [551]. As the main circulating vitamin D metabolite, the concentration of 25(OH)D in serum reflects total body stores derived from food, supplements, and endogenous cutaneous synthesis and is the generally accepted measure of an individual's overall vitamin D status. Vitamin D metabolism and sources of vitamin D are illustrated in Fig. 15.1.

In response to parathyroid hormone (PTH), 25(OH)D is hydroxylated in the kidney to the active hormonal form, 1,25-dihydroxyl vitamin D (also known as calcitriol) [551]. It is now apparent that 1,25-dihydroxyl vitamin D can also be synthesized in many tissues that express the enzyme 1-alpha-hydroxylase (including the placenta and maternal decidua [552]), dependent

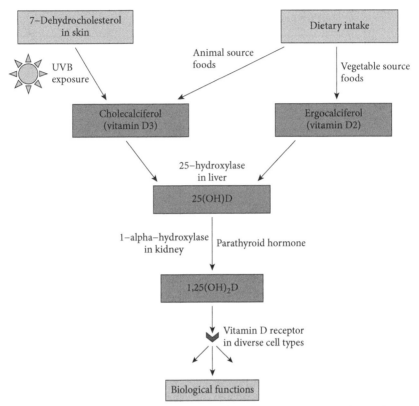

**Fig. 15.1** Vitamin D metabolism and sources of vitamin D. Vitamin D can be synthe-sised in the skin from 7-dehydrocholesterol in response to ultraviolet B (UVB) radia-tion, or can be ingested from animal and vegetable food sources (e.g. salmon, liver, eggs for cholecalciferol; mushrooms, yeast for ergocalciferol). These inactive forms are hydroxylated in the liver to 25-hydroxyvitamin D (25(OH)D) and then in the kidney to the active form, 1,25 dihydroxyvitamin D (1,25(OH)2D).

on the availability of its precursor 25(OH)D [553]. 1,25-Dihydroxyl vitamin D binds to the vitamin D receptor and acts as a transcription factor, its primary target tissues being bone, intestine, and kidney. Vitamin D receptor expression is widespread, however, accounting for the pleiotropic activities of vitamin D. One IU of vitamin D is defined as the activity of 0.025 µg of vitamin $D_3$, so the biological activity of 1 µg of a vitamin D supplement is 40 IU.

## Vitamin D deficiency

The active form of vitamin D promotes intestinal calcium absorption. When vitamin D levels are low, the absorption of calcium and phosphorous becomes less efficient, triggering an increase in the production of PTH. The consequent secondary hyperparathyroidism causes calcium to be resorbed from bone and stimulates increased renal clearance of inorganic phosphate, resulting in lower serum phosphate levels. Severe vitamin D deficiency manifests as rickets in children and osteomalacia in adults.

In addition to skeletal defects associated with low vitamin D and consequent elevated PTH levels, there may also be effects on the nervous system and the immune system, [550] leading to peripheral neuropathy and an impaired response to infection, respectively, and on glucose metabolism and insulin sensitivity [554, 555]. Vitamin D may also have a direct positive effect on insulin sensitivity and beta-cell function, as low levels have been associated with reduced beta-cell response [556]. Low vitamin D intakes in childhood have been associated with increased risk of type 1 diabetes [557]. Other consequences of mild to moderate vitamin D deficiency include possible increased risks of various cancers, infections, autoimmune disorders, asthma, hypertension, and cardiovascular disease [550, 558, 559]. Some of these increased risks are thought have their initial induction in early life and possibly in utero [560, 561].

## Definition of vitamin D deficiency

With the development of better assays for the various forms of vitamin D in serum, a number of studies have suggested that subclinical vitamin D deficiency is much more common than previously considered. In turn this has led to a flurry of research and not inconsiderable controversy. No consensus has been reached regarding what level of 25(OH)D renders a person vitamin D replete.

The US Institute of Medicine (IOM), which sets nutrient dietary reference intakes, recently issued new recommendations [562]. These guidelines state that individuals are at risk of vitamin D deficiency when their serum 25(OH)D levels are <30 nmol/L (<12 ng/mL) and that some are at risk with serum 25(OH)D levels between 30 and 50 nmol/L (12–20 ng/mL). The IOM considers that most people are vitamin D replete when their levels are >50 nmol/L, citing concern that treating individuals with serum 25(OH)D levels above this value with high doses of vitamin D might have unknown long-term effects. The IOM recommendations of 25(OH)D reference levels for vitamin D deficiency and insufficiency were based primarily on considering the role of vitamin D in bone health. The IOM deficiency reference threshold is disputed, however, with many experts calling for an upward revision, considering 75 nmol/L (30 ng/mL) as the minimum circulating level needed to maintain bone health [563, 564].

There are a number of factors to consider in relation to optimal circulating 25(OH)D levels. The efficiency of calcium absorption is said to be maximized and serum PTH levels maximally suppressed when 25(OH)D levels reach approximately 80 nmol/L, above which regulation of absorption is no longer limited by vitamin D status [553, 565, 566]. Yet, a meta-analysis of studies of vitamin D supplementation for fracture prevention considering over 83,000 subjects found that fracture risk continued to decline linearly with 25(OH)D levels up to 112 nmol/L (45 ng/mL) [567], far higher than the IOM report's view of a beneficial level.

Some studies of extra-skeletal effects of vitamin D suggest that the threshold for adequacy might be even higher. There have been reports of beneficial effects of vitamin D on reducing cancer risk at serum 25(OH)D levels around 125 nmol/L (50 ng/mL) [568]—effects not seen at levels below 100 nmol/L. However there are concerns about the potential for vitamin D toxicity at very high chronic exposures.

While these analyses are informative, it is important to consider the specific evidence for what vitamin D levels are required to optimize outcomes in pregnancy and in neonates. Evidence is mounting that women should attempt to maintain a level around 75 nmol/L of circulating 25(OH)D to ensure optimal pregnancy outcomes for both themselves and their offspring. The evidence in our view supports a higher (75 nmol/L or 30 ng/mL) rather than a lower (50 nmol/L) cut-off when assessing adequate supplementation.

## Vitamin D in pregnancy

The importance of vitamin D for both fetal and childhood skeletal development is well recognized. During gestation, the fetal skeleton accumulates a total of approximately 30g of calcium from maternal stores, most of which crosses from the placenta in the third trimester. The fetal requirement for calcium in late pregnancy is mostly met by an increase in the efficiency of intestinal calcium absorption and enhanced transport across the placenta, rather than by increased maternal calcium intake [569]. This increase in absorption is mediated by maternal 1,25-dihydroxyl vitamin D, which also increases during the third trimester as a result of the enhanced placental metabolism of 25(OH)D [570]. The change in absorption efficiency and calcium transfer to the fetus does not appear to result in a net loss in maternal bone mineral content in well-nourished women [569].

It is, however, well known that maternal vitamin D deficiency leads to poor fetal skeletal mineralization in utero that can manifest as rickets, craniotabes (soft skull bones), and osteopenia in newborns. Deficient maternal serum 25(OH)D levels are associated with classic, severe vitamin D deficiency rickets in the offspring [571]. Beyond classical rickets, several studies have demonstrated impaired bone mass accrual in otherwise healthy newborns associated with maternal vitamin D status <50 nmol/L [572] or <37.5 nmol/L [573].

There has been some reported evidence to suggest that the environment in utero, and in particular the mother's vitamin D status, may have a long-term impact on bone health later in life. Cord blood 25(OH)D levels are closely correlated to maternal levels in late pregnancy and at birth. Studies of the long-term effects of low maternal concentrations of serum 25(OH)D in pregnancy on offspring bone development have thus far produced inconsistent results [574].

In addition to skeletal effects, women with very low vitamin D status face increased risks of other adverse pregnancy outcomes and possible long-term effects on their own health and that of their offspring [575]. These include greater risks of pre-eclampsia and having low-birthweight offspring, as well as possible effects on the development of allergy in offspring [576].

The relationship between serum 25(OH)D concentrations and total intake of vitamin D is non-linear [577]; further, sun exposure confounds the interpretation of dose–response data for vitamin D intake. When determining an optimal dose for an individual, it is important to consider the baseline status, as the increment of 25(OH)D response to an oral dose is inversely related to the starting level [566]. Giving additional amounts to someone who already has enough, or not giving enough to someone whose levels are too low to show a response, will not produce a positive result.

To optimize a supplemental dose of vitamin D, an individual's relative adiposity also needs to be considered. Vitamin D is fat soluble, meaning it is absorbed and sequestered in adipose tissue. As a consequence, serum 25(OH)D levels decrease with increasing BMI, reflecting decreased bioavailability rather than decreased total body stores [578]. Conversely, serum 25(OH)D levels have been shown to rise when obese individuals lose body fat [579, 580].

Obese individuals exhibit lower responses both to UV irradiation in terms of cutaneous vitamin $D_3$ synthesis, and to oral supplementation with vitamin $D_2$ [581]. The BMI should therefore be taken into account when estimating the vitamin D intake needed to raise serum 25(OH)D to an appropriate level. A dose 2–3 times higher than that required for normal-weight women may be necessary to maintain a sufficient circulating 25(OH)D level in obese individuals [582]. Interestingly, recent data suggest that even when their vitamin D levels are replete, obese women appear to transfer a lower proportion of vitamin D to their infants during pregnancy than do normal-weight women [583], suggesting they may require an even higher level of circulating 25(OH)D during pregnancy. This may be because fat sequesters vitamin D.

## Vitamin D insufficiency in pregnancy

Vitamin D deficiency or insufficiency is now considered to be very common in pregnancy, especially among certain high-risk groups. Some reports indicate that African American women are eight times as likely as Hispanic women, and twenty times as likely as Caucasian women, to have vitamin D deficiency [584–586]. Ethnic groups at risk of vitamin D deficiency include those from the Indian subcontinent, South Asia, the Caribbean, and the Middle East, contributed to by the use of body-covering clothing.

A recent US study indicated that over 50 per cent of pregnant women had 25(OH)D levels below 75 nmol/L and 15 per cent had levels below 50 nmol/L (considered deficient), despite taking standard supplements (400 IU/day) for at least 180 days during their pregnancies [587]. While there may be biases in the study, it appears that for a large proportion of women, supplementing vitamin D intake with 400 IU/day is ineffective at maintaining sufficient levels during pregnancy. We are aware of a number of other as yet incompletely published studies, including some on maternal vitamin D status in Asian and UK populations, which reach not dissimilar estimates of the frequency of deficiency.

## Vitamin D insufficiency and pre-eclampsia

While there is some variance in the reported data, the evidence would suggest that inadequate vitamin D status is associated with a moderate increase in the risk of pre-eclampsia. This conclusion is supported by several small case–control studies which have shown a relationship between low serum 25(OH)D levels (<50 nmol/L) and an increased risk of pre-eclampsia [588–590]. While other studies have shown no such association [591–593], there are observational data in support of this association. A recent longitudinal study [594] in ~700 women found that risk of pre-eclampsia correlated with lower vitamin D levels at 24–26 weeks but not at 12–18 weeks gestation, perhaps suggesting that vitamin D may be involved in modulating the peripheral vascular phase of pre-eclampsia. Similarly, in a large cohort analysis in ~23,000 pregnant nulliparous women [595], supplementation with 10–15 μg (400–600 IU) vitamin D/day in the first 22 weeks of gestation was associated with a 25 per cent reduction in the risk for pre-eclampsia.

## Vitamin D levels and atopic disorders

It would appear that both low and very high maternal vitamin D levels are associated with risk of atopic disease in the offspring. Such U-shaped relationships are frequently found with micronutrients—with both low and high levels having adverse consequences [596]. A longitudinal study using a UK birth cohort [597] found the risk of infantile eczema to be higher in children whose mothers had been in the top quartile of the 25(OH)D concentration range (>75 nmol/L) during pregnancy, as compared with the bottom quartile. There is evidence from animal studies that vitamin D supplementation is associated with sustained proliferation of allergy-inducing Th2 cells; thus excess vitamin D could lead to an increased prevalence of allergy [598].There was a similar trend for increased risk of asthma at 9 years in the offspring of mothers with the highest 25(OH)D levels. In contrast, other studies have found that low, rather than high, 25(OH)D levels were associated with increased risk of eczema [599] and predisposed children to asthma [559–601] and allergic rhinitis [558].

## Vitamin D insufficiency and risk of infection

A link between vitamin D status and infection risk in pregnant women and infants has been suggested. Low 25(OH)D levels (<30 nmol/L) are strongly associated with bacterial vaginosis during pregnancy [602], particularly among HIV-infected women [603]. In infants, low, cord blood levels <25 nmol/L were associated with a greater than twofold increase in risk for respiratory or other infections in the first 3 months of life [601]. A prospective study observed that newborns with cord blood 25(OH)D levels <50 nmol/L had a significantly greater risk of developing respiratory syncytial virus-associated lower respiratory tract infections, as compared with newborns whose cord blood 25(OH)D levels were ≥75 nmol/L.

## Vitamin D and glucose regulation/gestational diabetes

Vitamin D deficiency has been linked to impaired glucose metabolism [604], and therefore the impact of vitamin D status on the risk of gestational diabetes mellitus (GDM) has been explored. The data suggest an adverse association between lower vitamin D levels and the risk of GDM [605–607], providing further support for considering closer attention to vitamin D status in pregnancy than has generally been the case. Improving vitamin D status may also be beneficial in women with established GDM. A recent small randomized controlled trial in which women with GDM received two doses of 50,000 IU vitamin D over a 6-week period in pregnancy found improvements in glycemic status and serum total and LDL cholesterol, as compared with women who received placebos [608].

## Vitamin D insufficiency in low birthweight, and infant and childhood adiposity

Intrauterine growth restriction and consequent low birthweight can negatively impact neonatal health, with sequelae that may persist into adulthood. Evidence is mixed regarding the impact of maternal vitamin D status on infant birthweight, but the data generally suggest a positive association between vitamin D status and birthweight. A recent large retrospective cohort analysis of >2,100 women reported that low vitamin D status (<37.5 nmol/L) in early pregnancy was associated with a higher risk of small-for-gestational-age offspring, with a positive correlation between maternal vitamin D levels and the weight of off-spring at birth [609]. Similarly a study of >4,200 pregnant women showed a significant association between vitamin D deficiency status (<30 nmol/L) in early pregnancy and a greater risk of having low-birthweight infants and a high risk of having small-for-gestational-age infants [610]. In a longitudinal follow-up study of offspring from 977 women in the Southampton Women's Survey cohort, mothers with low vitamin D levels in pregnancy more often gave birth to infants with low fat mass, although at 6 years of age these children had higher fat mass than those who were exposed to adequate vitamin D in utero and had higher fat mass at birth [611].

## Vitamin D and fertility

The effect of vitamin D on fertility has not been extensively studied in humans. However, the vitamin D receptor is expressed in ovaries and testes [612, 613]. Data have been inconsistent with regard to the association of vitamin D status with IVF outcome, with some indicating higher 25(OH)D serum levels correlating with increased chance of pregnancy, and others showing an adverse effect of high vitamin D status on embryo quality and IVF success. Similarly, conflicting results have been reported for vitamin D effects on semen quality and sperm count and motility in males [614]. At this point, no specific recommendations can be made with regard to optimal vitamin D status for conception. However, the other considerations given above suggest the importance of ensuring all women of reproductive age have adequate vitamin D status and that the presumption of normality cannot be made without serum testing.

## Vitamin D sources

The most potent source of vitamin D is the sun. Vitamin $D_3$ is produced in relatively large quantities in the skin by photochemical synthesis following exposure to UVB rays in sunlight. Some reports suggest that at tropical lati-tudes, 30 minutes of skin exposure per day (arms and face) in summer is suf-ficient to provide the body with all the vitamin D it needs [578, 615, 616]. However, several factors influence the amount of vitamin D that an individual produces. Having dark skin significantly reduces the cutaneous synthesis of vitamin D by reducing UVB penetration; a similar effect results from the use of sunscreens or protective clothing. Individuals living at latitudes that experi-ence fewer daylight hours in winter, spring, and autumn (i.e. north or south of 33°), will not have sufficient UVB exposure to synthesize the required amount of vitamin D. Modern lifestyles and cultural factors reduce UVB exposure further, as a result of clothing styles and cultures, and in general spending more time indoors.

Excessive sunlight exposure does not cause vitamin D toxicity because UVB converts excess vitamin $D_3$ to biologically inert isomers. However, the dermatology community discourages UVB exposure as a means of maintaining high vitamin D status because of the risk of skin damage and cancer [617]. If an individual follows current advice regarding sun protection, he or she is unlikely to achieve a level of vitamin D that is considered sufficient (if this is taken to be a serum 25(OH)D level above 75 nmol/L) from sun exposure alone. To avoid deficiency, vitamin D must be ingested from dietary sources or supplements.

Dietary sources of vitamin D include oily fish, liver, and egg yolks for vitamin $D_3$, and yeast and fungi (mushrooms) for vitamin $D_2$. With the exception of some fish [571], the vitamin D content of unfortified food is low. These natural sources do not generally provide enough vitamin D to render the average individual replete through diet alone, and supplementation is often required.

Because natural food sources do not contain large quantities of vitamin D, some countries have chosen to fortify foods, including milk, cheeses, margarine, breakfast cereals, and orange juice, with vitamin $D_2$ or vitamin $D_3$. In the US, milk is fortified with 385 IU/L, and some breakfast cereals and fruit juices are fortified with vitamin D. Infant formula and margarine have statutory vitamin D supplementation in the UK. Individuals with high milk intake in these regions may have relatively high vitamin D intake, but based on a nutrient intake survey [618] the highest intake levels were only 688 IU (17.2 µg)/day for women [71].

Although food fortification is controversial, it seems clear that most people will not exceed the tolerable upper intake level with dietary intake unless they also consume an unusual and very large amount of a particular fish (like Atlantic herring) and/or take excess supplements. Fortified foods can, however, be a useful mode of supplementing intakes of vitamin D. For example, consumption of 1,000 IU/day of vitamin $D_3$ in 240 mL fortified orange juice was shown to maintain levels >90 nmol/L and was as effective as oral supplement tablets at raising 25(OH)D levels [619].

Vitamin $D_3$ is more potent than vitamin $D_2$ [620] and, as a supplement, is more effective in raising serum levels of 25(OH)D [621]. Because vitamin D is fat soluble, supplements are most efficiently absorbed when consumed with foods containing fat. A recent study showed that taking vitamin D supplements with a large meal increases absorption by up to 50 per cent [622].

## Vitamin D supplementation

### Vitamin D supplementation during pregnancy

Multivitamin supplements (including prenatal vitamins) have traditionally contained 400 IU of vitamin D [623], but this dosage has been increasing in view of the evidence given above. Supplements in a range of dose levels (1,000–5,000 IU vitamin $D_3$/dose) are now available in the US. A number of randomized trials have been performed to determine the level of vitamin D supplementation required to achieve or maintain adequate vitamin D status in pregnant women, but many of these trials have suffered from methodological problems [624–630].

Overall, women supplemented with vitamin D during pregnancy had significantly higher concentrations of 25(OH)D at the end of pregnancy. Compared with placebo or no intervention, vitamin D supplementation during pregnancy did not have significant effects on length and weight at birth, but children born to women who received vitamin D supplements during pregnancy had a larger head circumference at birth than infants born to women who did not receive supplements (however, given that only two studies reported on this outcome, this result should be interpreted cautiously). It should be noted that even with supplementation, vitamin D sufficiency (defined as 25(OH)D ≥50 nmol/L) was achieved in only 30 per cent of treated women [629].

The results suggest that a daily dose of 800 IU vitamin $D_2$ may be inadequate during pregnancy. A recent study [585] examined a much higher dose of 4,000 IU/day of vitamin $D_3$ and showed no safety concerns. This dosage level was considered by the investigators to be the minimal level for suppressing secondary hyperparathyroidism and for optimal intestinal calcium absorption and bone mineral density [631]. The study concluded that 4,000 IU/day starting at 12–16 weeks gestation was most effective in achieving vitamin D 'sufficiency', defined as 25(OH)D ≥80 nmol/L.

### Vitamin D and breastfed infants

Maternal vitamin D status is an important factor for the development of rickets in newborns, particularly in breastfed infants [632]. Breast milk typically contains very little vitamin D [571, 633], unless the nursing mother is adequately supplemented or exposed to enough sunlight [634]. The level of maternal vitamin D intake required during pregnancy to ensure adequate vitamin D status in a full-term neonate may not be sufficient to satisfy the ongoing vitamin D needs of fully breastfed infants.

Most cases of rickets occur in babies who are exclusively breastfed, and who themselves are not exposed to sunlight or supplemented with vitamin D [635].

A 25(OH)D concentration below 27.5 nmol/litre (11 ng/mL) is considered to be consistent with vitamin D deficiency in infants and young children [562, 571, 636]. The adequate intake (AI) recommendation of the IOM has been raised from 200 IU to 400 IU/day and is now consistent with recommendations from the American Academy of Pediatrics (AAP) and the Pediatric Endocrine Society [562, 637].

## Vitamin D supplementation for breastfeeding mothers

In general, studies evaluating the effectiveness of maternal supplementation on the vitamin D status of breast milk suggest that much higher than standard supplementation doses are needed for infants whose only source of vitamin D is breast milk [638]. The data suggest that high doses of vitamin D would be required to substantially increase the 25(OH)D content of breast milk. A supplementation dosage of 6,400 IU/day has been suggested for lactating women if breast milk is to be the source of vitamin D [639]. A study of Caucasian mother–infant pairs in South Africa showed that maternal supplementation with either 500 or 1,000 IU/day was less effective in maintaining infant 25(OH)D levels than supplementing the infants themselves with 400 IU/day [640]. Thus, although supplementing lactating women with high doses of vitamin D is a possible option to increase the vitamin D intake of breastfed infants, it is clear that direct supplementation to infants is more suitable for ensuring optimal vitamin D status.

## Vitamin D supplementation for infants

Several studies indicate that a daily vitamin D dose of 400 IU, either as an oral supplement or in formula feed, maintains normal vitamin D status and activity, especially in low-birthweight infants [641, 642] and can prevent rickets in areas of high prevalence [636]. While this level of supplementation increases infant 25(OH)D levels, the effect on bone mineral content or circulating PTH is minimal in breastfed infants who had 'optimal' vitamin D status at birth [643]. It is clear that the effect of supplementation to infants is dependent on their initial vitamin D status, with a more pronounced effect seen in infants who have deficient or insufficient 25(OH)D levels at birth [644, 645]. Thus, low-birthweight and/or premature neonates may receive equal benefit from lower doses of ~200 IU/day [642, 646].

# Risks of excess vitamin D

Part of the controversy surrounding vitamin D supplementation and fortification of food is the perceived possibility of toxicity. However, the risk of toxicity of oral vitamin D supplementation of 1,000–4,000 IU per day is negligible.

Excess vitamin D increases calcium absorption in the intestine, resulting in high blood calcium levels. This can lead to calcium deposits in soft tissues such as the heart and lungs, confusion and disorientation, kidney stones and kidney damage, nausea, vomiting, constipation, poor appetite, weakness, and weight loss.

The physiological limit for serum 25(OH)D concentrations in humans appears to be approximately 220 nmol/L (88 ng/mL) because this approximates the top of the range of values reported for humans who are well exposed to UV light [647]. Indigenous populations in East Africa have been found to have average serum 25(OH)D levels around 115 nmol/L, and levels of 150 nmol/L are normal during pregnancy [648]. The lowest 25(OH)D concentration causing toxic effects appears to be greater than 500 nmol/L (200 ng/mL) [649]

## Agency guidelines for vitamin D intake

There are diverse expert recommendations regarding vitamin D supplementation of pregnant women, with a median of 400 IU (10 µg)/day [267]. The National Institute for Health and Clinical Excellence (NICE) in the UK recommends that pregnant and lactating women take a vitamin D supplement of 400 IU daily and that health professionals inform all pregnant women about the importance of this for their health and the future health of their baby. The recent IOM guidelines define the recommended dietary allowance (RDA) for vitamin D for pregnant women to be 600 IU (15 µg)/day [562]. The RDA is an intake that is intended to cover the requirements of most pregnant women (97–98%) and was set based on a target 25(OH)D level of 50 nmol/L (Box 15.1). These intakes represent an increase from the previous recommendation for an AI of 200 IU/day [571] but this recommendation still appears to many to be

## Box 15.1 US Institute of Medicine recommended dietary allowances for vitamin D

Infants 0–12 months (adequate intake) = 10 µg/day (400 IU)

Children 1–3 years = 15 µg/day (600 IU)

Females 14+ years = 15 µg/day (600 IU)

Pregnancy = 15 µg/day (600 IU)

Lactation = 15 µg/day (600 IU)

Tolerable upper intake level (including pregnancy and lactation) = 100 µg/day (4,000 IU)

Source: Institute of Medicine, *Dietary Reference Intakes for Calcium and Vitamin D*, National Academy Press, Washington, DC, copyright © 2012. [562]

unduly conservative. The Endocrine Society suggests that pregnant and lactating women require a vitamin D intake of at least 600 IU/day, although they also propose that to maintain a 25(OH)D serum level above 50 nmol/L, an intake of 1,500–2,000 IU/day may be required [582].

The IOM also increased the tolerable upper intake level to 4,000 IU (100 µg/day), indicating what the board views as the highest average intake that is likely to pose no risk of adverse effects. It has also been argued that supplementation with 4,000 IU per day of vitamin D in adults is comparable to the amount of vitamin D acquired through natural sun exposure and thus should be regarded as a physiological intake [553]. A recent randomized control trial found that women receiving 4,000 IU/day achieved an average serum 25(OH)D level of 111 nmol/L [585].

The Endocrine Society recommends screening for vitamin D deficiency in individuals at risk for deficiency [582], with pregnant and lactating women being included as a risk group. The American Congress of Obstetricians and Gynecologists (ACOG) suggests that women with other risk factors, particularly those with medical conditions such as chronic kidney disease, hepatic failure, malabsorption syndromes (e.g. inflammatory bowel disease), and granulomatous disorders (e.g. sarcoidosis, tuberculosis, and histoplasmosis) should be screened, as well as dark-skinned individuals, those with veiled/covered modes of dress, or those living at latitudes above or below 33° [650]. In the UK, the NICE guidelines for antenatal care were updated in 2008 to incorporate an additional recommendation on informing women of the importance of maintaining adequate vitamin D stores in pregnancy, particularly for those at greatest risk of vitamin D deficiency (women of South Asian, African, Caribbean or Middle Eastern family origin, women who have limited exposure to sunlight, women who eat a diet particularly low in vitamin D, and women with a pre-pregnancy BMI above 30 kg/m$^2$). The recommendation is to take a multivitamin supplement containing 400 IU (10 µg)/day, and physicians are advised to carefully monitor women at greatest risk to ensure that they are taking the recommended supplements [651].

In contrast to these recommendations, a 2012 WHO guideline document does not recommend supplementation in pregnancy except in cases of documented vitamin D deficiency, when supplements of 200 IU (5 µg)/day (the WHO/FAO reference nutrient intake level) are advised [652]. The recommendation cited a lack of quality evidence from interventional studies for either the efficacy or safety of vitamin D supplementation of pregnant women for various outcomes, including pre-eclampsia and low birthweight. For lactating women, the recent IOM report does not propose an increase over the 600 IU/day recommendation for pregnancy but recommends an intake of 400 IU/day for infants [562]. The Endocrine Society suggests that lactating women should, at minimum, take a multivitamin containing 400 IU of vitamin D along with an additional vitamin D supplement of ≥ 1,000 IU daily [582].

Both the IOM and the AAP recommend supplementation of infants rather than relying on provision of adequate vitamin D through breast milk. The AAP recommends that infants <6 months should be kept out of direct sunlight [653] and therefore considers that all breastfed infants require supplementation, as well as formula- or mixed-fed infants consuming less than 1 L/day of infant formula. The 400 IU/day recommendation originated because this is the approximate amount of vitamin D found in a teaspoon of cod liver oil, which is known to both prevent and treat rickets. In a 1987 statement from the European Society of Paediatric Gastroenterology and Nutrition a vitamin D dosage of 800 to 1,600 IU/day, more than double the AAP/IOM level, was recommended for infants [654]. This recommendation does not appear to have been updated.

Bolus supplementation of 50,000 IU is recommended by some Australian health care providers for infants born to vitamin D deficient mothers (defined as 25(OH)D levels <75 nmol/L) [655]. This would appear to be extreme considering both their definition of deficiency and the high suggested dose. We will not further discuss treatment of severe vitamin D deficiency, but note that a position statement for Australia and New Zealand recommends 150,000 IU bolus vitamin $D_2$ to be given to infants <1 month of age for treatment of 'moderate to severe' vitamin D deficiency (<25 nmol/L) [656].

## Our recommendations for vitamin D intake during pregnancy and lactation

Despite observational evidence that maintaining high vitamin D status (25(OH)D) >75 nmol/L) in pregnant women is desirable, the current data do not support the claim that high-dose vitamin D supplementation is necessary for all pregnant women. However, intakes of between 1,000 and 2,000 IU/day, which are in line with the Endocrine Society and ACOG recommendations, are likely to be beneficial and not harmful. Physicians should consider monitoring the vitamin D status (by measuring the 25(OH)D levels) of their pregnant patients, particularly those at risk for deficiency, including women who are dark-skinned or veiled, those who avoid the sun or regularly use sunscreens and/or protective clothing, live at high or low latitudes, eat vegan or vegetarian diets, or are obese. Women taking medications or having disorders affecting calcium and vitamin D metabolism should routinely be screened.

At a minimum, all pregnant women should take a supplement of 400 IU/day, in addition to maintaining sensible sun exposure and increasing their intake of oily fish during pregnancy, both of which will have other benefits for their own health as well as for that of their babies. However, our view is that all women should have their vitamin D status evaluated before or during pregnancy and supplemented in an individualized fashion. In general, the aim should be to maintain serum vitamin D levels between 75 and 110 nmol/L. In the absence of measurements, the data would suggest that pregnant women should receive dietary and supplementary vitamin D on the order of 1,000 to 2,000 IU/day. Fully breastfed infants should receive supplementation (400 IU/day) beginning shortly after birth.

# Chapter 16

# Vitamin K in pregnancy and breastfeeding

## Vitamin K functions

Vitamin K is a fat-soluble micronutrient that is essential for the functioning of several proteins involved in blood clotting. The pro-coagulation proteins, factors II (prothrombin), VII, IX, and X, as well as the anticoagulation proteins C and S, are all activated by vitamin K-dependent gamma-carboxylation of specific glutamic acid residues, forming gamma-carboxyglutamate (Gla) residues. This post-translational modification confers affinity for calcium, which is required for the function of these vitamin K-dependent proteins [657, 658]. If sufficient vitamin K is not available for carboxylation, proteins lacking Gla residues are produced. These under-carboxylated (or descarboxy) proteins have reduced or no activity. After the formation of coagulation factors, the reaction product vitamin K epoxide is enzymatically converted back to active vitamin K by the enzyme vitamin K epoxide reductase [659]. Thus, a lack of vitamin K leads results in a hypocoagulable state, associated with a high risk of bleeding events. Poor vitamin K status is also associated with an increased risk of osteoporotic bone fractures [660]. Other vitamin K-dependent proteins, including activated osteocalcin and matrix Gla protein, have roles in bone and other tissues.

## Indicators of vitamin K status

Functional bleeding time assays such as prothrombin time are not considered to be sensitive for detecting subclinical vitamin K deficiency, since the prothrombin time can be in the normal range even when the prothrombin concentration is 50 per cent of normal [661]. Direct measurements of vitamin $K_1$ (phylloquinone) in plasma, or of urinary Gla excretion, which reflects turnover of vitamin K-dependent proteins, have been considered as markers of vitamin K status [661]. However, the presence of under-carboxylated species of vitamin K-dependent proteins in blood is a more sensitive indicator of deficiency. The most commonly used of these markers is an under-carboxylated form of prothrombin known as protein induced by vitamin K absence or antagonist-II

(PIVKA-II). PIVKA-II assays can detect subclinical vitamin K deficiency before standard coagulation markers are altered or haemorrhage occurs [662]. PIVKA-II is also present in patients using warfarin for anticoagulation. The assessment of the degree of under-carboxylation of osteocalcin correlates well with PIVKA-II and plasma vitamin $K_1$ concentrations [661]. Osteocalcin appears to be the first Gla protein to appear in under-carboxylated form as intake of vitamin K decreases and thus may be the most sensitive marker of vitamin K status [660].

## Vitamin K deficiency

Vitamin K deficiency results in impaired blood clotting. Deficiency is rare among adults, because vitamin K is widely available in foods and is conserved via recycling by vitamin K epoxide reductase. It is also produced by intestinal anaerobic bacteria [663]; thus, long-term treatment with antibiotics can lead to vitamin K deficiency and hypoprothrombinaemia, due to the elimination of such vitamin K-producing intestinal microflora [664].

## Vitamin K in pregnancy and lactation

The placenta transmits lipids and vitamin K relatively poorly, leading to a general vitamin K deficiency in full-term neonates. The concentrations of vitamin $K_1$ in cord blood are typically too low to be accurately measured and are usually between 20- and 40-fold lower than in maternal blood. This apparent barrier to placental transfer is relatively unresponsive to maternal vitamin K supplementation [665].

The neonatal liver has immature prothrombin synthesis, rendering the newborn particularly vulnerable to the effects of low vitamin K levels. Deficiency can lead to intracranial haemorrhage following birth trauma, or classic vitamin K deficiency bleeding (also known as haemorrhagic disease of the newborn), which manifests as unexpected bleeding in the first week of life. Vitamin K deficiency may be exacerbated by prematurity, intrauterine growth restriction, or traumatic delivery [666].

Breastfeeding has been considered a 'risk factor' for vitamin K deficiency, because the short half-life of vitamin K means the levels in newborns can drop rapidly, as the vitamin K content of human milk is minimal (2.5 μg/L) compared with that in cow's milk (5,000 μg/L). Infant formulas are supplemented with vitamin K, and formula-fed infants have substantially higher vitamin K status than do breastfed infants. In addition, maternal use of anticonvulsant therapy during pregnancy significantly increases the risk of vitamin K deficiency in infants [667]. Such deficiency could be prevented by supplementation with 10 mg/day of vitamin K by pregnant women on anticonvulsants from 36 weeks onward [668].

The risk of neonatal vitamin K deficiency is also increased if the mother has taken coumarin anticoagulants. Coumarin derivatives are vitamin K antagonists that are known to act as teratogens, increasing the risk of CNS defects caused by microhaemorrhages in neuronal tissues. The abnormalities are known as warfarin embryopathy, or fetal warfarin syndrome [669]. A more recent study compared the pregnancy outcomes of 666 women exposed to coumarin anticoagulants with a control group of 1,094 unexposed pregnant women and confirmed a significantly increased risk of major birth defects with exposure in the first trimester. Prenatal exposure was also related to higher rates of miscarriage, preterm birth, and low birthweight [670]. In the absence of prophylactic vitamin K administration, the prevalence of vitamin K deficiency bleeding is up to tenfold higher in South East Asia than in Europe [666].

## Vitamin K sources and metabolism

Vitamin K derived from the diet is in the form of vitamin $K_1$. Vitamin $K_2$ (menaquinone) is synthesized by bacteria in the intestinal tract. The main dietary sources of vitamin $K_1$ are green leafy vegetables, such as kale, spinach, turnip greens, collards, Swiss chard, mustard greens, parsley, romaine, and green leaf lettuce. These sources contain >200 μg vitamin $K_1$ per 100 g (turnip greens contain as much as 650 μg/100 g). Soybean oil and canola oil are rich sources, containing >100 μg/100 g. Other vegetable sources are Brussels sprouts, broccoli, cauliflower, and cabbage. Fish, liver, meat, eggs, and cereals contain smaller amounts. Green tea contains >700 μg/100g, but black tea does not contain vitamin K. High concentrations of vitamin $K_2$ are found in yogurt, cheese, and butter, and fermented soybeans [671].

Dietary vitamin K is absorbed in the small bowel following the typical pathway of dietary lipids and is incorporated into chylomicrons for release into the lymphatic system and circulation [672]. The efficiency of absorption has been reported as 40–80 per cent [673]. Dietary fat enhances the absorption of vitamin $K_1$ from food, such that absorption of the vitamin from vegetable oil is significantly higher than from vegetables themselves. Consumption of spinach with butter can increase the availability of vitamin $K_1$ threefold [674]. The bioavailability of vitamin $K_2$ is higher than that of vitamin $K_1$ [675].

Vitamin K has a short half-life. Vitamin $K_1$, the most abundant dietary form, is poorly retained in the body. There is also a wide variation in response to vitamin K from the diet. Some of this variation is accounted for by polymorphisms in the apolipoprotein E gene, which is involved in lipoprotein transport of vitamin $K_1$, and uptake into liver and bone [676].

## Risks of excess vitamin K

Natural vitamin $K_1$ taken orally is not toxic, even in large amounts. Because of a lack of reported adverse effects of high intake of vitamin K, no tolerable upper intake level has been set [260]. Synthetic vitamin $K_3$ (menadione) can be toxic in large doses and is generally not available in supplement form. Vitamin K from food sources is not toxic.

## Agency guidelines for vitamin K intake

There are insufficient data available to determine recommended dietary allowances for vitamin K, so daily adequate intake (AI) recommendations are used instead. These are set based on the average intakes of healthy individuals [260]. The AI for infants 0–6 months is 2 µg/day. Infants 6–12 months require 2.5 µg/day, increasing to 30 µg/day for children 1–3 years of age (Box 16.1). There is no recommended increase in the AI for pregnancy and lactation. Adolescents 14–18 years, including those who are pregnant or breastfeeding, should consume 75 µg/day; women over 19 years should consume 90 µg/day. For men over 19 years, the AI is 120 µg/day [260].

The American Academy of Pediatrics recommends that all breastfed infants should receive 1.0 mg of vitamin K oxide intramuscularly after the first feeding is completed and within the first 6 hours of life [677]. Oral vitamin K is not recommended as sufficient. It may not provide the adequate stores of vitamin K necessary to prevent haemorrhage later in infancy in breastfed infants unless repeated doses are administered during the first 4 months of life [678].

---

### Box 16.1  US Institute of Medicine recommended dietary allowances for vitamin K

Infants 0–6 months (adequate intake (AI)) = 2.0 µg/day
Infants 7–12 months (AI) = 2.5 µg/day
Children 1–3 years = 30 µg/day
Females 14–18 years = 75 µg/day
Females 19+ years = 90 µg/day
Pregnancy and lactation 14–18 years = 75 µg/day
Pregnancy and lactation 19+ years = 90 µg/day

Source: Institute of Medicine, *Food and Nutrition Board, Dietary Reference Intakes for Vitamin A, Vitamin K, Arsenic, Boron, Chromium, Copper, Iodine, Iron, Manganese, Molybdenum, Nickel, Silicon, Vanadium, And Zinc*, The National Academies Press, Washington DC, copyright© 2011. [260]

## Our recommendations for vitamin K intake during pregnancy and lactation

It is important to maintain adequate vitamin K status throughout pregnancy in order to avoid added risk to the neonate at birth and in the first few weeks of life. Green leafy vegetables should be eaten with some dietary fats (e.g. vegetable oil, butter) during pregnancy to maintain or increase vitamin K stores. Supplementation of newborns by intramuscular injection should be universal.

# Chapter 17

# Vitamins C and E and other antioxidants in pregnancy and breastfeeding

## Antioxidant functions

Normal metabolism produces oxidizing free radicals that can damage cellular components such as polyunsaturated fatty acids (PUFAs), proteins, and DNA. Free radicals generated by environmental pollutants (e.g. cigarette smoke, emissions) and photo-oxidants (UV and gamma irradiation, ozone) have the same effect. A complex antioxidant defence system normally protects cells from the destructive effects of free radicals, particularly reactive oxygen species (ROS), but the balance can be critical [679]. In pregnancy and other health states involving high or altered metabolic demands, endogenous antioxidants may provide insufficient protection from the persistent and inevitable challenge by ROS, leading to oxidative stress. Hence, dietary antioxidants have an important role in maintaining human health.

The most prominent representatives of dietary antioxidants are vitamin C, vitamin E, carotenoids, and polyphenols (flavonoids). Vitamin C enhances the endogenous synthesis of glutathione, a powerful antioxidant that is also present in fresh fruits and vegetables [680]. Zinc, selenium, and manganese also have antioxidant properties [681–683], as they are required for the function of endogenous antioxidant enzymes, including selenium-dependent glutathione peroxidases (for which glutathione is a substrate), thioredoxin reductases, selenoprotein-P, and copper/zinc and manganese superoxide dismutases. These trace elements are discussed in chapters 23, 25, and 26.

## Antioxidants in pregnancy

The state of pregnancy can be considered one of oxidative stress, wherein high metabolic demands are accompanied by heightened oxygen requirements in tissues [684, 685]. The placenta contains endogenous antioxidant enzymes that control lipid peroxidation to some extent in normal pregnancies, but because of its high PUFA content, it is also a source of reactive lipid peroxides [686]. Several metabolic disturbances that can complicate pregnancy (in particular, placental disorders such as pre-eclampsia, but also gestational diabetes and hypertension) are characterized by enhanced oxidative stress. Antioxidant activity is attenuated in pre-eclamptic pregnancies [687, 688], and increased ROS activity has been observed in association with pregnancy-induced hypertension [689]. Plasma levels of some dietary antioxidant nutrients are also reduced in women with pre-eclampsia, possibly because these nutrients are utilized to a greater extent in such pregnancies to offset ROS-mediated disturbances, resulting in lower observed plasma antioxidant levels [690]. Interestingly, one study found that higher plasma vitamin E levels correlated with an increased rather than decreased risk of pre-eclampsia [691].

## Oxidative stress and diabetes in pregnancy

Pregnant women with type 1 diabetes are at increased risk for pre-eclampsia and low antioxidant status. Diabetes in pregnancy is also associated with an increased risk of congenital malformations, and the involvement of ROS has been suggested in this teratogenicity [692]. Hyperglycaemia in pregnancy is linked to a deficit in the detoxification of reactive carbonyl compounds derived from oxidative reactions. This causes chemical modification of proteins and results in an accumulation of advanced glycation end products [693]. The binding of these proteins to cell surface receptors induces an intracellular oxidative stress response, leading to lipid peroxidation and tissue damage [694]. Animal studies suggest that fetal exposure to high glucose or a diabetic in utero environment causes enhanced ROS production and lipid peroxidation and that maternal treatment with antioxidants can prevent ROS-mediated damage [695]. In humans, however, supplementation with vitamins C and E has not been shown to reduce the complications of diabetes in pregnancy, except in women with very low antioxidant status [696].

## Oxidative stress and fetal growth restriction

Disruption of fetal growth is a hallmark of maternal exposure to ROS during pregnancy, possibly caused by vasoconstriction and diminished placental blood flow [697]. Markers of oxidative stress have been observed early in pregnancies that were later affected by fetal growth restriction or that resulted in small-for-gestational-age births [698]. These markers may reflect early placental changes that affect fetal growth. Oxidative damage to DNA occurs in pregnancy as a result of low dietary antioxidant status in the face of rapid fetal growth and metabolic demands and is associated with increased risk of poor pregnancy outcome [697].

## Oxidative stress and the fetal immune system

Oxidative stress has additional deleterious effects on the immune system. Inadequate intake of dietary antioxidants is believed to contribute to T-cell differentiation favouring the T-helper cell type 2 (Th2) phenotype, which is predominant in allergic disorders [699]. Various animal models support the hypothesis that maternal antioxidant status is linked to the risk of allergic disorders and asthma in offspring; however, data in human pregnancy is limited and inconsistent. The 'Westernization' of Asian diets is thought to be reducing the overall intake of antioxidants, thereby increasing the susceptibility to oxidative damage and airway inflammation and thus increasing the prevalence of asthma among Asian populations. In a recent Japanese study, low maternal intakes of foods rich in antioxidants during pregnancy, including green and yellow vegetables and citrus fruit, were associated with an increased risk of infant and childhood eczema [700]. Although dietary changes may be effective, other recent data have not supported a role for antioxidant supplementation in pregnancy to reduce the risk of asthma, rhinitis, and eczema in the offspring [701].

# Dietary antioxidants

Antioxidants occur naturally in diets that are rich in fruits and vegetables, which are sources of the antioxidant vitamins C and E as well as carotenoids and polyphenols (mainly flavonoids). The antioxidant capacity of such natural compounds in foods is considered a key factor in the negative correlation between a fruit- and vegetable-rich diet and chronic illnesses, potentially through their ability to supplement cellular defence systems. A significant positive correlation exists between saturated fat intake, or diets rich in fats and poor in fruits and vegetables, and excretion of markers of oxidative stress [697].

## Polyphenols (flavonoids)

Polyphenols, a group of compounds that exhibit antioxidant activity, are abundant in the human diet. The two major types of polyphenols are flavonoids and phenolic acids. Flavonoids are widely available in fruits and vegetables, legumes, tea, and red wine. Phenolic acids are also present in fruits and vegetables and are abundant in chocolate and coffee. The total dietary intake of polyphenols is much higher than the intake of vitamin C, even though their concentration in the body is lower. Although the multiple ROS-scavenging properties of flavonoids have been demonstrated in vitro [702, 703], dietary flavonoids are poorly absorbed and are functionally altered in vivo. Contrary to popular belief, there is currently little evidence that flavonoids have significant antioxidant effects in the human body [704, 705]. In fact, it is appearing equally likely that polyphenols also act as pro-oxidants [706].

There is no evidence in the scientific literature of antioxidant benefit of consumption of polyphenols during pregnancy. Animal studies suggest that high maternal intake of polyphenol-containing foods (e.g. chocolate) may negatively affect fetal bone mineralization and angiogenesis [707]. There is also some evidence of fetal ductus arteriousus constriction resulting from maternal consumption of polyphenol-rich foods, including herbal teas in late pregnancy [708, 709], which was reversible upon restriction of intake [710]. Cautionary advice regarding consumption of herbal teas can be found in chapter 30.

## Carotenoids

Carotenoids are natural pigments that are synthesized by plants and are responsible for the red, orange, and yellow colours of fruits, flowers, and leaves. Some animals including birds, fish, crustaceans, and insects utilize carotenoids from their diets for their colour [711]. The most common carotenoid is beta-carotene, a precursor to vitamin A.

Carotenoids function as antioxidants, although this function is redundant and can be compensated by other antioxidant mechanisms [712]. Because of their lipid solubility and ability to scavenge singlet molecular oxygen and peroxyl radicals, carotenoids are thought to help maintain the integrity of lipid membranes. Like polyphenols, however, it has also been suggested that carotenoids, when supplemented in large amounts, can act as pro-oxidants [713]. When beta-carotene is present in excess, it loses its ability to protect against DNA damage and may even contribute to its cause [714–716]. Plasma levels or dietary intake of carotenoids have been assessed in pregnant women, along with other dietary antioxidants, in relation to pre-eclampsia and gestational hypertension, although results are somewhat inconsistent [691, 717]. The current evidence does not suggest that supplementation with carotenoids such as beta-carotene is beneficial in reducing the risk of pre-eclampsia or other pregnancy complications induced by oxidative stress.

## Vitamins C and E

Vitamins C and E are powerful non-enzymatic antioxidants that are essential for optimal performance of antioxidant defences, and adequate intake of these vitamins is important in pregnancy. Because various disorders of pregnancy are characterized by a reduction in antioxidant activity, it has been hypothesized that maternal supplementation with antioxidants, particularly vitamins C and E, may be beneficial in preventing their occurrence. However, the balance of evidence indicates that supplementation with these vitamins does not reduce the rate of adverse maternal or perinatal outcomes related to oxidative stress, and taking high doses in pregnancy is not recommended.

# Vitamin C

Vitamin C (ascorbic acid) is an essential water-soluble antioxidant vitamin that is required for normal metabolic functioning. Vitamin C scavenges reactive oxidants in activated leukocytes, lung, and gastric mucosa and protects against lipid peroxidation. It is a cofactor for hydroxylase and oxygenase metalloenzymes involved in the biosynthesis of collagen, carnitine, hormones, and amino acids. In the diet, vitamin C promotes absorption of non-haem iron from foods. Adequate levels of vitamin C are important for immune function and vasodilation and may play a role in the prevention of cancer and cardiovascular disease. Severe vitamin C deficiency results in the life-threatening disease scurvy [718].

The brain maintains one of the highest vitamin C concentrations in the body, suggesting an important function. In animals (guinea pigs), vitamin C has been shown to play a role in the regulation of neuronal development, and in particular, the development of the hippocampus. Maternal vitamin C deficiency results in a reduction in postnatal hippocampal volume, irrespective of vitamin C repletion in the neonate immediately after birth. This reduction is associated with diminished spatial memory ability [719].

Ascorbic acid occurs naturally in plants and most animals but is considered as a vitamin in humans because of our inability to synthesize it. This is the result of a mutation in the gene encoding L-gulono-gamma-lactone oxidase, an enzyme needed for vitamin C synthesis. Loss of activity of this enzyme was not deleterious in our ancestors, whose diets were replete in vitamin C and other antioxidants [8]. Attention to dietary vitamin C intake is therefore essential to human health and protection against oxidative damage-mediated diseases, including those brought on by the demands of pregnancy and lactation.

## Requirements in pregnancy and lactation

Vitamin C deficiency in pregnancy is implicated in increased risk of infections and complications, including pre-eclampsia, premature rupture of membranes (PROM), and preterm birth [720]. However, supplementation with vitamin C has not been shown to reduce the incidence of these disorders (see 'Supplementation trials of vitamins C and E in pregnancy'). Maternal plasma vitamin C concentration decreases over the course of pregnancy as a result of active transfer to the fetus, as well as haemodilution. As long as there are appreciable amounts of ascorbic acid in the maternal circulation, the fetus accumulates the nutrient to meet its needs, regardless of maternal requirements. To compensate for this, the calculated increased requirement for pregnancy is 10–15 mg/day higher than for non-pregnant women [718].

Breast milk supplies large quantities of vitamin C to the growing infant. In women not taking supplements, the content of vitamin C in milk is reported to vary between ~30 and 80 mg/L. With supplementation of between 45 to >1,000 mg/day, the content can be from 45 mg/L to 115 mg/L [721]. Infantile scurvy, which is characterized by haemorrhage around connective tissue and bone, impaired bone development, listlessness, loss of appetite, and weight loss, has not been observed in breastfed infants even when maternal vitamin C intake is low. However, formula-fed infants can develop infantile scurvy if the formula is lacking in vitamin C [718]. To compensate for the excretion of vitamin C into breast milk, lactating women require an additional 35 mg/day above the pregnancy requirement [718]. Consuming high doses of supplemental vitamin C does not result in higher vitamin C concentrations in breast milk; maternal vitamin C intake in excess of 200 mg/day resulted in increased urinary excretion of vitamin C but did not increase the breast milk content of the vitamin [721]. After weaning, the vitamin C intake of infants declines significantly—this is reflected in the US Institute of Medicine (IOM) adequate intake recommendations for older infants.

## Sources and metabolism of vitamin C

Vitamin C is available in many fruits and vegetables. Major dietary sources of vitamin C include citrus fruits, bell peppers (capsicum), green beans, strawberries, papaya, guava, kiwi fruit, potatoes, broccoli, and tomatoes. Intestinal absorption of vitamin C occurs by a saturable and dose-dependent process, such that very high intakes from supplements are not absorbed. Ascorbic acid is absorbed and efficiently metabolized at doses up to 80 mg/day, but at higher doses the renal excretion of unmetabolized ascorbic acid increases proportionately with increasing dose. At very high doses, unabsorbed ascorbic acid is degraded in the intestine, which may account for the intestinal discomfort that sometimes accompanies ingestion of large doses [722].

## Risks of excess vitamin C

The most common adverse effects associated with intake of high doses of vitamin C are gastrointestinal disturbances. Although not a common concern in pregnancy, excess vitamin C may be harmful in the presence of pathological iron overload (haemochromatosis), as it increases the mobilization of iron from the spleen and its deposition in liver, enhancing the deleterious effects of excess iron [723]. High-dose vitamin C supplementation in pregnancy may be associated with poorer pregnancy outcomes (see 'Supplementation trials of vitamins

C and E in pregnancy'). The IOM has set an upper tolerable intake level of 2,000 mg/day for pregnancy and lactation in women aged 19 years and older, and 1,800 mg/day for those aged 14–18 years.

## Agency guidelines—vitamin C

The IOM recommended intakes for vitamin C are based primarily on prevention of deficiency and not chronic disease prevention or optimal health promotion. For pregnant women aged 19 years and older, the recommended dietary allowance (RDA) is 85 mg/day (80 mg/day for pregnant women under 19 years of age) [718] (see Box 17.1).

Cigarette smoke affects vitamin C metabolism, decreasing its availability in the circulation in a manner that is independent of dietary vitamin C intake. According to an analysis of data from the second US National Health and Nutrition Examination Survey, smokers have a threefold increased risk of marginally or severely deficient vitamin C status, and approximately 130 mg of additional dietary vitamin C per day would be required to overcome the adverse effect of cigarette smoking on vitamin C levels [724]. Smoking should be avoided in pregnancy; however, in individuals who smoke, the RDA is increased by 35 mg/day to account for the increased oxidative stress caused by toxins in cigarette smoke [718].

## Box 17.1 US Institute of Medicine recommended dietary allowances for vitamin C

Infants 0–6 months (adequate intake (AI)) = 40 mg/day
Infants 7–12 months (AI) = 50 mg/day
Children 1–3 years = 15 mg/day
Females 14–18 years = 65 mg/day
Females 19+ years = 75 mg/day
Pregnancy 14–18 years = 80 mg/day
Pregnancy 19+ years = 85 mg/day
Lactation 14–18 years = 115 mg/day
Lactation 19+ years = 120 mg/day
Tolerable upper intake level (including pregnancy and lactation)
14–18 years = 1,800 mg/day
19+ years = 2,000 mg/day

Source. Institute of Medicine, Food and Nutrition Board, *Dietary Reference Intakes for Vitamin C, Vitamin E, Selenium and Carotenoids*. Dietary Reference Intakes, The National Academies Press, Washington, DC, Copyright © 2000. [718]

The recommended nutrient reference values for Australia and New Zealand are notably lower than those of the IOM, except for young children, for whom they are higher (35 mg/day) [725]. The recommendation for pregnant women aged 14–18 is 55 mg/day, and for those aged 19+ years it is 65 mg/day, which is below the IOM recommendations for non-pregnant women. The Australia/New Zealand recommendations for lactating women are equivalent to the IOM recommendations for non-pregnant, non-lactating women (80–85 mg/day).

## Vitamin E

The major biological role of vitamin E is to protect PUFAs, other components of cell membranes, and low-density lipoprotein from oxidation by free radicals. Vitamin E renders free radicals unreactive by donating the hydrogen from the hydroxyl group on its ring structure. Vitamin E is lipophilic, and as the major fat-soluble antioxidant, it acts synergistically with vitamin C [726]. Primarily located in cell and organelle membranes, vitamin E is transported in the blood by plasma lipoproteins and erythrocytes.

Vitamin E is involved in regulating the atherosclerotic process, both by controlling oxidative damage and via other functions not related to its antioxidant capacity. Smooth muscle cell proliferation is inhibited by a protein kinase C-dependent mechanism that requires vitamin E. Additional roles for vitamin E include inhibition of platelet aggregation, adhesion, and release [727]. Numerous studies have examined the effect of vitamin E for prevention or treatment of cardiovascular disease and have found that, although an adequate intake decreases disease risk, supplemental intake in those already at risk of cardiovascular disease does not reduce the incidence of cardiac events [728]. In general, adequate long-term dietary vitamin E intake has been found to be associated with lower risk of chronic disease [729].

Overt vitamin E deficiency generally does not occur except in cases of protein–energy malnutrition or fat malabsorption syndromes, or in individuals with genetic defects affecting the vitamin E transport protein tocopherol transfer protein alpha. The main symptom is peripheral neuropathy [730]. However, marginal vitamin E intake is common; the third National Health and Nutrition Examination Survey found that at least 30 per cent of the US population had serum levels below 20 µmol/L, a level corresponding to increased risk of cardiovascular disease [731]. The average intake of vitamin E in the US continues to be below the recommended level [732].

There are multiple forms of vitamin E, including four tocopherols and four tocotrienols. Of these, gamma-tocopherol is the most abundant form in the human diet, but alpha-tocopherol has the greatest nutritional significance and is the only form that is maintained in the body [718]. For dietary purposes, vitamin E activity is expressed as alpha-tocopherol equivalents (alpha-TEs). One alpha-TE is the activity of 1 mg *RRR*-alpha-tocopherol ((+)-alpha-tocopherol), which is the naturally occurring form. One milligram (+)-alpha-tocopherol is equivalent to ~1.49 IU (or 1 IU = 0.67 mg). The synthetic form of alpha-tocopherol, (±)-alpha-tocopherol, is less bioavailable: 1 mg = 1.1 IU (1 IU = 0.9 mg). To estimate the alpha-TE of a mixed diet containing natural forms of vitamin E, the number of milligrams of beta-tocopherol should be multiplied by 0.5, gamma-tocopherol by 0.1, and alpha-tocotrienol by 0.3.

## Vitamin E in pregnancy and lactation

As serum lipids increase, so do the concentrations of lipid-soluble vitamins such as vitamin E [733]. The hyperlipidemic state of pregnancy is associated with an increase in maternal plasma vitamin E concentration [734], unlike other micronutrient levels, which tend to decrease as a result of haemodilution and placental transfer. Placental transfer of vitamin E to the fetus is constant throughout pregnancy.

It is assumed that an adequate maternal antioxidant status should protect the maternal–fetal unit from damage, allowing appropriate fetal growth. Low vitamin E status was reported to be associated with higher incidence of low-birthweight or small-for-gestational-age infants in some studies [735], although others have not found a relationship [736]. A prospective study in a group of women at high risk for adverse pregnancy outcomes found that higher circulating alpha-tocopherol levels correlated with increasing birthweight [737]. Nonetheless, supplementation studies have not reported a positive influence of vitamin E on birth outcomes, including birthweight, and in some studies showed a negative influence (see 'Supplementation trials of vitamins C and E in pregnancy'). There is no evidence that vitamin E requirements in pregnancy or lactation should be different from those of other adults. It is generally assumed that increased energy intake during these periods can compensate for the increased needs for infant growth and milk synthesis [738].

## Sources and metabolism of vitamin E

Most vitamin E is found in foods containing fat. Vegetable oils are high in vitamin E but also contain PUFAs which deplete the body of vitamin E. Palm oil has a higher vitamin E:PUFA ratio than soybean or safflower oil. Avocado oil and olive oil are considered to be good dietary sources. Nuts, seeds, fruits, vegetables, and grains also contain vitamin E.

The efficiency of vitamin E absorption is low in humans. Vitamin E is absorbed from the intestinal lumen and secreted in chylomicrons, to be distributed to circulating lipoproteins. Mechanisms of lipoprotein metabolism (e.g. uptake via the LDL receptor or HDL-mediated delivery systems) determine the delivery of vitamin E to tissues [718].

## Risks of excess vitamin E

Animal studies indicate that excess vitamin E prolongs prothrombin times, thus increasing the risk of haemorrhage [739]. A meta-analysis of 19 randomized controlled human trials of high-dose vitamin E supplementation concluded that intake of ≥400 IU (~440–600 mg) vitamin E/day as supplements increased all-cause mortality and should be avoided [740]. Some research indicates that taking even less than the RDA of vitamin E as a supplement during pregnancy can increase the risk of congenital heart defects [741]. However the study had methodological flaws, and vitamin E intake was based on maternal recall of pre-conception and pregnancy diet when the child was 16 months old. A study of the use of high-dose vitamin E in early pregnancy found no association with major congenital malformations but was suggestive of an effect of vitamin E on reducing birthweight [742]. Potential negative effects of prenatal vitamin E supplementation, concomitant with vitamin C, are discussed below.

## Agency guidelines—vitamin E

The IOM RDA for vitamin E is 15 mg per day, including during pregnancy [718]. In general, well-nourished pregnant women consume adequate vitamin E in the diet, and supplementation is not required. There is a slight increase in the requirement during lactation, to 16 mg/day (Box 17.2).

The IOM recommendations indicate a tolerable upper intake level for adults of 1,000 mg of supplementary alpha-TE, including for pregnant or lactating women 19 years or older. Pregnant or breastfeeding adolescents are advised to consume no more than 800 mg/day. Infants up to 12 months of age should not be supplemented; intake of vitamin E should be from breast milk, formula, or food only. Children 1–3 years should not take more than 200 mg/day of supplementary alpha-TE [718]. UK guidelines from the Royal College of Obstetricians and Gynaecologists (RCOG) recommend against supplementation with high doses of vitamin E in pregnancy [743].

As for vitamin C, the vitamin E nutrient reference values for Australia and New Zealand are lower than those of the IOM, except for infants [744]. The recommendation for pregnant women aged 14–18 is 8 mg/day, and for those aged 19+ years it is 7 mg/day (these are unchanged from the recommendation for non-pregnant women of the same ages). The Australia/New Zealand recommendations for

> ## Box 17.2  US Institute of Medicine recommended dietary allowances for vitamin E
>
> Infants 0–6 months (adequate intake (AI)) = 4 mg/day alpha-TE (6 IU)
> Infants 7–12 months (AI) = 5 mg/day alpha-TE (7.5 IU)
> Children 1–3 years = 6 mg/day alpha-TE (9 IU)
> Females 14+ years = 15 mg/day alpha-TE (22.4 IU)
> Pregnancy = 15 mg/day alpha-TE (22.4 IU)
> Lactation = 16 mg/day alpha-TE (23.9 IU)
> Tolerable upper intake level (including pregnancy and lactation)
> 14–18 years = 800 mg alpha-TE/day
> 19+ years = 1,000 mg alpha-TE/day
>
> Source: Institute of Medicine, Food and Nutrition Board, *Dietary Reference Intakes for Vitamin C, Vitamin E, Selenium and Carotenoids.* Dietary Reference Intakes, The National Academies Press, Washington, DC, copyright © 2000. [718]

lactating women incorporate an allowance for the vitamin E secreted in milk, reflected in an increase to 12 mg/day for women aged 14–18, and 11 mg/day for those aged 19 or older. The recommended upper level of intake is much lower than that of the IOM, at 300 mg/day.

## Supplementation trials of vitamins C and E in pregnancy

Vitamins C and E interact to maximize antioxidant activity. In addition, vitamin C helps recycle oxidized vitamin E [745]. The two vitamins are often used together as an antioxidant supplement, and most trials in pregnant women have used the combination of 1,000 mg/day of vitamin C and 400 IU/day of vitamin E.

### Supplementation with vitamins C and E for the prevention of pre-eclampsia or gestational hypertension

In general, studies of the effect of providing supplementary vitamin C and E to improve pregnancy outcomes have been inconsistent or have shown no positive effect. Although one single-centre study showed a significant reduction in pre-eclampsia risk in women identified as being at high risk [746], larger, multicentre trials have not confirmed such results. For example, a 2009 WHO trial of supplementation with vitamins C and E for pregnant women who were considered to be at high risk for pre-eclampsia found no association of supplementation with maternal or infant outcomes [747]. In this randomized trial, 687 women received vitamin C at 1,000 mg/day and vitamin E at 400 IU/day from ~18 weeks gestation until delivery, and 678 women received placebos. No reduction of pre-eclampsia, eclampsia, gestational hypertension, or any other maternal outcome was observed. Rates of low-birthweight infants, small-for-gestational-age infants, and perinatal deaths were also unaffected.

Another randomized trial (the VIP trial) of 2,404 women identified as being at increased risk of pre-eclampsia provided the same dosages of vitamins C and E or placebo. This study also found that concomitant supplementation with vitamin C and vitamin E did not prevent pre-eclampsia in women at risk but did increase the incidence of low birthweight. The results indicate that the use of these high-dose antioxidants is not justified in pregnancy [748]. This recommendation is echoed in results of a later study conducted by the INTAPP group as a multicentre randomized controlled trial involving 2,363 women. Vitamin C and E supplementation did not reduce the rate of pre-eclampsia or gestational hypertension but increased the risk of fetal loss, perinatal death, or PROM [749]. A larger multicentre trial in nearly 10,000 nulliparous women at low risk for pre-eclampsia also observed no effect on adverse maternal or perinatal outcomes related to pregnancy-induced hypertension in the high-dose vitamin C and E supplemented group but did not report a similar increase in rates of low birthweight or still birth [750].

It is possible that no effect was seen because the women in these studies already had adequate vitamin C and E status before receiving the high-dose supplements, as most were taking prenatal multivitamins containing amounts of vitamin C that provide near maximal tissue saturation. However, the previous WHO study also showed no benefit of antioxidant vitamin supplements in women who were in developing countries and were at high risk for pregnancy complications because of their nutritionally deficient status [747]. A prospective observational study of over 57,000 women in the Danish National Birth Cohort assessed vitamin intake based on a food frequency questionnaire completed in gestational week 25, in relation to the development of pre-eclampsia. The general incidence of pre-eclampsia was not correlated with dietary vitamin C and E intake, although incidence of severe pre-eclampsia, eclampsia, or HELLP syndrome declined with increasing dietary vitamin C intake [751].

## Supplementation with vitamins C and E for the prevention of PROM or preterm birth

Antioxidants have postulated benefits for fetal membrane integrity. It is suggested that antioxidants might inhibit the damage to fetal membrane integrity caused by ROS, thereby lessening the likelihood of PROM [752]. A randomized trial examined the effect of maternal supplementation with vitamin C at a dose of 100 mg/day, beginning before 20 weeks gestation, on the incidence of PROM and preterm birth compared with placebo. Plasma vitamin C decreased during pregnancy in both placebo and vitamin C groups as a consequence of haemodilution, but leukocyte vitamin C increased in the supplemented group and declined in the non-supplemented group. The incidence of both PROM and preterm birth were lower in the group receiving supplemental vitamin C [753]. However, conflicting results have also been reported. Another trial (n = 223 women) examined the effects of vitamins C and E given from midgestation to delivery on fetal membrane biomechanics, with membranes studied both in vivo and in vitro. Supplementation did not alter the normal remodelling process; in fact, incubation with vitamin C in vitro had an unexpected weakening effect on fetal membranes (vitamin C was expected to counteract the normal weakening process) [754].

A recent systematic review found convincing evidence that there is no gain from vitamin C supplementation for the prevention of preterm birth but did not suggest that it should be limited for other indications [755]. A study of a Hungarian cohort (of 38,151 newborns with congenital defects, representing 1.8 per cent of all Hungarian births between 1980 and 1996) specifically examined the effects of maternal vitamin E supplementation. The study showed a nearly 30 per cent reduction in preterm births in pregnant women who received vitamin E treatment. These results do not agree with those of other studies, and several confounding factors could have influenced the results, including the fact that vitamin E intake was recorded by retrospective recall in 37 per cent of the women [756].

## Supplementation with vitamins C and E on infant/chilhood respiratory outcomes

The effect of maternal vitamin C and E supplementation on offspring respiratory outcomes has also been studied. A randomized trial of high-dose antenatal vitamin C and E (1,000 mg vitamin C + 400 IU alpha-tocopherol/day) found that supplementation did not improve infant respiratory outcome up to 2 years of age, and was associated with increased health care utilization and cost of care [757]. However, a recent assessment of the impact of maternal antioxidant intakes on infant allergic outcomes reported that maternal dietary vitamin C intake (assessed by food frequency questionnaire) was associated with a reduced risk of diagnosed allergic disease at 1 year for the highest vs the lowest quartile [758]. No relationship was observed between allergic outcomes and maternal intake of vitamin E, zinc, or beta-carotene.

## Summary and recommendations for antioxidant intake

Traditionally, plant-based, antioxidant-rich foods formed the basis of the human diet. The western diet of today is relatively poor in such foods, and supplements are often considered to compensate for a low dietary intake. Although the risks of poor antioxidant status are even greater in pregnancy, the evidence for a beneficial effect of supplementation with antioxidant micronutrients is thus far unconvincing.

Recently, new avenues of evidence have suggested that, although free radicals may be dangerous in some contexts, they may actually beneficial in others, triggering a stress response that initiates repair processes. Every antioxidant is in essence an oxidation–reduction agent—protecting against ROS is some situations and promoting their generation in others. While antioxidants are clearly necessary to maintain a normal level of cellular defence against ROS, most evidence points to high-dose antioxidants as being more harmful than beneficial [759].

This has been borne out in numerous studies of antioxidant supplementation in pregnancy. Based on multiple studies showing a lack of effect of supplementation of vitamins C and E for the prevention of pre-eclampsia, gestational hypertension, PROM, and fetal growth restriction, the UK National Institute for Clincal Excellence (NICE) and RCOG recommend against supplementation with high doses of these vitamins during pregnancy [760, 761]. The NICE guideline specifically states that antioxidants (vitamins C and E) should not be recommended for the purpose of preventing hypertensive disorders of pregnancy [761].

## Our recommendations for antioxidant intake during pregnancy and lactation

Vitamins C and E and other antioxidants are necessary in pregnancy and should ideally be obtained from food sources. Most prenatal multivitamin supplements contain vitamin C in the range of 50–70 mg, which can complement dietary intake of fruits and vegetables to help meet vitamin C needs. Additional intake of vitamin C-containing supplements is not necessary in most cases, and is not recommended. Despite mounting evidence that high levels of vitamin E are not beneficial (and in fact are potentially harmful) to pregnancy outcomes, women should not be concerned about vitamin E obtained from food sources. However, supplementation during pregnancy is not recommended.

# Chapter 18

# Calcium in pregnancy and breastfeeding

## Calcium functions

Calcium is the most abundant mineral in the body, and 99 per cent of it is present in bones and teeth, where it contributes to structural integrity as a component of hydroxyapatite, a crystallizable salt compound. The average adult female skeleton contains approximately 1 kg of calcium, or ~25 per cent of the skeleton's dry weight. The skeleton serves as a reservoir for ionized calcium, storing it for use in other tissues, where it mediates signalling pathways for vascular contraction and vasodilation, muscle contraction, nerve transmission, and glandular secretion of hormones. As calcium is essential for the maintenance of healthy teeth and bones, its requirement is most critical during phases of rapid bone growth and tooth formation—that is, fetal development and infancy, early childhood, and the adolescent 'growth spurt'. While the skeleton is growing and maturing, it accumulates calcium at an average rate of 150 mg/day [762].

Calcium cannot be stored in excess in bone; increasing calcium intake beyond the amount required for optimal bone mass will not result in more bone accumulation. Below the threshold intake, bone formation is positively (and linearly) correlated with calcium intake and therefore limited by the amount of calcium ingested. Above the threshold, bone maintenance is not related to calcium intake. Hence, calcium requirements are based on levels correlating with maximal calcium retention, which differ depending on the life stage [562]. Calcium retention (with respect to intake) is generally positive during growth phases, neutral in adults, and negative in the elderly as an adaptation to reduced mechanical loading of bone. There is a consistent relationship between bone mass and calcium intake in both children [763] and adults [764], but different ethnic groups have different equilibrium levels. People of African descent generally have lower calcium intake but absorb and retain calcium more efficiently and therefore have stronger skeletons than Caucasians or Asians [765].

In addition to the key role that calcium plays in bone maintenance, ionized calcium in extracellular fluid is critical to many physiological functions, and its concentration is therefore tightly regulated (primarily by the calcium-sensing receptor, parathyroid hormone, and the active form of vitamin D—1,25-dihydroxyvitamin D (calcitriol)) [766]. When calcium levels decrease, the calcium-sensing receptor triggers parathyroid hormone secretion from the parathyroid glands to stimulate the conversion of 25-hydroxyvitamin D to 1,25-dihydroxyvitamin D, which raises serum calcium levels via mobilization from bone stores and increases smooth muscle contraction. Low calcium also triggers the release of renin from kidneys, leading to vasoconstriction and fluid/sodium retention, and is associated with hypertension [767]. Serum concentrations of free ionized calcium vary above or below a very narrow 'normal' range only in extreme circumstances such as severe malnutrition or hyperparathyroidism.

## Indicators of calcium status

Total calcium measured in blood is the common test used to screen for, diagnose, and monitor conditions relating to calcium status. The normal reference range for adults is 8.6–10.2 mg/dL (2.15–2.55 mmol/L). Total blood calcium does not provide an indication of bone calcium status and is primarily a measure of free, rather than bound calcium. Ionized calcium concentration is the preferred indicator in individuals with blood protein abnormalities such as low albumin, which can affect the ratio of free to bound calcium. Measurement of urine calcium is used to determine whether renal calcium excretion is adequate [768].

## Calcium in pregnancy

The fetal skeleton accumulates ~30 g of calcium by the end of gestation. Most of this uptake occurs during the third trimester, when fetal bone growth is at its peak. The extra demand for calcium by the fetus during pregnancy is balanced by increased intestinal calcium absorption in the mother, such that additional dietary calcium is usually not required if pre-pregnancy intake is adequate.

### Calcium and bone turnover in pregnancy

Correlating with this peak in maternal-fetal calcium transfer, the rate of maternal bone turnover doubles in late pregnancy, observed as changes in markers of bone resorption and formation [769, 770]. Despite this increase, compensatory changes in endogenous hormone levels occur to prevent extreme calcium loss from the maternal skeleton. Specifically, serum calcitonin levels increase, opposing the effects of parathyroid hormone, and synthesis of 1,25-dihydroxyvitamin D increases, enhancing intestinal absorption and limiting the mobilization of calcium from bone. Although total serum calcium declines as a result of a haemodilution-induced reduction in serum albumin (which binds calcium), the physiologically relevant fraction—free ionized calcium—remains constant throughout pregnancy [771]. Bone loss is minimized if calcium intake is maintained at 1,000–1,200 mg/day during pregnancy. This intake level builds up calcium stores in early pregnancy for increased fetal transfer in the third trimester.

There are situations in which bone loss may increase during pregnancy. In pregnant adolescents whose bones are still growing, bone mineral density (BMD) declines by ~10 per cent during gestation [772]. Women carrying multiple fetuses also experience negative calcium balance during pregnancy, as do those taking heparin (for prevention of deep vein thrombosis), as it inhibits the synthesis of 1,25-dihydroxyvitamin D [772].

Some of the compensatory mechanisms that come into play to maximize calcium absorption during pregnancy also operate in individuals on calcium-deficient diets. The effect of low calcium intake is accentuated in pregnant women and is manifested in higher rates of calcium absorption, and reduced excretion [569, 773]. Even with this apparent intestinal and renal adaptation to low calcium consumption, chronically low dietary intakes (<500 mg/day) may still not meet maternal and fetal needs during pregnancy. Low calcium intake during pregnancy has been associated with reduced bone mineral content (BMC) in newborns [774].

Because active (vitamin D-dependent) calcium absorption is increased under calcium-deficient diets, the requirement for vitamin D is also likely to be greater. Vitamin D regulates not only calcium absorption but also plasma calcium homeostasis, and deficiency or inadequacy of this vitamin limits the body's adaptive responses to low calcium intake. Thus, calcium intake may need to be adjusted for certain dietary factors, including vitamin D intake, and for sun exposure, since both can affect calcium absorption and retention [231] (see chapter 15 for details on vitamin D).

## Bone outcomes—trials of calcium supplementation during pregnancy

### Maternal outcomes of calcium supplementation during pregnancy

Although resorption of calcium from the maternal skeleton into the circulation is known to increase during pregnancy, particularly in women with low calcium intakes, few randomized studies have evaluated the effect of supplemental calcium on bone mass and density in pregnant women. Short-term studies of calcium supplementation of 1–1.2 g/day for 7–10 days in late pregnancy resulted in a reduction in the expression of markers of bone turnover in women consuming low-calcium diets [775, 776]. In China, supplementation with milk or milk plus calcium (600 mg/day) increased calcium in the diet of women with habitually low intakes from ~530 mg/day to ~880 mg/day with milk alone, and to ~1,360 mg/day with milk plus calcium. A dose-dependent increase in maternal BMD was observed with increasing calcium intake [777].

Interestingly, in Gambian women with very low calcium intakes (<355 mg/day), supplementation with 1,500 mg calcium/day from 20 weeks gestation until delivery did not result in significant differences in total-body BMC, BMD, or bone area at 2 weeks postpartum, as compared with placebo. In fact, in the supplemented women, the decreases seen in these bone measures at specific sites (lumbar spine, distal radius, and hip) were significantly greater than those in unsupplemented mothers, up to 52 weeks postpartum. It is possible that this increase in calcium intake during pregnancy disrupted the adaptive mechanisms established in these women who were accustomed to very low levels of calcium in their normal diets [778].

## Infant outcomes of calcium supplementation during pregnancy

Data are relatively scarce regarding the effect of maternal calcium supplementation during pregnancy on bone mineralization in the fetus. Studies have mainly evaluated growth parameters such as birthweight and length, and intrauterine growth restriction (small for gestational age at birth), and often these were studied as secondary end points to the effect of supplemental calcium on hypertensive disorders in pregnancy (see 'Calcium intake and pre-eclampsia/high blood pressure'). An early supplementation trial in India using 300 or 600 mg calcium lactate/day (from between 18 and 22 weeks gestation until delivery) found an increase in BMD in neonates born to supplemented mothers in both groups, compared with those born to unsupplemented mothers [779]. Another trial found that, overall, total calcium intake was positively associated with total-body BMC in infants [774].

A recent study of women consuming a low-calcium diet (<600 mg/day) in Argentina reported no effect of supplementation on fetal somatic or skeletal growth [780]. This is consistent with the results seen in the offspring of Gambian women who were similarly supplemented. The Gambian diets were lower in calcium, and, similar to the effect seen in the women themselves, the infants of supplemented mothers exhibited a slower rate of bone accretion (slower increase in bone area and BMC) in the first year of life compared with those born to women who had not received supplements during pregnancy [781]. The effect of maternal calcium intake on infant bone outcomes during breastfeeding has been more extensively studied and is discussed in 'Calcium in lactation.'

## Calcium intake and pre-eclampsia/high blood pressure

Pre-eclampsia is characterized by vascular endothelial dysfunction and placental insufficiency during pregnancy. Epidemiological evidence has shown an inverse relationship between calcium intake and hypertensive disorders of pregnancy, and the consequent higher risk of preterm birth. Populations with high-calcium diets have low incidence of pre-eclampsia and eclampsia (e.g. historically in Ethiopia and in the Mayan Indians of Guatemala) [782].

Numerous studies have evaluated the relationship between calcium intake and the risk of pregnancy-induced hypertension and pre-eclampsia, and the effect of calcium supplementation in reducing this risk. Meta-analyses indicate an overall protective effect of supplemental calcium on pre-eclampsia in populations with low calcium intake [783, 784]. A systematic review and meta-analysis of 13 studies concluded that, with calcium supplementation of at least 1 g/day, the average risk of gestational hypertensive disorders was reduced by 35 per cent, and the average risk of pre-eclampsia was reduced by 55 per cent. The effects of calcium supplementation on the risk of pre-eclampsia were greatest for 'high-risk' women and those with low calcium intake [783]. Focusing on developing countries, a meta-analysis of ten randomized controlled trials found that calcium supplementation (1,500–2,000 mg/day) during pregnancy reduced the risk of all gestational hypertensive disorders in women with low baseline calcium intakes [784]. The reduction in risk was greatest in the subgroup of women whose pre-pregnancy risk of developing hypertensive disorders was highest.

Calcium supplementation to women with low dietary intakes (<600 mg/day) was found to reduce the risk of severe pre-eclamptic complications by 25 per cent in a WHO multicentre trial, although no effect on gestational hypertension was observed [785]. However a 2007 US FDA review considered the evidence to be insufficient to support the use of calcium supplements for the purpose of reducing gestational hypertensive disorders in the US, where baseline calcium intake is relatively high [786].

## Calcium intake and preterm delivery

Preterm delivery is commonly associated with hypertensive disorders in pregnancy. Calcium supplementation was found to reduce the average risk of preterm birth in a meta-analysis of clinical trials on the prevention of hypertensive disorders in pregnancy [783]. In a WHO-sponsored randomized trial in 8,325 women with calcium intakes <600 mg/day, the risk of early preterm delivery (<32 weeks of gestation) was statistically significantly lower in the calcium group (2.6%) than in the placebo group (3.2%) [785]. Supplementation of pregnant adolescent women (≤17 years; n = 94) in the US with 2 g/day elemental calcium resulted in a significant reduction in the incidence of preterm delivery compared with placebo (7.4% vs 21.1% for the placebo group) [787]. A pooled analysis of data from five trials in developing countries (where baseline calcium intake was low) reported a significant reduction in preterm births in women who received 1,500–2,000 mg supplemental calcium from around 20 weeks gestation [784].

## The effect of maternal calcium intake on childhood blood pressure

As calcium appears to have an influence on blood pressure in pregnant women, the effect of maternal calcium intake on blood pressure in infants and children has also been analysed. A systematic review of studies of maternal calcium intake and offspring blood pressure reported that higher maternal calcium was associated with a reduction in offspring systolic blood pressure up to 9 years of age [788]. However, the benefit of maternal supplementation is most evident in offspring of mothers who had high blood pressure during pregnancy, which is an independent risk factor for high blood pressure in children.

## Calcium intake and lead exposure

Calcium intake may modify the impact of maternal lead exposure during pregnancy, protecting the fetus from toxic exposure. High calcium intake during pregnancy and lactation helps to minimize bone demineralization, and consequently, slows the release of lead from bone into the maternal circulation. The impact of lead exposure in pregnancy is discussed in detail in chapter 30.

## Calcium in lactation

Because the concentration of calcium is tightly regulated (referred to as 'calcium economy'), maternal calcium intake has little effect on the amount that is secreted in breast milk. This appears to apply even in women consuming very little dietary calcium, such as those in Gambia, where supplementation had little effect on the amount of calcium present in breast milk [789]. The mean concentration of calcium in breast milk is approximately 260 mg/L. Based on an observed average breast milk consumption of ~780 mL/day, and using a conservative estimate of absorption, the estimated calcium intake by fully breastfed infants is around 200 mg/day [562]. This level is considered adequate for most infants, assuming that vitamin D is also present in sufficient quantity.

The absorption of calcium from breast milk is high compared with calcium absorption from solid foods. Infants who were fed a mixed diet of breast milk and solid food in a study using stable calcium isotopes retained more of the calcium derived from breast milk than from solids [790]. Calcium absorption from infant formula is also lower than from breast milk, but formula-fed infants absorb more calcium overall because of the higher calcium content of formula [791].

BMC and bone mass accretion was significantly higher during the first 6 months of life in infants fed formula containing 510 mg/L calcium and 390 mg/L phosphorous, compared with infants fed breast milk containing 300 mg/L calcium and 150 mg/L phosphorous (calcium:phosphate ratios of 1.3:1 for formula vs 2.0:1 for breast milk). This high-phosphate, high-calcium formula resulted in low serum calcium levels in the first few weeks of life. Despite the early faster accretion in formula-fed infants, breastfed infants who began consuming formula at 6 months of age had a greater increase in bone mass during the second 6 months of life than those who had been fed formula from birth [792].

A number of studies conducted in women with relatively high calcium intakes found no association between maternal calcium intake and changes in either bone mineral status or biochemical indicators of calcium metabolism in women during lactation [793, 794]. Yet, as indicated by markers of bone turnover and bone mass in breastfeeding women and after weaning, BMD decreases in the first 6 months postpartum and returns to normal 6 months after weaning in women with an average daily intake of ~1,200 mg/day [795]. It appears that, in general, calcium supplementation has little effect on lactation-induced changes in the calcium economy.

## Prevalence of calcium deficiency

The incidence of calcium deficiency is high in regions such as Africa and Asia, where the prevailing diets consist of few or no dairy products and grains are dietary staples. Low calcium exacerbates the effects of vitamin D deficiency and increases the risk of rickets [796], and there are also reports of rickets occurring in children with adequate levels of vitamin D [797, 798]. Low calcium intake combined with high protein intake also results in calcium deficiency, manifesting in increased rates of bone fracture [799]. Clinical signs of vitamin D deficiency—rickets and osteomalacia—are still common in tropical and subtropical countries, where people are exposed to abundant sunlight. It is suggested that the low-calcium/high-cereal diets typical of some of these regions (where susceptibility to rickets remains high) might alter the efficiency of vitamin D utilization. Calcium deficiency has been shown to enhance the degradative metabolism of 25-hydroxyvitamin D [800]. Absorption of calcium from the gut in people with minimal calcium intake cannot be enhanced if vitamin D status is also deficient. It is important to bear in mind that vitamin D deficiency aggravates the consequences of low calcium, and vice versa.

In Canada, the prevalence of inadequate calcium intake in adult women ranges from 48–87 per cent, depending on the age group [801]. In the US, the average dietary intakes of calcium are well below the recommended dietary allowance (RDA; 1,000–1,300 mg/day; see 'Agency guidelines for calcium intake'), especially for adolescent females, as a result of replacing the main source of calcium—milk—with soft drinks [571]. A survey of 250 pregnant women in the UK in 2006 indicated that 40 per cent failed to meet the UK guidelines for calcium intake [802]. In India, in both rural and urban populations, dietary intake is low relative to the Indian Council of Medical Research RDA of 400 mg/day [803] (a low RDA compared with US recommendations). Urban women in India have an average daily calcium intake of 306 mg/day, and rural women average 262 mg/day.

## Calcium sources

In Western countries, milk and milk products are the major source of dietary calcium, with cereal products (where flour is fortified) and fruits and vegetables making a smaller contribution. Milk contains ~115 mg calcium/100 g, and cheeses range between 60 and 1,200 mg/100 g. Raw spinach contains ~170 mg calcium/100 g but also contains oxalic acid, which inhibits calcium absorption. Asian diets provide calcium in the form of leafy green vegetables such as bok choy, chinese cabbage, broccoli, spinach, kale, and mustard greens, as well as fish that are eaten whole, such as anchovies (or *ikan bilis*—dried anchovies), sardines, and canned salmon. Soy products (e.g. tofu and soy milk) are also good sources of calcium, containing 500–1,400 mg/100 g.

A number of dietary factors influence calcium balance. Oxalic acid present in spinach, beetroot, sweet potatoes, and other vegetables (as well as some fruits, nuts, grains, and legumes) also limits the bioavailability of calcium present in the same foods. Sodium intake affects calcium excretion; it is estimated that for every 2,300 mg of sodium excreted, there is an approximate calcium loss in urine of 40 mg [804]. A diet high in processed food will therefore provide less useable calcium than a diet that is lower in sodium but contains equal amounts of calcium. A high intake of animal protein also increases urinary calcium excretion [805]. Phytate, the storage form of phosphorus founds in grain fibre, inhibits the absorption of calcium in the gut [806]. Consumption of a high-fibre diet was associated with calcium deficit in lactating women in rural Mexico (who consumed 32 g fibre/day and 750 mg calcium/day) as a result of impaired intestinal absorption [807], although another report indicated that chronic wheat dextrin consumption did not inhibit calcium absorption in the gastrointestinal tract in women [808].

Sufficient calcium can be obtained by eating four servings of dairy products or other calcium-rich foods (e.g. sardines, dark green vegetables, or tofu) per day. Taking calcium together with iron (either in the diet or as a supplement) is not recommended, since calcium inhibits iron absorption [809]. It should be noted that diets high in animal protein and/or phytates would possibly render an individual more calcium deficient than their calcium intake alone would indicate.

## Risks of excess calcium

It is unlikely that ingestion of calcium from foods would result in excess serum calcium; however, high use of supplements and medications containing calcium (e.g. antacids) has been known to cause hypercalcaemia and/or hypercalciuria in some cases. Serum calcium levels of 10.5 mg/dL (2.63 mmol/L) or higher signify hypercalcaemia, with clinical signs varying depending on the rapidity and magnitude of the elevation. Symptoms of hypercalcaemia include weight loss, anorexia, fatigue, polyuria, heart arrhythmia, and soft tissue calcification. Ultimately, hypercalcaemia can lead to renal failure.

The tolerable upper intake level set by the US Institute of Medicine (IOM) for pregnant women is 3,000 mg/day for adolescents and 2,500 mg/day for women over 18 years of age. Infants should not consume more than 1,000 mg/day for the first 6 months of life, and more than 1,500 mg/day between 6 and 12 months [562]. These levels are relatively close to the intake levels corresponding to nutritional adequacy, so care should be taken when advising the use of calcium supplements such that the upper limit is not exceeded. A recent meta-analysis suggested that calcium supplementation modestly increased the risk of cardiovascular events in middle aged women taking supplements for the prevention of osteoporosis [810, 811], but many experts disagree with the data analysis and conclusions and continue to recommend calcium supplementation in postmenopausal women [812–814].

## Agency guidelines for calcium intake

The IOM Food and Nutrition Board in the US based their calcium intake recommendations on the criteria of 'maximal calcium retention'—threshold values above which the calcium balance does not further improve as intake increases [562]. The dietary reference intakes put forth by the IOM are also endorsed by Health Canada. The recommendations for pregnant women and infants are shown in Box 18.1.

## Box 18.1 Institute of Medicine recommended dietary allowances for calcium

Infants 0–6 months (adequate intake (AI)) = 200 mg/day
Infants 7–12 months (AI) = 260 mg/day
Children 1–3 years = 700 mg/day
Females 14–18 years = 1,300 mg/day
Females 19–50 years = 1,000 mg/day
Pregnancy 14–18 years = 1,300 mg/day
Pregnancy 19+ years = 1,000 mg/day
Lactation 14–18 years = 1,300 mg/day
Lactation 19+ years = 1,000 mg/day
Tolerable upper intake levels
Pregnancy and lactation 14–18 years = 3,000 mg/day
Pregnancy and lactation 19+ years = 2,500 mg/day

Source: Institute of Medicine, *Dietary Reference Intakes for Calcium and Vitamin D*, The National Academies Press, Washington, DC, copyright © 2011. [562]

The recommendations for pregnant and lactating women over the age of 18 do not differ from those for non-pregnant women, because the body adapts to the increased calcium demand by increasing calcium absorption and retention. Pregnant adolescents require a higher calcium intake to compensate for the dual demands of the fetus and their own continued bone growth. These RDAs reflect the view that no additional health benefits are achieved at intakes above these levels. The IOM recommendations are endorsed by the American Pregnancy Association [815]. According to WHO guidelines, in regions where dietary calcium intake is low, calcium supplementation during pregnancy (at doses of 1.5–2.0 g elemental calcium/day) is recommended for the prevention of preeclampsia in all women, but especially those at high risk of developing preeclampsia [816].

## Our recommendations for calcium intake during pregnancy and lactation

Pregnant and lactating women consuming a diet including sufficient amounts of dairy products and vegetable calcium sources do not require supplemental calcium during pregnancy. All women should be encouraged to achieve or maintain a dietary calcium intake between 1,000 and 1,300 mg/day by increasing their intake of calcium-rich foods. Women consuming low amounts of calcium (<600 mg/day), and those at risk for hypertensive disorders, should be encouraged to increase their intake by an additional 1 g of calcium per day throughout pregnancy in order to reduce their risk of pre-eclampsia and related adverse pregnancy outcomes. Increasing dietary calcium is preferable to supplementation, but if there is a possibility of inadequate dietary intake, supplements should be taken at a dosage of 1–1.5 g/day.

Because vitamin D is essential for the adaptive calcium homeostatic mechanisms that occur during pregnancy and lactation, it is important to ensure that vitamin D is also present in sufficient amounts (see chapter 15). Calcium supplementation is also recommended for pregnant and lactating women with a history of environmental or occupational lead exposure, to reduce both circulating lead levels in the mother and lead exposure to the developing fetus and nursing infant. Infants can obtain their full calcium requirement (200 mg/day) through breast milk in the first 6 months of life, or from calcium-fortified infant formula.

# Chapter 19

# Iodine in pregnancy and breastfeeding

## Iodine functions

Iodine is a key component of the thyroid hormones, thyroxine (also known as T4) and triiodothyronine (also known as T3), which regulate a number of physiological processes, including growth, development, and reproductive function, the maintenance of metabolic rate, cellular metabolism, and the integrity of connective tissue. All biological actions of iodine are attributed to thyroid hormones, although there may be a role for elemental iodine in early brain development [817]. Development of the fetal brain and nervous system are dependent on thyroid hormones supplied by the mother during gestation [818]. The requirement for thyroid hormone production is substantially increased in the first trimester. Thyroid hormones are important for myelination of the CNS, which is most active late in pregnancy and shortly after birth. Because the fetal thyroid system does not mature until the late third trimester, the increased demand for thyroid hormones, and therefore for iodine, is sustained throughout the full term of pregnancy. There is also a significant increase in renal iodide clearance during pregnancy reflecting increased thyroid hormone production. This results in a shortfall of ~20 µg iodine per day [819]. Women with adequate iodine intake before conception (~150 µg/day) can adapt to the increased demand for thyroid hormones during pregnancy, because the thyroid gland adjusts its hormonal output [820], but this depends on sufficient availability of dietary iodine, and the integrity of the thyroid gland.

## Indicators of iodine status

Almost all iodine is excreted in urine, so urinary iodine concentration (UIC) is often used as a surrogate measure of iodine intake in populations [821]. Iodine sufficiency in pregnant women is defined as UIC >150 µg/L. Iodine nutrition status is considered optimal in a population at urinary levels between 150–249 µg/L; levels ≥500 µg/L are reflective of excessive iodine intake. For lactating women, a median UIC of ≥100 µg/L indicates adequate intake and optimal iodine status. However, the UIC test is not appropriate to diagnose iodine deficiency in individuals. Urine iodine levels are variable from day to day in a given individual, because they reflect only recent intake, whereas the thyroid can store relatively large amounts of iodine. The body of a healthy adult contains 15–20 mg of iodine, of which 70–80 per cent is found in the thyroid. In chronic iodine deficiency, the iodine content of the thyroid might fall to less than 20 μg. Measurement of UIC therefore has a low predictive value for iodine deficiency [822].

Blood levels of free T4 or thyroid stimulating hormone (TSH) have also been used to estimate iodine status. In the first trimester of a normal pregnancy, serum TSH levels are lower than before conception, but during the second half of gestation, TSH levels return progressively to pre-pregnancy values and remain stable. Because of the normal changes in thyroid hormone levels and TSH during pregnancy, measurements of free T4 and free T3 are used to assess thyroid status in early gestation. In later gestation (from 16 weeks), a low TSH is a sensitive measure of adequate thyroid status [823].

## Iodine deficiency in pregnancy

In women with suboptimal pre-pregnancy iodine stores, thyroid adaptation in pregnancy is impaired. If iodine intake continues to be inadequate in pregnancy, it triggers a progressive increase in serum TSH that enhances thyroid gland stimulation and increases thyroid volume, leading to goitre [824, 825]. Typically, plasma levels of the biochemically active thyroid hormones T4 and T3 fall, while TSH increases, sometimes to very high levels.

### The effects of iodine deficiency on preterm delivery, placental abruption, miscarriage, and fetal/infant mortality

Approximately 2–5 per cent of pregnant women are affected by subclinical hypothyroidism (defined as normal circulating free T4 and elevated TSH), which can result from inadequate iodine intake. In a large prospective analysis of pregnant women who were screened for abnormal thyroid function in the first half of pregnancy, there was a twofold higher incidence of preterm delivery at or before 34 weeks gestation, and a threefold higher incidence of placental abruption among women diagnosed with subclinical hypothyroidism [826]. High maternal TSH has also been associated with miscarriage [827] and an increased risk of fetal death [828].

Maternal iodine supplementation in areas of severe iodine deficiency has been shown to decrease the rates of stillbirth and neonatal and infant mortality. Oral administration of iodized oil to mothers before or during pregnancy reduced the rate of prematurity, stillbirth, and spontaneous abortion compared with that for untreated mothers in an area of endemic goitre in Algeria [829]. In addition, iodination of irrigation water reduced infant mortality in an area of severe iodine deficiency in China [830].

## The effects of iodine deficiency on birthweight and fetal/infant growth

In iodine-deficient areas, repletion of iodine in pregnancy resulted in higher birthweights and increased head circumference in newborns [831]. Children born to mothers treated with iodized oil in pregnancy had a 200 g higher mean birthweight than those born to untreated mothers [829]. Birthweight and infant growth were positively correlated with maternal use of iodized salt in an analysis of iodine intakes in several Asian countries [832].

## The effects of iodine deficiency on neurodevelopment

The brain is particularly vulnerable to deficiencies of iodine and thyroid hormones during development. A lack of maternal iodine disrupts the development of the brain and myelination of the CNS. In infants, an elevated concentration of TSH reflects an insufficient supply of maternal and/or fetal thyroid hormones to the developing brain and indicates a risk of irreversible brain damage [833]. In severe form, congenital hypothyroidism resulting from iodine deficiency can manifest in major neurocognitive deficits and cretinism, which can have multiple forms, including deaf–mutism, motor abnormalities, and myxoedematous cretinism. Moderate iodine deficiency in pregnancy is associated with lower learning capacity, reduced IQ, hearing impairment, and increased risk of attention deficit hyperactivity disorder [834]. Two meta-analyses of observational studies of the effect of iodine deficiency on cognitive development found that the IQs of children from areas with moderate to severe iodine deficiency were on average 12–13.5 points lower than those of children from non-iodine-deficient areas [835, 836]. Undiagnosed hypothyroidism in pregnant women may have the same effects, which suggests that screening for thyroid deficiency in pregnant women is warranted [837].

The severity of neurodevelopmental damage depends on the timing and severity of iodine deficiency during gestation. In the first trimester, the cerebral vesicles, from which the cerebral cortex will form, begin developing. Even mild iodine deficiency during this period of neocortical proliferation can affect neurological development. If iodine supplementation is delayed until after the first 12–14 weeks of gestation in women with mild dietary iodine deficiency, their offspring are at increased risk for poor gross and fine motor coordination, and socialization problems. These adverse effects are amplified if women are not supplemented with iodine at all, as compared with being supplemented later in pregnancy [838]. Iodine supplementation before the third trimester predicted higher psychomotor test scores for children than did iodine supplementation later in pregnancy or postnatally. Women and children in iodine-deficient regions may be given iodinated oil as depot injections [831].

In Europe only 15–30 per cent of women receive iodine supplements, and consumption of iodized salt varies. A study conducted in Spain, where iodine intake is below recommended levels, evaluated neurocognitive function in infants aged 3–18 months whose mothers received 300 µg potassium iodide in pregnancy or no supplement. Children whose mothers received iodine daily from the first trimester performed better on psychomotor evaluation than those from unsupplemented mothers, suggesting benefits can be gained by maternal iodine supplementation in areas of mild to moderate deficiency [839].

## Iodine in lactation

Iodine continues to be vital for brain development in the newborn infant through to 3 years of age. Maternal iodine is the only source of iodine for infants after birth, unless they receive formula or supplements. The iodine demand of newborns is partly supported by iodine accumulated in the fetal thyroid gland during gestation [840]. The recommended intake for infants in the first 6 months is 110 µg/day and between 7 and 12 months is 130 µg/day.

The concentration of iodine in breast milk is 20–50 times higher than that in plasma [841]. The sodium iodide symporter mediates iodide uptake by the mammary gland, and its expression increases during lactation [842]. Iodine in breast milk varies in response to short-term changes in dietary iodine intake. A study in which healthy pregnant women ingested 600 µg of potassium iodide showed a measurable rise in breast milk iodine concentrations, peaking 6 hours after ingestion [843]. The iodine concentration in colostrum following delivery is approximately 200–400 µg/L, but decreases to between 75 and 200 µg/L in breast milk [841]. Breastfeeding women require increased dietary iodine intake to compensate for this iodine loss.

## Iodine supplementation in pregnancy

Although universal iodine supplementation during pregnancy remains controversial, the benefits of correcting iodine deficiency are generally considered to outweigh the risks of supplemental iodine. This is particularly true in areas known to have iodine-deficient soils and a moderate to high risk of deficiency.

A large number of studies have examined the effects of iodine supplementation on pregnancy outcomes.

## Interventional studies—severe iodine deficiency in pregnancy

Five randomized controlled trials in low-income countries have shown that iodine supplementation before or during pregnancy reduces the incidence of cretinism in areas of high prevalence [844]. An early trial of intramuscular iodinated oil supplementation (vs saline injection) in a region of endemic cretinism in Papua New Guinea found that cretinism did not occur in offspring from women who received iodinated oil before conception [845]. In addition, studies on cognitive development showed that iodine treatment before or during pregnancy improved development scores in the offspring by 10–20 per cent [844]. In an area of severe iodine deficiency (4% cretinism rate) in Zaire, pregnant women were randomized to receive injections of either iodized oil or vitamins at around 28 weeks gestation. Psychomotor development scores at 6 years of age of the offspring from women in the iodine group were significantly higher than those of offspring from the group that did not receive iodine [846]. Other studies conducted in Zaire, Peru, and Ecuador have shown similar results [847].

## Interventional studies—mild/moderate iodine deficiency in pregnancy

Multiple studies in areas of mild to moderate iodine deficiency have examined measures of maternal (and sometimes infant) thyroid function following iodine supplementation in pregnancy. Healthy pregnant women in Italy were given 120–180 μg iodine as iodized salt or a placebo daily, beginning in the first trimester. Thyroid volume increased in placebo recipients but not in those receiving iodine (n = 35; median UIC: 31–37 μg/L) [848]. Similarly, in a randomized trial of pregnant women in Denmark (n = 54) in which women received either 200 μg iodine/day as a potassium iodide solution or no supplement from 17 weeks to term, maternal thyroid volume increased by 16 per cent in the treated group and by 30 per cent in the control subjects [849]. Other studies also indicate that supplementation of women with low iodine intakes resulted in smaller thyroid volumes and improvement in both maternal and infant thyroid parameters, as compared with unsupplemented controls [850, 851].

However, data are limited with regard to the effect of iodine supplementation to mildly iodine-deficient mothers on the developmental outcomes of their offspring. Despite many agencies recommending routine iodine supplementation for pregnant women, a recent systematic review of randomized controlled trials has suggested this may not be without risk to the fetus in women with adequate iodine status [852]. As there is some disagreement on safe levels of supplementation, further investigation is necessary in areas of mild to moderate iodine deficiency as well as in areas of iodine sufficiency, to assess the benefits and risks according to background iodine status.

A possible side effect of iodine supplementation is aggravation of subclinical autoimmune thyroid disease, which is common in pregnant women and can develop into postpartum thyroid dysfunction. Subclinical autoimmune thyroid disease is diagnosed by the detection of antibodies against thyroid peroxidase. A placebo-controlled, randomized, double-blind trial of women positive for antibodies against thyroid peroxidase examined whether supplementation increased the risk of autoimmune thyroid disease but found no significant increase in postpartum thyroid dysfunction in women given 150 μg iodine per day during pregnancy and postpartum, or during pregnancy only, as compared with unsupplemented controls [853].

## Iodine sources

The total body iodine requirement must be derived exogenously. Iodine is present in seawater, igneous rocks, and some soils. Food sources of iodine can vary greatly in their iodine content, depending mainly on the natural or supplemented (fertilizer) iodine content of the soil they are grown in, or the content of the food eaten by animal sources. The amount of iodine in soils varies considerably around the world, translating to a wide variation in iodine content of similar crops grown in different regions [260]. The soil in many regions is very low in iodine, and deficiency is a risk if locally grown foods are primarily consumed.

Seaweed (e.g. kelp, nori, kombu, and wakame) is an excellent source of iodine, although the content can vary from 16 μg to nearly 3,000 μg iodine per 1 g serving [260]. Many seafoods are also high in iodine. Dairy products in some areas (including the US) may have relatively high iodine content due to the use of iodine feed supplements, and contamination from iodine-containing disinfectants in milk tankers and milking equipment (although this is declining in some countries). The transfer of iodine from feed into milk from dairy cows is approximately 30–40 per cent, compared to transfer from feed into meat from pork or beef, which are both less that 1 per cent. Iodine transfer from feed into eggs is also much higher (10–20%) than from feed into meat [854]. Some bread has high iodine content because of the use of iodate conditioners in the baking process. Iodine for infants is supplied by breast milk for the first six months, or iodine-fortified formulas. However, there is a wide variation in iodine content in infant formulas.

## Areas of concern for iodine availability

According the WHO, over half the population of Europe lives in areas of iodine deficiency [855]. The Eastern Mediterranean, Africa, Himalayas, Andes and the Western Pacific are also regions of concern, although many other areas also have suboptimal iodine nutrition. Inland, mountainous regions are generally most affected, as iodine leaches from the soils due to snow, water movement, and heavy rain. The reasons for iodine deficiency in different regions is therefore primarily geological rather than socioeconomic. Correction of deficiency in a region has to be achieved by supplying iodine from an external source.

Salt iodization programmes have been instituted in various countries to combat this problem and have had some success in reducing the prevalence of iodine deficiency. A 2009 report by the UN Standing Committee on Nutrition indicated that, at that point, control of iodine deficiency via fortification of salt covered an estimated 70 per cent of households worldwide, and it was calculated that ~2 billion people would have shown signs of iodine deficiency without this intervention [236]. However, iodized salt as a source of iodine may not be sufficient or appropriate for pregnant women. Even in iodine-sufficient regions (based on salt iodization), significant numbers of pregnant women still have insufficient iodine intake (e.g. Iran [856], China [857], Italy [858], and Turkey [859]). The ten most iodine-deficient countries in 2011 (assessed as those with the greatest numbers of school-aged children with insufficient intake) were Ethiopia, Sudan, Russian Federation, Afghanistan, Algeria, Angola, the UK, Mozambique, Ghana, and Morocco [860].

## Risks of excess iodine

It is important to monitor the risk of thyroid disease due to an excessive consumption of iodine, as well as that due to deficiency. The range between the required amounts of iodine and the tolerable upper intake level (UL) is only about 1:3, depending on the life stage. According to the WHO, the UL for pregnancy (500 μg/day) is only twice the required intake (250 μg/day). Iodine is therefore categorized as a trace element with a high risk of deficiency, but also with high risk of excess. Symptoms of acute iodine toxicity include diarrhoea, with alternating periods of hyperactivity, weakness, convulsions, and death. Sub-chronic toxicity symptoms include reduced weight gain and haemolysis, in addition to specific inhibitory effects on thyroid function [861]. A recent cross-sectional study in China (n = 384 pregnant women) found that women with excessive iodine intake were more likely to have thyroid disease, particularly subclinical hypothyroidism [862].

Iodine readily crosses the placenta and is secreted in breast milk. Fetal exposure to excess iodine in utero via placental transfer, or infant overexposure via breast milk, can cause neonatal hypothyroidism. This has been reported in Japan, where dietary iodine intake is very high from consumption of seaweed (kombu) [863], and in the US in cases of maternal consumption of tablets containing 12.5 mg iodine per day during pregnancy [864]. Women in some Asian cultures (particularly Korea and North China) consume seaweed soup to promote breast milk supply, and this practice has been linked to iodine-induced neonatal hypothyroidism [865].

## Agency guidelines for iodine intake

The US Institute of Medicine (IOM)'s recommended dietary allowance (RDA) for iodine in pregnancy is 220 µg/day, and during lactation the RDA is 290 µg/day. This is an increase from 150 µg/day for non-pregnant, non-lactating women [260]. The IOM UL is 1,100 µg/day for all adults, and 900 µg/day for adolescents 14–18 years of age. No UL has been established for infants or children. According to the IOM, the adequate intake (AI) level for infants aged 0–6 months is 110 µg/day of iodine, which can be acquired through breast milk if the mother's iodine intake is sufficient. Between 7 and 12 months of age, infants require 130 µg/day of iodine; complementary foods and/or iodine-fortified formula should be added to the diet at this point. For children between the ages of 1 and 8 years, the RDA is 90 µg/day, increasing to 120 µg/day for children 9–13 years of age [260]. Other government agencies, including the Australian National Health and Medical Research Council [866] and the New Zealand Ministry of Health, have made similar recommendations, that is, iodine intakes of 220 µg/day in pregnancy and 270 µg/day during lactation, to be achieved by consuming iodine supplements of 150 µg/day in addition to dietary sources [143]. The recommendations of the IOM are in general agreement with those of the International Council for the Control of Iodine Deficiency Disorders and UNICEF, and are shown in Box 19.1.

The WHO, UNICEF, and the International Council for the Control of Iodine Deficiency Disorders, all of which focus on the developing world, all advise women who are pregnant or breastfeeding to take a daily oral iodine supplement, so that the total daily intake is 250 µg [867]. A daily intake greater than 500 µg/day is considered unnecessary, as it would not provide any additional benefit for health and may be associated with impaired thyroid function. The WHO recommends fortification of salt at 20–40 mg iodine/kg salt. This level assumes no iodine in the usual diet pre-fortification and that salt is consumed at 10 g/day, and it is designed to provide an intake that is adequate

## Box 19.1 US Institute of Medicine recommended dietary allowances for iodine

Infants 0–6 months (adequate intake (AI)) = 110 µg/day

Infants 7–12 months (AI) = 130 µg/day

Children 1–3 years = 90 µg/day

Females 14+ years = 150 µg/day

Pregnancy = 220 µg/day

Lactation = 290 µg/day

Tolerable upper intake level during pregnancy and lactation, 14–18 years = 900 µg/day

Tolerable upper intake level during pregnancy and lactation, 19+ years = 900 µg/day

Source: Institute of Medicine, *Food and Nutrition Board, Dietary Reference Intakes for Vitamin A, Vitamin K, Arsenic, Boron, Chromium, Copper, Iodine, Iron, Manganese, Molybdenum, Nickel, Silicon, Vanadium, and Zinc*, The National Academies Press, Washington, DC, copyright © 2001. [260]

for non-pregnant adults (150 µg/day). Pregnant and lactating women would need to consume approximately 6–15 g per day of iodized salt to receive the recommended 250 µg iodine. However, the WHO also recommends a salt intake of <5 g/day to reduce the risk of cardiovascular diseases—this may be insufficient during pregnancy in terms of iodine intake.

The Endocrine Society recommends an intake of 150 µg/day for women of childbearing age, with an increase to 250 µg/day as soon as possible before or during pregnancy. This level of intake should be maintained through breastfeeding—breast milk should provide 100 µg/day to the infant. The Society's view is that iodine intake during pregnancy and breastfeeding should not exceed twice the daily recommended nutrient intake for iodine, that is, 500 µg iodine per day [868]. The Endocrine Society recommends iodine supplementation beginning prior to conception if possible, and continuing through pregnancy and lactation. Once-daily prenatal vitamins should contain 150–200 µg iodine in the form of potassium iodide or iodate, the content of which is verified to ensure that all pregnant women taking prenatal vitamins are protected from iodine deficiency. The American Thyroid Association supports the recommendation of 250 µg/day for pregnant and lactating women [869]. To meet this daily intake requirement, supplements containing 150 µg iodine are recommended. Prenatal multivitamins should include iodine (in the form of potassium iodide—at least 197 µg), which will ensure that these vitamins contain 150 µg of supplemental daily iodine (potassium iodide contains ~76% iodine) [870]. However only about half of the prenatal vitamins available in the US contain iodine [871].

The WHO recommendation for infants is 15 µg/kg/day for those born full term, and 30 µg/kg/day for preterm infants. Based on the assumption of an average body weight of 6 kg for a child of 6 months, 15 µg/kg/day corresponds approximately to an iodine intake and requirement of 90 µg/day. The iodine requirement of preterm infants is twice that of term infants because of a much lower retention of iodine by preterm infants [231]. The WHO, UNICEF, and the International Council for the Control of Iodine Deficiency Disorders advise an increase in the iodine content of infant formulas to 100 µg/L from the former recommendation of 50 µg/L for term infants, and to 200 µg/L for preterm infants.

## Our recommendations for iodine intake during pregnancy and lactation

Throughout gestation, the fetus is dependent on the maternal supply of iodine, and a lack of iodine in pregnancy is the most common cause of preventable brain damage in infants. Pregnant and breastfeeding women therefore need to increase their dietary iodine intake (from 150 µg/day before conception to 250 µg/day in early pregnancy and throughout lactation) because of the increased requirements during pregnancy and breastfeeding. We recommend that women have an adequate iodine intake of 150 µg/day before conception to avoid triggering thyroid hypertrophy during pregnancy. If pre-pregnancy iodine intake or stores are suboptimal, iodine supply should be increased as soon as possible during pregnancy, continuing through gestation and breastfeeding. The goal is to restore and maintain balanced iodine status.

It is likely that the use of iodized salt will still not meet the needs of most pregnant women, if they follow advice on sodium reduction. We therefore recommend that pregnant women take a daily multivitamin that contains 150 µg of iodine, unless they regularly consume concentrated food sources of iodine. Because of the narrow therapeutic window for iodine, care should be taken when ingesting iodine from seaweed or kelp supplements during pregnancy, to avoid excess iodine intake. The risk of iodine deficiency needs to be assessed locally and monitored over time, because of regional differences in iodine intake.

# Chapter 20

# Iron in pregnancy and breastfeeding

## Iron functions

Most iron in the body is present as haemoglobin in red blood cells, where it serves as a carrier of oxygen from the lungs to tissues. Iron-containing enzymes in mitochondria, the cytochromes, play key roles in energy transfer during oxidative metabolism. Iron in myoglobin facilitates oxygen use and storage in muscle. Disruption of these functions because of lack of iron leads to anaemia and other serious adverse health consequences. Iron deficiency affects physical working capacity (especially endurance activities), brain function, and behaviour. Conversely, excess iron accumulation produces reactive oxygen species that can cause multiple organ dysfunction [71, 872]. Because of the negative impact of both high and low iron levels, the systemic availability of iron is tightly regulated [873].

## Iron homeostasis

Iron is reversibly stored in ferritin complexes in the liver, and to a lesser extent in insoluble complexes with phosphate and hydroxide (haemosiderin). Absorption of iron in the intestine, and transfer into the circulation, is mediated by the export protein ferroportin. Hepcidin, a peptide produced in the liver, binds ferroportin and down-regulates its function by targeting ferroportin for degradation [874]. Overproduction of hepcidin decreases iron absorption and results in iron deficiency, whereas underproduction results in increased iron absorption and iron overload. Hepcidin is thus considered to be the main hormone regulating iron metabolism, and mutations in genes encoding hepcidin or its regulators are responsible for the iron-overload disorder hereditary haemochromatosis [875].

Under normal circumstances, extracellular iron is sequestered and maintained in a redox-inert state by the protein transferrin, which transports iron between body compartments when it is needed. As such, plasma transferrin is the key physiological source of iron. The soluble transferrin receptor (sTfR) mediates cellular uptake of iron by binding transferrin for internalization in endosomes, where iron is released and sTfR is recirculated. Unlike other metals, iron is not eliminated through the kidneys or liver; rather, it is lost through bleeding and exfoliation of skin and mucosal cells.

## Indicators of iron status and deficiency

Measurement of sTfR in serum by various immunoassay methods provides an indication of bone marrow iron stores and is useful in the clinical diagnosis of iron-deficiency anaemia [876]. Elevated serum sTfR ($\geq$2.0 mg/L) is indicative of iron-deficient erythropoiesis. The fractional saturation of transferrin by iron is often used as a measure of functional iron status, representative of the iron-binding capacity of serum [877]. Serum ferritin levels, on the other hand, are indicative of the status of iron stores, which become exhausted before serum iron levels are affected. Serum ferritin is therefore a more sensitive index of early iron deficiency than assays based on transferrin [878]. Measurement of hepcidin level is being considered as an additional marker of iron status [879]. The diagnosis of anaemia is generally based on haemoglobin levels or haematocrit [880], although the sensitivity and specificity of these measurements are low [881].

A serum ferritin level of <12 μg/L is indicative of depleted iron stores, and when transferrin saturation is <16 per cent in the presence of depleted stores, the individual is considered to be iron deficient. Pregnant women are considered anaemic if their haemoglobin concentration (at sea level) is lower than 110 g/L. Iron deficiency as the cause of the anaemia is confirmed by low ferritin levels, because anaemia can also be caused by deficiencies in folate, vitamin B$_{12}$, or vitamin A [882]. The severity of iron deficiency can thus be separated into three stages: (1) depletion of iron stores (serum ferritin <12 μg/L); (2) iron deficiency without anaemia (serum ferritin <12 μg/L, transferrin saturation <16%); and (3) iron-deficiency anaemia (serum ferritin <12 μg/L, transferrin saturation <16%, and haemoglobin <110 g/L).

## Iron in pregnancy

Iron requirements increase approximately 2.5-fold by the end of pregnancy. This is the largest relative increase in nutrient requirements for pregnant women. During pregnancy there is a rise in plasma volume, red blood cell mass, and haemoglobin mass, resulting from an increased need for oxygen transport. This requires an increased iron intake of ~450 mg over the course of pregnancy (for a 55 kg woman). In addition, the growing fetus requires ~270–300 mg, and more is required for the placenta and to compensate for maternal blood losses at birth. Thus the total additional requirement during gestation is ~1,000–1,240 mg [883–885], equating to an additional 9–12 mg of iron per day above pre-pregnancy needs in the third trimester, when the majority of the iron stores in the fetus are accumulated. Even with this additional iron intake, women need to enter pregnancy with iron stores of approximately 500 mg to be able to fully meet the demands of pregnancy.

Homeostatic regulatory mechanisms operate during pregnancy to partially protect the fetus from deficiency, such that maternal and neonatal stores are correlated only if maternal iron status is very low [886]. Maternal iron absorption decreases in the first trimester, when needs are lower because of the respite from menstrual losses, but absorption increases during the second trimester and continues to rise until the end of term. Maternal iron absorption remains elevated for the first few months after delivery, to restore body iron levels [883].

Despite these regulatory mechanisms, the prevalence of iron deficiency and iron-deficiency anaemia is very high among pregnant women. The WHO estimates that 42 per cent of pregnant women worldwide are anaemic, the majority from iron deficiency [887]. The prevalence is highest in Africa, where it is estimated that 57 per cent of pregnant women have iron-deficiency anaemia. Chronic parasitic worm infections, common in South East Asia, contribute to iron-deficiency anaemia [888]. Iron deficiency and anaemia in pregnancy is still common in the US, particularly in low-income and minority groups [889].

## Iron deficiency in pregnancy and infancy

Most maternal iron deficiency is caused by inadequate intake, poor iron absorption, or blood loss. When maternal iron status is suboptimal, fetal iron needs are also compromised [890]. Other conditions can influence fetal iron status, such as maternal hypertension or cigarette smoking, both of which restrict placental nutrient flow and can result in fetal iron deficiency. Vasculopathy associated with gestational diabetes impairs iron acquisition by the fetus [891]. Low pre-conception iron stores, and iron-deficiency anaemia in pregnancy, are associated with an increased risk of premature birth, low birthweight, and infant and child mortality, as well as impaired neurobehavioural development.

### The effects of iron deficiency on gestational length and birthweight

Low maternal haemoglobin correlates with risk of premature birth and low birthweight. This may be due to maternal and fetal hypoxic stress associated with anaemia [892]. Pregnant women with low haemoglobin levels were found to have double the risk of premature delivery and low birthweight [893, 894].

Preterm infants themselves have low iron stores, as most iron is transferred in late pregnancy. In addition, low birthweight infants have insufficient iron stores to meet requirements for rapid catch-up growth. Maternal anaemia is also associated with increased placental weight and volume; [895] the combination of low birthweight and high placental weight are risk factors for high blood pressure in adult life [896]. A recent study of dietary iron intakes in pregnant British women found a positive correlation between intake of non-haem iron and infant birthweight [897].

## The effects of iron deficiency on neurobehavioural development

There are many iron-dependent enzymes with critical functions in the CNS, including those involved in dopamine neurotransmission, which regulates motion, cognition, emotion, and hormone release [898]. Iron is supplied to the brain during an early phase of brain development, so early deficiency may lead to irreversible damage [899]. Animal studies have shown abnormal development of brain structures and altered brain myelination resulting from lack of iron in utero [900, 901]. In humans, iron deficiency in infancy is associated with poor cognitive function [902] and deficits in social–emotional behaviour [903]. Iron deficiency in early infancy has been shown to have long-term effects on auditory and visual functions that are not fully corrected by iron repletion [904]. The normal development of sleep patterns has also been shown to be disrupted in infant with iron-deficiency anaemia, with long-lasting neuro-functional effects [905].

## Other effects of iron deficiency

Iron deficiency impairs thyroid metabolism and blunts the efficacy of iodine prophylaxis, which is important in pregnancy. Maternal plasma iodine declines in pregnancy and the postpartum period as it is transferred to the growing fetus via the placenta and is secreted in breast milk (see chapter 19). Further impairment of thyroid function resulting from iron deficiency is therefore of significant concern during pregnancy and breastfeeding, and iron supplementation may be warranted in women with low iodine status. Iron supplementation has been shown to improve the efficacy of iodized oil supplementation in goitrous children with iron-deficiency anaemia [906].

## Groups at high risk of iron deficiency

Low body iron stores are more prevalent in pregnant adolescents than in adult pregnant women [907]. Women carrying multiple fetuses generally have lower iron stores than do those with singleton pregnancies, because of the increase fetal demand [908, 909]. A short interpartum period and high parity also increase the likelihood of low maternal iron stores. Higher rates of iron deficiency have been noted in overweight adults [910, 911], adding to the risks that overweight and obesity carry for pregnant women. Women with gestational diabetes or hypertension convey an increased risk of iron deficiency to their babies, because of poor nutrient transfer [891].

## Infant iron requirements

Breast milk contains little iron, but the full-term newborn infant has iron stores of ~250–300 mg, which is sufficient for the first 4–6 months of life. Through the remainder of the first year, infants have very high iron requirements relative to body size (0.7–0.9 mg/day) [370]. From ~6 months, breastfed infants require an additional source of iron in their diets, such as lean red meat or iron-fortified infant cereal (30g cereal provides a daily requirement). Foods rich in vitamin C (fruits) enhance iron absorption from cereal. Late introduction of complementary foods was found to be the most significant risk factor for iron-deficiency anaemia in children 1–2 years of age in a study in Pakistan [912]. Iron absorption is significantly higher from human milk than from cow's milk, as casein binds iron and severely limits its absorption [260].

## Iron supplementation during pregnancy

### Iron supplementation in pre-pregnancy

Because of the importance of adequate pre-pregnancy iron stores, recent WHO guidelines [887] recommend intermittent supplementation (once per week) with both iron (60 mg elemental) and folic acid (2.8 mg) as a public health intervention in all non-pregnant women of reproductive age living in regions with a high prevalence of anaemia ($\geq$ 20%, as in most developing countries). Intermittent dosing may improve iron absorption efficiency and minimize interference with absorption of other minerals (e.g. zinc), as well as minimizing the adverse effects of daily iron and improving compliance. These recommendations are based on a systematic review of 21 randomized controlled trials in Latin America, Asia, Africa, and Europe involving over 10,200 menstruating women who received weekly iron supplementation (alone or in combination with folic acid or other micronutrients) or placebo. Supplemented women had higher haemoglobin and ferritin concentrations and were less likely to develop anaemia than non-supplemented women [913].

Iron deficiency is exacerbated in malaria-endemic areas, as malaria causes iron to be shifted from haemoglobin to storage forms, resulting in anaemia. However, iron deficiency may also be protective against infection, by limiting critical nutrients to the infectious agent. Iron deficiency associated with malaria is due to iron delocalization rather than an overt lack of iron, so supplementation may not be helpful [914]. In malaria-endemic areas, supplementation with iron needs to be administered in conjunction with appropriate malaria prevention, diagnosis, and treatment measures.

## Iron supplementation during pregnancy

Daily or weekly iron supplementation during pregnancy decreases the prevalence of maternal anaemia at term [915]. Meta-analyses of multiple trials could not detect any significant effect on other adverse outcomes including low birthweight, delayed development, preterm birth, infection, or postpartum haemorrhage [915, 916], although some individual studies have reported a positive effect of iron supplementation on infant birthweight. The effect of iron supplementation appears to be dependent on the degree of baseline anaemia in the population. In well-nourished women who are not anaemic, iron supplementation does not appear to affect outcomes. Nonetheless, a modelling study sponsored by Health Canada concluded that a supplement of 16 mg/day throughout pregnancy would be effective and safe for pregnant women who are in good health. When added to the iron obtained from a mixed (non-vegetarian) diet, women taking such a supplement would have sufficient iron needed for pregnancy [917, 918]. However, some studies have found that supplementation with low-dose iron (18 mg/day) could not prevent depletion of maternal stores at term [919].

In women with multiple micronutrient deficiencies, supplementation with iron alone may adversely impact the absorption of other nutrients. The prenatal supplement UNIMAP (for UN Multiple Micronutrient Preparation), formulated by WHO and UNICEF for trials in developing countries, contains 14 additional micronutrients in addition to 30 mg iron (folic acid; vitamins A, C, D, E, $B_1$, $B_2$, $B_6$, $B_{12}$, and niacin; zinc; iodine; selenium; and copper) [920]. Additional micronutrients have not been found to have a significant impact on the prevalence of anaemia, but a meta-analysis of 13 trials in developing countries found that multi-micronutrient supplementation reduced the risk of low birthweight compared with iron plus folic acid supplementation [921]. Long-term follow-up of controlled iron intervention trials in Nepal reported a 31 per cent decrease in mortality in the first 7 years of life in children born to supplemented mothers [922].

## Iron supplementation in preterm infants

Because preterm infants miss the critical period in late pregnancy when the bulk of fetal iron is supplied, supplementation is generally recommended. Iron supplementation of preterm infants improves haemoglobin levels and iron stores and lowers the risk of developing iron deficiency anaemia. However, supplementation does not have clear long-term benefits on neurodevelopmental outcomes in preterm infants [923]. There appears to be no benefit in exceeding the 'standard' dose to infants (2–3 mg/kg/day) for those born preterm. Supplementation of low birthweight infants from 6 weeks to 6 months of age did not affect cognitive functions at 3.5 years but did reduce behavioural problems [924].

## Iron sources and metabolism

Iron is present in the diet in two forms—haem and non-haem iron. Haem iron is a component of haemoglobin and myoglobin, and its main dietary sources are meat, poultry, and fish. Non-haem iron is obtained from cereals, pulses, legumes, fruits, and vegetables. The iron content of vegetables, fruits, breads, and pastas ranges from 0.1–1.4 mg/serving. Some fortified breakfast cereals contain up to 24 mg iron per cup. The haem iron content of meat is between 1.5 and 3 mg/serving, with pork, fish, and chicken ranging between 0.5 and 2 mg haem iron per serving. Haem iron is degraded to non-haem iron if food is cooked at high temperatures for long periods of time [260].

Although non-haem iron makes up a greater portion of iron content in most diets, it is not absorbed as efficiently as haem iron, and its absorption is inhibited by phytates present in some of the same foods. Iron absorption is also inhibited by calcium, and polyphenols from tea and coffee. However, diet modification can improve the absorption of non-haem iron. When consumed with foods containing phytates or calcium, vitamin C (ascorbic acid) improves iron absorption by releasing iron that is bound to these inhibitors. For example, a glass of orange juice can help minimize the effect of phytate in breakfast cereal and calcium in milk. Meat, fish, and poultry can also improve non-haem absorption. Even modest amounts of these foods can improve the absorption of non-haem iron in a meal [71, 925].

The recommended iron intake for pregnant women (recommended dietary allowance (RDA) 27 mg/day; see 'Agency guidelines for iron intake') is difficult to achieve even with the most optimal diets. Typical Western diets provide approximately 5–7 mg iron per 1,000 kilocalories; consuming 2,500 kcal/day would provide 12.5–17.5 mg iron/day. Analyses of intakes of middle- and upper-income pregnant women in the US found that 90 per cent had intakes below the estimated average requirement (EAR) of 22 mg/day, which is a level that is deemed to be satisfactory for around 50 per cent of the population [369, 926]. An even higher percentage would fail to meet the RDA, which was exceeded in one study only by women who regularly consumed high iron-fortified breakfast cereals [369].

In order to meet iron requirements for the latter half of pregnancy, iron usually needs to be mobilized from iron stores, or absorbed from supplemental iron. Absorption of iron is significantly lower with vegetarian diets because of a lack of meat and fish that provide haem iron and enhance non-haem iron absorption [927]. It is estimated that 10 per cent of iron is absorbed from a lacto–ovo–vegetarian diet, compared with 18 per cent from Western diet, so the iron requirement is 1.8 times higher for vegetarians [260].

## Risks of excess iron

Iron supplementation is associated with adverse effects including heartburn, constipation, diarrhoea, nausea, and vomiting [928]. In various clinical studies, iron supplements of 50–60 mg/day resulted in moderate to severe gastrointestinal adverse effects in a substantial proportion of participants [929, 930]. Lower dose supplements had fewer side effects [930]. Data from studies in Canada suggested that avoidance or discontinuation of iron-containing prenatal multivitamins (and switching to folic acid + multivitamins without iron) improved symptoms of nausea and vomiting in pregnancy [931] and that adherence to and tolerability of prenatal vitamins for women with pre-existing gastrointestinal conditions was better using small tablets with low-dose iron [932]. Some of the negative gastrointestinal effects of iron supplementation may be due to increased intestinal permeability. [933]

High levels of iron in blood may have harmful effects on pregnant women. Iron overload leads to metabolic alterations that contribute to insulin resistance and increased risk of type 2 diabetes [934]. According to a recent prospective study in a cohort of 3,158 pregnant women in the US and Sweden, dietary intake of high levels of haem iron (but not total iron or non-haem iron) prior to conception and in early pregnancy were associated with an increased risk of gestational diabetes [935]. However, daily iron supplementation (60 mg/day of non-haem iron) during pregnancy was not found to affect the prevalence of gestational diabetes in a cohort of 1,164 women in China [936].

Haem iron intake was positively associated with development of type 2 diabetes in the Nurses' Health Study, which followed over 85,000 healthy women for 20 years. Women who regularly consumed >2.25 mg/day of haem iron had a significantly higher risk of developing diabetes than did women who consumed <0.75 mg/day [937]. Iron supplementation also increases the risk of zinc and copper deficiency, by competing for absorption of these minerals.

In non-anaemic women, iron supplementation can increase risk of maternal hypertension and of newborns being small for gestational age [938].

Excess free iron can generate reactive oxygen species that cause oxidative damage to tissues. Epidemiological studies support this link, showing a correlation between excess iron and increased risk of cardiovascular disease [939] and various cancers [940]. Preterm infants are particularly susceptible to the effects of reactive oxygen species because their antioxidant defence systems are immature. They are therefore at increased risk of oxidative injury from excess iron [941].

In infants who are iron replete, provision of iron-fortified formula may not be beneficial. In a small recent study, children who had high haemoglobin levels at 6 months of age and were fed iron-fortified infant formula (12.7 mg iron/L formula) had lower cognitive and visual–motor test scores at 10 years of age than children who had similar haemoglobin levels in infancy but did not receive additional iron. Those with lower baseline haemoglobin levels in the fortified group had higher scores. In other words, children who were lacking iron and received it did well, but those who received iron that they did not need did worse [942]. Although this small study needs to be replicated, the results suggest that haemoglobin levels should be tested before iron supplementation and that benefits of additional iron are dependent on baseline iron status.

Excess iron supplementation to newborns may also increase the risk of infection. Intramuscular iron dextran given prophylactically to infants in the 1970s in New Zealand (2 injections containing 50 mg each in the first week of life) resulted in a substantial increase in the incidence of *E. coli* septicaemia and meningitis until this practice of prophylactic treatment was stopped [943]. In extreme cases, excess iron can be fatal in children. Before the introduction of safety measures such as childproof caps and unit-dose blister packaging, iron supplements were the single most frequent cause of accidental ingestion fatalities in children in the US [944]. All iron-containing supplements in the US now carry the warning: 'Accidental overdose of iron-containing products is a leading cause of fatal poisoning in children under 6' [945].

## Agency guidelines for iron intake

Iron requirements typically exceed intake during infancy, and in adolescent girls and pregnant women. The US Institute of Medicine (IOM) RDAs for iron intake are shown in Box 20.1. Recommendations differ somewhat between agencies and countries, reflecting the typical status of women and children and the prevalence of iron deficiency within their target audiences.

## Box 20.1  US Institute of Medicine recommended dietary allowances for iron

Infants 0–6 months (adequate intake (AI)) = 0.27 mg/day
Infants 7–12 months (AI) = 11 mg/day
Children 1–3 years = 7 mg/day
Females 14–18 years = 15 mg/day
Females 19–50 years = 18 mg/day
Pregnancy = 27 mg/day
Lactation 14–18 years = 10 mg/day
Lactation 19+ years = 9 mg/day
Tolerable upper intake level (including pregnancy and lactation) = 45 mg/day

Source: Institute of Medicine, *Food and Nutrition Board, Dietary Reference Intakes for Vitamin A, Vitamin K, Arsenic, Boron, Chromium, Copper, Iodine, Iron, Manganese, Molybdenum, Nickel, Silicon, Vanadium, and Zinc,* The National Academies Press, Washington, DC, copyright © 2001. [260]

### Iron intake guidelines for pregnant women

The IOM advises pregnant women of all ages to consume 27 mg iron/day, an increase from pre-pregnancy of 15 mg/day for adolescents and 8 mg/day for adults [260]. If this intake is not achieved in the diet, iron is mobilized from maternal stores. In many women in developing countries iron stores are insufficient or do not exist. The WHO recommends that these women should be given 60 mg/day of supplemental iron (between meals) from 16 weeks gestation. Larger doses (~100 mg/day) are advised in cases of anaemia [946]. The IOM recommends supplementation for iron deficiency in pregnant women whose serum ferritin level is <12 µg/L [260].

In the US, the CDC has recommended screening for anaemia in all women of childbearing age, and low-dose iron supplementation for pregnant women [947]. The American Congress of Obstetricians and Gynecologists Practice Bulletin also recommends that all pregnant women take prenatal supplements containing iron, and advocates universal screening for anaemia, with additional iron supplementation to anaemic pregnant women [948]. The most recent publication of the Dietary Guidelines for Americans recommends that pregnant women consume dietary iron from haem sources (meat) in addition to taking an iron supplement [949]. The IOM considers a supplement of 30 mg iron/day in the second half of pregnancy to be appropriate for women consuming a diet with reasonable levels of bioavailable iron [883]. For women who consume a strictly vegetarian diet, the RDA of 27 mg iron/day (EAR 14.5 mg/day) applies even for non-pregnant women. Because of this higher requirement, the iron supplementation recommendation is even stronger for pregnant vegetarian women [260].

The UK guidelines differ from those in the US and Canada, in that routine supplementation of all pregnant women is not recommended [266, 738]. The guidelines indicate that pregnant women should screened for anaemia by full blood count in early pregnancy and at 28 weeks gestation and supplemented only following diagnosis of anaemia (defined as haemoglobin <110 g/L in the first trimester, <105 g/L in the second and third trimesters, and <100 g/L post-partum). All women should be given dietary advice to maximize iron intake and absorption [950].

## Iron intake guidelines for lactating women

For lactation, the requirement drops 10 mg/day for mothers 18 years and younger, and 9 mg/day for those over 19 years. The same advice is given by the Australian National Health and Medical Research Council (<http://www.nrv.gov.au/nutrients/iron.htm>). The lower postpartum recommendation reflects the fact that secretion of iron into breast milk is not affected by maternal iron intake, unless maternal stores during pregnancy are very low. Supplementation is not generally recommended.

## Iron intake guidelines for infants

The IOM has set an adequate intake level of 0.27 mg/day of iron for infants up to 6 months of age, an amount that is obtainable from breast milk and is sufficient for full-term infants born with replete iron stores. No supplementation is required for such breastfeeding infants in the first 6 months, although iron-fortified formula is recommended for those receiving formula [260]. However, after 6 months, sufficient intake of iron-rich foods (meat products or iron-fortified foods) should be ensured.

The American Academy of Pediatrics (AAP) recommends supplementation of breastfed infants from 4 months of age with 1 mg/kg oral iron supplement until iron-rich complementary foods are introduced [951]. The RDA for infants 7–12 months of age is 11 mg/day (EAR 6.9 mg/day). This is much higher (in mg/kg bodyweight terms) than other stages; after 1 year the iron requirement drops to an RDA of 7 mg/day (EAR of 3 mg/day) for children up to 3 years of age. The European Community Committee on Food guidelines state that full-term infants require an intake of 6 mg iron/day from between 4 and 6 months, up to 12 months, which equates to 0.7–0.9 mg iron/day based on an estimated bioavailability of 15 per cent [370]. More recent recommendations supported by the EURRECA (EURopean micronutrient RECommendations Aligned) network is that infants aged 6–12 months require 0.9–1.3 mg/kg body weight per day, equivalent to 7.8–11 mg/day dietary iron intake [952].

For preterm neonates, the AAP recommends supplementation with 2 mg/kg/day of enteral iron from 1 month of age, either as an iron mixture or in the form of iron-fortified formula [951]. Infant formula in Europe is usually fortified with 4–7 mg iron/L; in the US it is 12–13 mg/L. However, agencies have called for the development of a global standard [953].

## Tolerable upper intake levels for iron

It is important to avoid excess iron intake. The IOM tolerable upper intake level for pregnancy is 45 mg of iron/day, which is the same as for non-pregnant women [260]. For infants and children to 13 years of age, the tolerable upper intake level is 40 mg/day. This upper limit may not be protective against iron overload in individuals with hereditary haemochromatosis, chronic alcoholism, alcoholic cirrhosis, other liver diseases, or iron-loading abnormalities (e.g. thalassaemias), in whom a lower intake is required.

# Our recommendations for iron intake during pregnancy and lactation

Iron deficiency is the most common nutritional deficiency worldwide, and its prevalence is particularly high among pregnant women. Deficiency is more common in populations where malaria is endemic. Maternal iron deficiency may result in cognitive and motor deficits in the infant that may be irreversible. Prevention of deficiency is therefore critical.

Women should be advised to build or maintain sufficient iron stores prior to conception if possible. There is no international consensus on iron prophylaxis for pregnant women. During pregnancy, iron needs increase from an EAR of 8.1 mg/day for non-pregnant women to 22 mg/day, and the RDA increases from 15–18 mg/day to 27 mg/day. Pregnant women cannot normally obtain adequate iron from diet alone to meet the very high demands of the second half of pregnancy; therefore, supplementation should be considered, particularly if dietary intake of meat is low. Vegetarian women should be offered iron supplements at a recommended dosage of 30 mg/day.

In vulnerable populations, iron supplementation should be started in early pregnancy or pre-conceptionally in order to prevent preterm birth and low birthweight. Infants born to well-nourished mothers do not require iron supplementation in the first 4–6 months of life. Their first introduced complementary foods should be iron rich, for example, lean meat, lean poultry, fish, or iron-fortified cereals.

# Chapter 21

# Magnesium in pregnancy and breastfeeding

## Magnesium functions

Approximately 50–60 per cent of magnesium in the body is present in bone; most of the rest is intracellular, with less than 1 per cent present in extracellular fluid [954]. All enzymes utilizing ATP require magnesium for substrate formation, and thus magnesium is critical to the activity of over 300 enzymes, including those involved in energy metabolism and neuromuscular signalling [955]. Magnesium acts as an allosteric activator for enzymes such as phospholipase C and adenylate cyclase, and of Na/K-ATPase, which regulates sodium and potassium transport in and out of cells. Magnesium also regulates ion channels for calcium transport, and, in addition to regulating calcium channel activity, magnesium is involved in several steps of calcium homeostasis. It is necessary for the calcium-triggered release of parathyroid hormone and for the action of parathyroid hormone on bone, kidney, and gut.

Magnesium deficiency is often accompanied by calcium deficiency, because impaired parathyroid hormone secretion caused by a lack of magnesium perpetuates low serum calcium levels. The expected rise in serum 1,25-dihydroxyvitamin D (the active form of vitamin D) that follows dietary calcium deprivation is attenuated under magnesium-deficient conditions, resulting in impaired intestinal calcium absorption. Individuals with hypocalcaemia and magnesium deficiency are resistant to pharmacological doses of vitamin D, and the hypocalcaemia cannot be corrected by administration of calcium—only supplementation with magnesium restores serum calcium to normal and improves calcium utilization [956].

Magnesium also affects potassium metabolism; the kidney cannot conserve potassium adequately if magnesium concentrations are low. Under magnesium-deficient conditions, potassium levels cannot be restored by supplementation with potassium alone—magnesium therapy is required [955]. Various conditions including diabetes, alcoholism, and malabsorption syndromes (e.g. Crohn's disease and coeliac disease) cause magnesium to be lost from the body.

## Indicators of magnesium status

Hypomagnesaemia is generally defined as serum magnesium <0.7 mmol/L (<1.7 mg/dL or <1.4 mEq/L). However, measurements of serum magnesium may not adequately reflect total physiological magnesium stores because <1 per cent of total body magnesium is represented in serum. There is no generally accepted test for magnesium status [957].

## Magnesium deficiency

Magnesium depletion results in neuromuscular hyper-excitability, and the first signs of deficiency are usually neuromuscular and neuropsychiatric disturbances. Other early signs of magnesium deficiency include loss of appetite, nausea, vomiting, fatigue, and weakness. This can be followed by numbness, tingling, spontaneous muscle contractions, and cramps (the latter are common in pregnancy).

Magnesium is a cofactor for enzymes involved in energy and carbohydrate metabolism, and low magnesium is associated with an increased likelihood of developing metabolic syndrome [958]. In particular, dyslipidaemia is strongly related to low serum magnesium levels. Supplemental magnesium may have beneficial effects in overweight individuals. Magnesium supplementation has been shown in some studies to improve dyslipidaemia and lower fasting glucose concentrations in overweight individuals and reduce markers of systemic and hepatic inflammation [959, 960].

Low magnesium levels are common in people with type 2 diabetes and can worsen insulin resistance. In the Nurses' Health Study/Health Professionals' Follow-up Study involving >85,000 women and >42,000 men, the risk of developing type 2 diabetes was higher in people with low dietary magnesium intake [961]. Particularly in overweight women, higher magnesium was associated with lower risk of type 2 diabetes [962]. The Atherosclerosis Risk in Communities Study, which involved >12,000 middle-aged participants, observed an inverse association between diabetes incidence and magnesium serum levels in Caucasian subjects but not subjects of African descent [963]. Magnesium supplementation (300 mg/day) has been shown to improve blood-glucose control in individuals with type 2 diabetes [964].

Magnesium status has an influence on cardiac function, and depletion is associated with various cardiac complications including arrhythmias, hypertension, cardiac ischaemia, and atherosclerosis. Among >7,700 women in the Atherosclerosis Risk in Communities Study, those who developed coronary heart disease had significantly lower serum magnesium levels than those who remained free of the disease, and there was a negative association between coronary risk factors and both serum magnesium and dietary magnesium intake [965]. Low dietary intake of magnesium (<200 mg/day) was associated with an increased incidence of hypertension in both men [966] and women [967] in large prospective nutritional survey studies.

Treatment with magnesium lowered blood pressure in women with mild to moderate hypertension [968]. Oral magnesium supplements of ~700 mg/day also improved exercise tolerance in small studies [969, 970]. Because of these associations, dietary changes are recommended to increase magnesium intake in individuals with or at risk for cardiovascular problems. A diet high in fruits and vegetables, which increased daily magnesium intakes from an average of 176 mg to 423 mg, significantly lowered blood pressure in non-hypertensive adults [971].

Magnesium depletion has been shown to cause a reduction in bone mass in animal models and is considered a risk factor for osteoporosis [972]. Observational data suggests a link between low magnesium intake [973] or low serum level [974] and osteoporosis [975]. Thus, supplementation may be helpful in preventing fractures.

## Magnesium in pregnancy

During pregnancy, magnesium is actively transferred from mother to fetus at an average rate of 4.5 mg/day, creating a magnesium gradient across the placenta, with fetal plasma levels higher than maternal levels. However, the gradient is not sufficient to protect the fetus from maternal deficiency; in deficiency states magnesium is retained by the mother at the expense of the fetus [976]. In normal pregnancies, there is a physiological decrease in magnesium levels in the myometrium over the course of gestation. This may play a role in the initiation of uterine contractions and labour at full term [977]. Chronic or excessive vomiting that occurs with severe morning sickness in pregnancy can result in magnesium depletion, and magnesium deficiency itself can exacerbate nausea and vomiting [978]. Replenishment of magnesium is recommended in such cases.

### The effects of magnesium on gestational diabetes and metabolic disturbances

Magnesium status is compromised in women with gestational diabetes [979], with decreased serum magnesium and increased urinary magnesium losses reported [980]. The effect of magnesium supplementation on the risk or severity of gestational diabetes has not been well studied, but the known effects of magnesium status on insulin resistance in non-pregnant individuals suggests that maintaining an adequate magnesium level during pregnancy would be helpful in women at risk, especially overweight and obese women. The negative impact of obesity on pregnancy outcomes suggests magnesium supplementation may help to reduce obesity-associated maternal and fetal pregnancy complications. A clinical trial is currently underway to test this (ClinicalTrials.gov Identifier NCT01510665).

## The effects of magnesium on pregnancy-induced hypertension and pre-eclampsia

In non-pregnant women, higher dietary magnesium intakes have been shown to be associated with a lower risk of developing hypertension [981]. No published studies have assessed dietary magnesium in pregnancy and the risk of pregnancy-induced hypertension (PIH), but a small recent study reported significantly lower serum magnesium levels in women who developed PIH than in pregnant women without hypertension [982]. A small study in China suggested that supplementation with low-dose magnesium gluconate (3 g/day (~165 mg/day elemental magnesium)) during pregnancy may help prevent PIH in high-risk women [983], but a larger study (n = 400) using 365 mg/day elemental magnesium (as magnesium aspartate HCl) found no difference in blood pressure between the supplemented and placebo groups of young, normotensive, primigravid women [984]. A meta-analysis that included both these studies concluded that there was not enough evidence to recommend oral magnesium supplementation during pregnancy for the purpose of lowering blood pressure [985].

Magnesium is, however, used pharmacologically during pregnancy. Magnesium sulphate infusion is considered the treatment of choice for the acute management of pre-eclampsia in the US. In a trial of >10,000 participants, magnesium sulphate treatment of women with pre-eclampsia halved the risk of developing eclampsia and prevented eclamptic convulsions [986].

## The effects of magnesium on preterm birth

Low serum magnesium correlated with a higher incidence of preterm birth and was associated with lower socio-economic class (and therefore probably poor diet) in a case–control study in India [987]. One study of magnesium supplementation (15 mmol/day (=369 mg/day)) provided to women prior to 16 weeks gestation reported a lower risk of preterm labour and delivery in women who received magnesium, compared with a placebo control group [988]. However, a review of trials of magnesium supplementation therapy after an episode of threatened preterm labour to prevent further preterm contractions did not find enough evidence to support the use of maintenance magnesium supplementation for this indication [989].

## The effects of magnesium on low birthweight

An epidemiological study in Taiwan found evidence of a relationship between high levels of magnesium in drinking water and a reduced risk of very low birthweight (<1,500 g) in newborns [990]. Most other evidence suggesting an effect of magnesium on birthweight comes from studies on magnesium in reducing preterm births; cohorts with lower incidence of preterm birth would naturally have higher mean birthweight. A meta-analysis of trials of oral magnesium supplementation during pregnancy found that treatment before the 25th week of gestation reduced the number of low-birthweight and small-for-gestational-age infants, but because the methodology of most studies was poor, supplementation could not be recommended [985]. There is no unequivocal evidence at this time that magnesium has a direct effect on intrauterine growth restriction.

## The effects of magnesium on neuroprotection in the fetus

Magnesium has neuroprotective effects via actions of the $N$-methyl-D-aspartate receptor (also known as the NMDA receptor). Neurodevelopmental problems including cerebral palsy are associated with preterm birth (<34 weeks) and very low birthweight (<1,500 g) as major obstetric risk factors [991]. Magnesium sulphate is administered pharmacologically to women in the US and other countries during threatened preterm labour to lower the risk of fetal neurological defects and improve neurodevelopment in preterm neonates. Multiple studies have assessed the efficacy and safety of magnesium sulphate administered antenatally to women at risk of preterm birth, and significant beneficial neuroprotective effects for preterm infants have been demonstrated [992].

Fetal hypoxic–ischaemic encephalopathy is a common obstetric problem in underdeveloped regions. A study of fetal outcomes of indigent Black women in South Africa found that daily supplementation with 256 mg elemental magnesium during pregnancy reduced the number of stillbirths compared with placebo but did not significantly reduce the incidence of hypoxic–ischaemic encephalopathy in this low socio-economic group, who are known to consume a diet deficient in magnesium. However, across the entire study cohort, women with red blood cell magnesium levels below the median (1.71 mmol/L) had a sevenfold increased risk of having a baby with hypoxic–ischaemic encephalopathy than those whose levels were above the median (red blood cell magnesium is considered a better reflection of total body magnesium than serum levels). Supplemental magnesium appeared to benefit the fetus in labour, reducing fetal distress and depressed respiration during birth, possibly by reducing or preventing the impaired uterine activity caused by low maternal magnesium [993].

## The effects of magnesium on skeletal development

There are no data directly linking magnesium deficiency to fetal skeletal defects or maternal bone resorption in pregnancy, although its involvement in calcium metabolism suggests that deficiency could lead to adverse bone outcomes during fetal development. A longitudinal study into the effect of the maternal diet on bone mineral density (BMD) in children found a positive association between maternal magnesium intake during pregnancy and total body BMD in the offspring at 9 years of age [994]. Similarly, a smaller longitudinal cohort study showed femoral neck BMD at 8 years of age was related to the magnesium and phosphorus content of the maternal diet in the third trimester of pregnancy [995]. Maternal magnesium intake remained positively associated with BMD in offspring at 16 years of age [996], supporting the idea that in utero magnesium exposure contributes to long-term bone mineralization responses and influences peak bone mass.

## The effects of magnesium on muscle cramps

Nocturnal leg cramps are a common occurrence during the second half of pregnancy. An early study found that supplementation with 360 mg/day (15 mmol) magnesium lactate/magnesium citrate was effective in relieving muscle cramps in pregnant women [997], but a more recent study of the same supplementation regimen did not find a significant effect on cramp frequency or intensity [998]. Another study using magnesium bisglycinate chelate at 3 daily doses of 100 mg demonstrated a 50 per cent reduction in cramp frequency [999]. The frequency and occurrence of leg cramps was found to be lower in a group of pregnant women who habitually consumed a high magnesium, plant-based diet compared with a control group consuming a standard Western diet [1000], suggesting that dietary changes may be at least as effective as supplementation in reducing leg cramps in pregnancy.

## Magnesium supplementation in pregnancy

Overall, trials of oral magnesium supplementation during high-risk or normal pregnancies have not shown definitive benefit for various maternal and infant outcomes including neonatal mortality, neonatal morbidity (low birthweight, preterm birth, and related measures), maternal morbidity, blood pressure, PIH, pre-eclampsia, and length of labour. A meta-analysis of seven magnesium supplementation trials concluded that there was not enough high-quality evidence to recommend the routine use of magnesium supplements during pregnancy [985]. Other observational data suggest that routine magnesium supplementation is not needed for populations of relatively good socio-economic status [1001].

## Magnesium in breast milk

Maternal serum magnesium does not change significantly during lactation, and excretion in breast milk also remains relatively constant. Despite this, magnesium concentrations in infant sera appear to increase with longer breastfeeding duration [1002]. No relationship has been found between intake of dietary magnesium supplements and the level of magnesium in breast milk. It is estimated that fully breastfed infants receive approximately 6.5 mg/kg/day of magnesium in early lactation [1003] and that the average concentration of magnesium in breast milk is approximately 31 mg/L [1004]. Mothers nursing multiple infants may require additional magnesium intake to account for the increased milk volume requirement [253]. Adolescent pregnancy is a risk factor for poor bone mineralization, and the magnesium content of breast milk from adolescent mothers is lower than that from adult mothers [1005].

## Sources of magnesium

Magnesium is present in the core of the chlorophyll molecule; thus, green vegetables such as spinach are good dietary sources. A half-cup serving of cooked spinach contains 78 mg of magnesium. Other good sources are whole grains (wheat bran), nuts, and legumes (beans and peas). On a weight basis, spices, nuts, cereals, and seafood are high in magnesium; however, on a calorie basis, green leafy vegetables have the highest amount. Coffee, tea, and cocoa are also magnesium rich, although coffee and tea are diuretic and therefore result in some magnesium loss.

Drinking water can also be a major source of magnesium, although the concentrations of magnesium in drinking water are highly variable. 'Hard' water is characterized by the presence of minerals and has a higher magnesium content than 'soft' water. Consumption of tap water containing magnesium can therefore significantly influence magnesium intake, contributing up to 40–100 mg/day [571], or up to 38 per cent of daily magnesium intake in hard-water communities [1006]. Regular consumption of magnesium-rich mineral water (110 mg/L) can also make a significant contribution to magnesium requirements [1007].

The calcium, phytate, and protein content of the diet can influence magnesium absorption. When magnesium intake is low, calcium supplementation may reduce magnesium absorption and retention. Low dietary protein intake (<30 g/day) also lowers magnesium absorption [1008, 1009], but protein intakes over 94 g/day may enhance magnesium excretion [1010]. Excess protein, calcium, phosphate, and phytate therefore increase the magnesium requirement, and the magnesium balance can be negative in pregnancy under diets that provide adequate amounts of these other nutrients [1011].

Refining and cooking foods diminishes their magnesium content. In particular, the refining of flour results in the loss of ~90 per cent of its natural magnesium content. Moreover, refined foods in general have the lowest magnesium content [571]. A diet that is high in green vegetables and whole, unprocessed grains, nuts, legumes, and seafood is beneficial from a standpoint of magnesium content and is recommended generally as an ideal pregnancy diet that has a positive impact on overall health. It should be noted, however, that predatory fish and seafood containing high levels of mercury or other toxins should be avoided (see chapter 30).

## Risks of excess magnesium

Magnesium intake from food does not pose a health risk. Pharmacological doses of magnesium supplements or high doses of magnesium-containing antacids and laxatives can cause diarrhoea and abdominal cramps. Single doses of elemental magnesium of 800–1,600 mg can produce a dose-limiting laxative effect. The kidney has a large capacity to excrete excess magnesium. However, people with kidney disease should not take magnesium supplements, as excretion of excess magnesium could be impaired [1012]. Hypermagnesaemia in the fetus can result from administration of magnesium sulphate to the mother for pre-eclampsia or threatened preterm labour. This can result in neuromuscular depression at birth and other possible adverse effects including anaphylaxis [976], although these effects are rare using current standard infusion protocols.

## Agency guidelines for magnesium intake

According to the US Institute of Medicine (IOM), the normal requirement for non-pregnant women is between 310 and 360 mg/day of magnesium, but requirements are elevated somewhat during periods of growth, including pregnancy. The IOM recommended dietary allowances (RDA) for pregnancy and lactation vary according to maternal age, as shown in Box 21.1.

The RDA represents an increase of 40 mg/day during pregnancy, returning to non-pregnancy requirements during lactation. The calculation is based on the assumption that women gain an average of 7.5 kg lean mass during pregnancy, and that the absorption efficiency of magnesium is ~40 per cent. This increase could be achieved through the consumption of green leafy vegetables, whole grains, and nuts. Throughout lactation, bone resorption and reduced urinary excretion compensate for the extra requirements for magnesium secretion in milk. However, women who are breastfeeding multiple infants will require additional intakes of magnesium-rich foods to account for their increased milk production requirement [71, 571].

## Box 21.1 US Institute of Medicine recommended dietary allowances for magnesium

Infants 0–12 months = not determined.
Children 1–3 years = 80 mg/day
Females 14–18 years = 360 mg/day
Females 19–30 years = 310 mg/day
Females 31+ years = 320 mg/day
Pregnancy 14–18 years = 400 mg/day
Lactation 14–18 years = 360 mg/day
Pregnancy 19–30 years = 350 mg/day
Lactation 19–30 years = 310 mg/day
Pregnancy 31+ years = 360 mg/day
Lactation 31+ years = 320 mg/day
Tolerable upper intake level = 350 mg/day supplemental magnesium

Source: Institute of Medicine, Food and Nutrition Board, *Dietary Reference Intakes for Calcium, Phosphorus, Magnesium, Vitamin D, and Fluoride*, Dietary Reference Intakes, The National Academies Press, Washington, DC, copyright © 1997. [571]

Because acute excessive intake of magnesium is possible from non-food sources, the IOM recommends a tolerable upper intake level of 350 mg/day of supplemental magnesium. Higher doses are prescribed for specific medical problems. There is no set upper level for magnesium intake from food [253, 571].

The UK National Institute for Clinical Excellence recommends against advising women to take magnesium supplements, with the aim of preventing hypertensive disorders during pregnancy [761]. The UK Royal College of Obstetricians and Gynaecologists (RCOG) recommends that pregnant women should not take supplemental magnesium unless advised to do so by their physicians following tests to identify possible deficiency. The American Pregnancy Association suggests that intake of supplemental magnesium in the form of antacids may be beneficial if taken in limited quantities, but should not be taken in high doses without the advice of a physician [1013].

Various clinical practice guidelines recommend administration of intravenous magnesium sulphate to women for fetal neuroprotection (reducing the risk of cerebral palsy) in situations of threatened preterm birth. (Australia [1014]; Canada [1015]; UK (RCOG) [1016]). The recommended adequate intake for infants up to 6 months of age is 30 mg/day, which can be acquired through breast milk in most cases. Infants 7–12 months of age require ~75 mg/day, some of which will need to come from solid food sources [71, 571].

## Our recommendations for magnesium intake during pregnancy and lactation

Current evidence does not support a requirement for specific magnesium supplementation for most pregnant women, although all women should strive to increase their consumption of magnesium-rich foods, such as green leafy vegetables, relative to high-fat and processed foods in the diet. Diets high in magnesium represent positive lifestyle modifications, particularly for individuals with hypertension, as they are often also high in dietary fibre and potassium. Consuming a magnesium-rich diet throughout pregnancy is recommended. Women who are overweight, have risk factors for hypertensive or metabolic disorders or malabsorption syndromes, or who are carrying multiple fetuses should pay particular attention to their diets and should be monitored for signs of magnesium deficiency.

# Chapter 22

# Potassium in pregnancy and breastfeeding

## Potassium functions

Potassium is an important electrolyte that is present in intracellular fluid at a concentration that is much higher than that outside cells. The ion concentration difference across the cell membrane generates a voltage gradient (membrane potential) that allows cells to transmit electrical signals important for muscle contraction, nerve impulse transmission, and cardiac function. The balance between intra- and extracellular potassium and sodium is maintained by the sodium–potassium pump Na/K-ATPase [1017].

Serum potassium less than 3.5 mmol/L is indicative of potassium deficiency (hypokalaemia), which is characterized by cardiac arrhythmias, blood pressure elevation, muscle weakness, and glucose intolerance. Blood pressure is closely associated with the sodium:potassium ratio, correlating inversely with potassium intake and directly with sodium intake [1018]. Glucose intolerance occurs in the presence of hypokalaemia because the capacity of the pancreas to secrete insulin is reduced. Thiazide diuretics used for the treatment of hypertension cause a reduction in serum potassium and have been associated with an increased risk of type 2 diabetes [1019]. Potassium bicarbonate acts as a buffer which neutralizes non-carbonic acids from the diet. When potassium is low, alkaline calcium salts are mobilized from bone matrix for acid neutralization, and bone demineralization occurs [1020].

Normal renal function protects against hyperkalaemia at high potassium intakes, but does not prevent deficiency at low intakes. High levels of potassium (hyperkalaemia) can also cause dangerous, even life-threatening arrhythmias. High serum potassium concentrations have been observed in people with sickle-cell anaemia, as deoxygenation of sickle cells induces potassium efflux, resulting in red blood cell dehydration. Potassium intake from supplements can cause gastrointestinal upset, although this is not observed with potassium intake from food [1017].

## Potassium in pregnancy

The fetus accumulates approximately 12 g (307 mmol) of potassium by the end of gestation. Very little information is available, however, about maternal potassium balance during pregnancy [1017]. A small study in Swedish women found that total body potassium decreased in pregnancy and was significantly lower at 6 months postpartum than in the pre-pregnant state [1021].

Conditions associated with pregnancy, such as severe vomiting or morning sickness, can cause potassium loss. Caffeine increases the renal excretion of potassium, and a high caffeine intake in pregnancy can cause a further reduction in serum potassium. Cases of hypokalaemia in pregnancy have been observed in women with heavy caffeine/cola consumption, resulting in extreme muscle fatigue [1022] and muscular paralysis [1023]. Hypokalaemia caused by excess caffeine and/or cola consumption can also manifest as myopathy [1024]. Similar hypokalaemic symptoms caused by eating clay (geophagia) during pregnancy have also been reported [1025].

Despite its role in cardiac function and blood pressure control, potassium intake has not been not associated with hypertensive disorders of pregnancy [1026]. There are no data available on the effect of potassium on bone mineralization changes during pregnancy and lactation. To date, there is insufficient evidence to suggest that the potassium requirement is increased during pregnancy, although a small increase in intake is needed for lactation. To maintain the normal potassium content of human milk (0.5 g/L (13 mmol/L)), an additional 0.4 g/day (10 mmol) is required, based on a milk output of 780 mL/day [1017].

## Potassium sources

Leafy green vegetables are good sources of potassium, as are root vegetables, beans and peas, fruits from vine-based plants (e.g. tomatoes, cucumbers, zucchini, eggplant, and pumpkin), and tree fruits. Dairy products, meats, and nuts have moderate potassium contents. Salt substitutes that are sometimes used in low-sodium diets contain between 440 and 2,800 mg potassium/teaspoon. High protein, low carbohydrate diets that are also low in fruit contain adequate potassium but result in mild metabolic acidosis. Long-term consumption of cola-based soft drinks or large amounts of coffee or other caffeinated beverages can result in hypokalaemia.

## Agency guidelines for potassium intake

The US Institute of Medicine recommends an adequate intake (AI) level for infants for the first 6 months of 0.4 g potassium/day (see Box 22.1), which

**Box 22.1 US Institute of Medicine recommended dietary allowances for potassium**

Infants 0–6 months (adequate intake (AI)) = 0.4 g/day

Infants 7–12 months (AI) = 0.7 g/day

Children 1–3 years = 3.0 g/day

Females 14+ years = 4.7 g/day

Pregnancy = 4.7 g/day

Lactation = 5.1 g/day

Source: Institute of Medicine, Food and Nutrition Board, *Dietary Reference Intakes for Water, Potassium, Sodium, Chloride, and Sulfate,* The National Academies Press, Washington, DC, copyright © 2005. [1017]

can be acquired from breast milk. Infants aged 7–12 months should consume 0.7 g/day, based on consumption of human milk and complementary foods [1017]. From the age of 14, the recommended AI level for both adolescents and adults is 4.7 g potassium/day [1017]. This is based on the protective effects of this potassium intake level on blood pressure, bone density, and risk of kidney stones. No increase in this requirement is advised for pregnant women, but lactating women need 5.1 g potassium/day.

## Our recommendations for potassium intake during pregnancy and lactation

Pregnant and lactating women should ensure adequate potassium in their diets by increasing their consumption of fruits and vegetables. Consumption of cola and caffeine should be minimized to reduce the risk of hypokalaemia. Reduction of cardiovascular risk factors and bone loss may be assisted by increasing potassium intake, and/or by dietary sodium reduction.

# Chapter 23

# Selenium in pregnancy and breastfeeding

## Selenium functions

Selenium is an essential trace mineral that is required in the diet in small amounts. It is a component of selenoproteins that act as antioxidant enzymes, preventing cell damage by neutralizing the deleterious effect of free radicals. Selenoproteins also regulate thyroid hormone metabolism [1027] and immune function [1028]. The main selenoprotein families include glutathione peroxidases, thioredoxin reductases, and iodothyronine deiodinases. The iodothyronine deiodinases are required for the conversion of thyroxine (also known as T4) to the biologically active thyroid hormone, triiodothyronine (also known as T3). Thyroid metabolism is thus sensitive to selenium in the diet, and selenium deficiency can exacerbate the effects of iodine deficiency [906].

Selenium deficiency is also associated with enhanced viral virulence. For example, Keshan disease myocarditis is a selenium deficiency disorder that occurs in regions where soil selenium, and therefore selenium intake from food, is very low (e.g. China). Keshan disease appears to involve activation of a normally quiescent virus via increased oxidative stress in the presence of low selenium [1029]. Vitamins A, E, and C can modulate selenium absorption. A combined deficiency of vitamin E and selenium leads to an increase in oxidative damage.

## Indicators of selenium status

Urinary selenium is used to assess selenium intake status, with a reference range of 15–50 µg/L. Daily excretion of <15 µg/L indicates insufficient selenium nutriture, and an output of >50 µg/L indicates excessive intake [1030]. Other frequently measured markers include plasma selenium, plasma selenoprotein P, and glutathione peroxidase, all of which are responsive to changes in selenium intake. However, all these markers exhibit some heterogeneity in responses to supplementation, and further research is required to optimize them as standard tests for selenium status [1031].

## Selenium and fertility

Several selenium-dependent proteins are important in male fertility. The selenoprotein glutathione peroxidase 4 is essential for sperm structure and function. In addition, the sperm mitochondrial capsule selenoprotein has both structural and enzymatic roles in sperm tail motility and integrity. A study in Glasgow (an area with low selenium intakes) found enhanced sperm motility in men receiving selenium supplements [1032]. A more recent randomized controlled trial in Iran found that supplementation of infertile men with 200 μg selenium and/or N-acetyl cysteine increased sperm count and sperm motility after 26 weeks of treatment [1033]. However, there is no indication of a link between selenium levels and fertility in females.

## Selenium in pregnancy

Selenium is important in pregnancy as an antioxidant, and low selenium status has been implicated in pregnancy complications that are associated with increased oxidative stress. During pregnancy, there is a decrease in maternal selenium concentrations in whole blood and plasma and in glutathione peroxidase activity in red blood cells, correlating with an increase in selenium concentration in cord blood, as selenium is actively transported to the fetus. An analysis of intakes of middle- and upper-income pregnant women in the US found that the usual intake in this group exceeded the estimated average requirement (49 μg/day) and generally met the recommended dietary allowance (RDA; 60 μg/day) [718]. Selenium levels are affected by alcohol consumption and tobacco smoking, both of which decrease selenium absorption.

### Selenium and miscarriage

Selenium deficiency is associated with idiopathic spontaneous abortion in farm animals [1034], and several studies have investigated the possible link between low maternal selenium levels and increased risk of miscarriage in humans; however, the results are inconsistent. One study reported that serum selenium levels were lower in women who miscarried in the first trimester when compared to those in women with viable pregnancies [1035]. Others found no difference in selenium levels in whole blood or plasma between women with viable pregnancies and those who had miscarried but noted a significantly lower activity of the selenoprotein glutathione peroxidase in red blood cells and plasma of women who had miscarried [1036]. Lower levels of selenium were also found in hair samples from women with recurrent miscarriage [1037]. However, all studies were small and therefore should be interpreted with caution.

## Selenium and preterm delivery

Low selenium concentrations in maternal and cord blood were observed in pre-term deliveries as compared with term births in two small case–control studies [1038, 1039]. It was suggested that decreased levels of selenium may be involved in the pathogenesis of retinopathy and respiratory distress syndrome in prema-ture infants, as oxidative stress is implicated in these preterm complications [1040]. Epidemiological evidence suggests that good maternal selenium status may be protective against the potentially toxic effect of oxidizing agents that can provoke preterm delivery.

## The effects of selenium on infection and viral transmission

In animals, blood selenium levels are inversely correlated with risk of infection from various bacterial agents. Selenium deficiency may be a risk factor for mother-to-child transmission of HIV, which can occur in utero, during deliv-ery, or through breastfeeding [1041]. It is possible that selenium deficiency accelerates HIV disease during pregnancy. There is evidence that viral shedding into the genital tract is increased in selenium-deficient women [1042].

Low selenium is also a risk factor for the progression of AIDS in children who were infected perinatally, leading to an increased risk of death by the age of 5. Children with selenium levels ≤85 µg/L died at a younger age, suggesting a more rapid disease progression [1043]. In HIV-infected pregnant women in Tanzania (n = 670), low maternal plasma selenium was not related to risk of in utero HIV transmission but did increase the risk of intrapartum transmission, and transmission through breast milk during early lactation [1041]. Selenium levels were also inversely correlated with risk of fetal death and child death in the first 24 months. This is supported by the results of a placebo-controlled intervention trial (randomized, double-blind) in 913 HIV-infected pregnant women, which showed improved child survival with maternal selenium sup-plementation. Selenium supplementation did not, however, delay maternal HIV disease progression or improve other pregnancy outcomes [1044]. A recent systematic review concluded that the evidence is currently insufficient to recommend selenium supplementation alone; multivitamin supplementation is recommended [1045].

## Selenium in breast milk

The selenium concentration and glutathione peroxidase activity of breast milk are positively correlated with maternal plasma selenium concentrations, indicating that the selenium content in breast milk is influenced by maternal selenium nutrition [1046]. Selenium decreases in breast milk over the course of lactation and is lower in the serum of lactating mothers compared with that of non-lactating mothers [1047]. Lactating women therefore require additional selenium intake in order to produce milk that meets their infant's selenium needs.

## Selenium sources

The selenium in crop foods is substantially affected by the amount of selenium in the soil in which they are grown. Brazil nuts are extremely high in selenium and should be eaten only occasionally or in small amounts. Other dietary sources include shellfish and other seafood, meat, poultry, and cereals. A recommended diet emphasizes intake of a variety of fruits, vegetables, whole grains, and reduced fat or fat-free dairy products, with a moderate intake of lean meats, poultry, fish, beans, and eggs. In the UK, cereals account for ~20 per cent of total selenium intake; 30–40 per cent comes from meat, poultry, and fish [1048].

## Risks of excess selenium

Selenium overload, or selenosis, results from excess selenium in soil and consequent elevated selenium intake in localized areas. High blood selenium ($\geq$100 µg/dL) occurs at intakes around 1.25 mg/day [1049]. Symptoms include garlic breath odour, gastrointestinal distress, hair loss and fingernail changes, fatigue, and irritability. Selenosis can also cause mild nerve damage. The Nutritional Prevention of Cancer Trial found that intake of selenium supplements of 200 µg/day in addition to usual dietary intake over a period of almost 8 years was associated with increased risk of type 2 diabetes, as compared with placebo [1050].

## Agency guidelines for selenium intake

Selenium has a very narrow safe intake range. Agency recommendations in the US and UK differ slightly. The UK reference nutrient intakes [738] for selenium are slightly lower for infants and slightly higher for adults, as compared with the US Institute of Medicine (IOM) recommendations [718] (see Box 23.1 for IOM recommendations). However, these agencies' recommendations are the same for pregnancy, at 60 µg selenium/day, and lactation, at 70 µg/day. These levels are increased from the 55 µg/day RDA for the non-pregnant state. European recommendations [370] are similar to those of the IOM. For infants 0–6 months of age, the UK reference nutrient intake is 10–13 µg/day, whereas the US adequate intake (AI) level is 15 µg/day. For those aged 7–12 months, the UK reference nutrient intake is 10 µg/day, whereas the US AI level is 20 µg/day. The

> ## Box 23.1  US Institute of Medicine recommended dietary allowances for selenium
>
> Infants 0–6 months (adequate intake (AI)) = 15 µg/day
> Infants 7–12 months (AI) = 20 µg/day
> Children 1–3 years = 20 µg/day
> Females 14+ years = 55 µg/day
> Pregnancy = 60 µg/day
> Lactation = 70 µg/day
> Tolerable upper intake level = 400 µg/day
>
> Source: Institute of Medicine, Food and Nutrition Board, *Dietary Reference Intakes for Vitamin C, Vitamin E, Selenium and Carotenoids*, Dietary Reference Intakes, The National Academies Press, Washington, DC, copyright © 2000. [718]

tolerable upper intake level is 400 µg/day for adults, 45 µg/day for infants aged 0–6 months, and 60 µg/day for those aged 7–12 months.

A report of a joint FAO/WHO expert consultation in 2001 [884] proposed a significant decrease in the suggested need for selenium for developing countries, based on a proportionally lower weight range than for most Western and developed communities, among other factors. Their recommendations for pregnant women were 28 µg/day in the second trimester and 30 µg/day in the third; these levels are approximately half that of the IOM recommendation.

## Our recommendations for selenium intake during pregnancy and lactation

Selenium supplements are usually not necessary to meet dietary needs, regardless of pregnancy or lactation status. More is not better, as excess selenium can be toxic. However, individuals with malabsorption syndromes may require supplementation, which should be supervised by a physician.

Because some foods differ widely in selenium content according to their geographical sources, a variety of foods should be eaten to ensure adequate intake and to avoid toxicity. Most pregnant women in developed countries will be able to meet selenium requirements through their usual diet. Taking selenium supplements in addition to adequate dietary intake is not recommended.

Chapter 24

# Copper in pregnancy and breastfeeding

## Copper functions

Copper is an essential trace mineral that readily accepts and donates electrons, which accounts for its central role in oxidation–reduction reactions. It is a component of oxidase metalloenzymes (cuproenzymes) with essential cellular functions. The copper-dependent ferroxidase enzyme ceruloplasmin, for example, plays a significant role iron transport and metabolism [1051]. Cytochrome C oxidase, another copper-dependent enzyme, catalyses the reduction of molecular oxygen to water, generating an electrical gradient involved in cellular energy production. Copper/zinc superoxide dismutase is important in antioxidant defence in cells exposed to oxygen [1052]. Other copper-dependent oxidases catalyse metabolic reactions in the formation and degradation of neurotransmitters, including norepinephrine, epinephrine, serotonin, and dopamine [260].

Copper is involved in connective tissue formation, as the cuproenzyme lysyl oxidase is required for collagen and elastin cross-linking. Reduced activity of this enzyme leads to fragility of connective tissue and blood vessels. Copper also plays a role in the disulphide bonding of keratin [1053]; one manifestation of copper deficiency is twisted, kinked hair [1054]. Most copper in the body, however, is found in bones, muscle, and liver.

## Indicators of copper status

Low levels of serum or plasma copper or ceruloplasmin and decreased erythrocyte dismutase activity are all indicators of copper deficiency but not of copper intake, as they are not sensitive to marginal copper status [1055]. In deficiency conditions, these markers respond to copper supplementation. A serum copper level below 10 µmol/L or ceruloplasmin below 180 mg/L is indicative of deficiency [260].

## Copper deficiency

Clinical deficiency for copper is uncommon but can result from malnutrition, a lack of trace metals in food sources, or genetic disorders. Nutritional copper deficiency has been increasing in prevalence, including in people consuming a Western diet [1056]. Genetic mutations in copper transporters or the copper-binding protein ceruloplasmin result in severe copper deficiency, with multiple serious health consequences including neurodegeneration [1057]. Marginal copper deficiency may compromise immune responses [1058]. Secondary copper deficiency can be induced by excess intake of zinc or iron and is sometimes seen in individuals taking supplements of these minerals. Conversely, alteration of the copper:zinc ratio during treatment for copper deficiency can precipitate zinc deficiency.

## Copper in pregnancy, lactation, and infant feeding

Copper requirements are increased in pregnancy, and a suboptimal supply may have adverse effects on developing tissues and organ systems, including lungs, skin, bones, and the immune system [1059]. Serum copper and ceruloplasmin concentrations increase in pregnancy as copper is mobilized from the liver. This normal increase in blood copper has the potential to mask copper deficiency in tissues.

The body of a full-term fetus contains approximately 13.7 mg of copper. Manifestations of deficiency in the newborn include oedema, anaemia, bone disease, and recurrent apnoea [1060]. The requirement of the fetus for copper must be met throughout gestation from the maternal diet and maternal tissue reserves; low birthweight or premature infants are at risk of copper deficiency because of their increased need of nutrients for growth and bone formation. Infants of very low birthweight require at least 1 μmol/kg of copper per day during parenteral and enteral feeding [1061]. Premature infants fed iron-fortified formulas lacking sufficient copper may also be at increased risk for deficiency conditions [1062]. The copper content of human milk is highest during early lactation and declines as lactation progresses, averaging approximately 250 μg/L during the first 6 months [260]. The recommended intake for infants is based on this breast milk concentration and average daily milk intake and is estimated at 200 μg/day for the first 6 months.

## Risks of excess copper

There is an adaptive response to high copper intake that limits absorption, although increased serum copper levels may lead to an increased risk of cardiovascular disease. Acute copper poisoning is rare, as excess copper is highly emetic, causing nausea and vomiting. Ingestion of >15 mg is toxic. Gastrointestinal irritation is seen at 5.3 mg/day. Ingestion of gram quantities is fatal [1063].

## Copper sources

Foods high in copper include organ meats, grains, shellfish (oysters), nuts, seeds, and cocoa products. Foods that are relatively low in copper but are consumed in substantial amounts include tea, potatoes, milk, and chicken, and these represent significant dietary sources for many populations. Fats and oils are notably low or completely lacking in copper. A higher percentage of copper is absorbed from animal sources than from plant sources [260]. Pure drinking water contains approximately 4–10 µg copper/L water and contributes 6–13 per cent of the average daily copper intake in the US [1064].

## Agency guidelines for copper intake

The US Institute of Medicine recommendation for adults (19+ years) is 900 µg/day copper, with a tolerable upper intake level of 10 mg/day from a combination of food, water, and supplements (see Box 24.1). For pregnant women of all ages, the recommended dietary allowance is 1 mg/day, increasing to 1.3 mg/day during lactation [260].

The Australian National Health and Medical Research Council and the New Zealand Ministry of Health recommend 1.3 mg/day for pregnant adults and 1.2 mg/day for pregnant adolescents (14–18 years) [1065]. The upper level of intake that is considered safe during pregnancy is 8–10 mg/day.

### Box 24.1 US Institute of Medicine recommended dietary allowances for copper

Infants 0–6 months (adequate intake (AI)) = 200 µg/day

Infants 7–12 months (AI) = 220 µg/day

Children 1–3 years = 340 µg/day

Females 14–18 years = 890 µg/day

Females 19+ years = 900 µg/day

Pregnancy = 1,000 µg/day

Lactation = 1,300 µg/day

Tolerable upper intake level 14–18 years = 8,000 µg/day; 19+ years = 10,000 µg/day

Source: Institute of Medicine, Food and Nutrition Board, *Dietary Reference Intakes for Vitamin A, Vitamin K, Arsenic, Boron, Chromium, Copper, Iodine, Iron, Manganese, Molybdenum, Nickel, Silicon, Vanadium, and Zinc*, The National Academies Press, Washington, DC, copyright © 2001. [260]

## Our recommendations for copper intake during pregnancy and lactation

Copper is an important micronutrient that is widely available in foods and drinking water. Although copper needs are increased in pregnancy, supplementation is generally not recommended. Women consuming high doses of iron and/or zinc supplements are at risk for marginal copper deficiency, and this should be taken into account in assessing the mineral supplement needs of pregnant women. An increased intake of foods high in copper, such as nuts, and a proportionate lowering of low-copper foods (e.g. fats/oils) may be advisable in women with potentially marginal copper status.

Chapter 25

# Zinc in pregnancy and breastfeeding

## Zinc functions

Zinc has important structural and functional roles in a number of enzyme systems that are essential for gene expression, cell growth and division, neurotransmission, and reproductive and immune functions [1066]. Loss of zinc from plasma membranes increases their susceptibility to oxidative damage [1067]. In infants and children, zinc is necessary for physical and neurobehavioural development, and protection against infection. It is crucial for periods of growth, including pregnancy and lactation, infancy, childhood, and adolescence.

## Indicators of zinc status

Although much is known about the effects of zinc and its deficiency, the ability to provide practical advice to individuals has been hampered somewhat by the lack of a sensitive marker of zinc status. The concentration of zinc in serum or plasma is used as a biomarker of zinc deficiency risk in populations, as on a population scale, it reflects dietary zinc intake and response to zinc supplementation. However, serum zinc does not consistently reflect the functional zinc status of an individual, and it is not recommended as a diagnostic indicator or to signal the need for supplementation on an individual basis [1068, 1069]. Marginal deficiency for zinc causes broad, and often non-specific, adverse effects due to its involvement in the normal function of a wide range of biochemical pathways. The diagnosis of zinc deficiency can therefore be difficult—there are no truly characteristic physical signs or appropriately sensitive laboratory indices.

## Zinc deficiency

Inadequate zinc intake often accompanies general protein/calorie malnourishment but is also seen in individuals consuming poor quality diets. It is estimated that 20–30 per cent of the global population are at risk of inadequate zinc intake, and deficiency is common in regions such as sub-Saharan Africa and South Asia, where the zinc content in the food supply may be inadequate to meet nutritional needs [1070]. Diets low in animal protein [1071] and/or those high in phytates (e.g. in whole grains or unleavened bread) [1072] provide limited amounts of bioavailable zinc. In addition to inadequate dietary intake, zinc deficiency occurs under conditions of abnormal mucosal uptake (e.g. coeliac disease), abnormal intestinal loss (e.g. Crohn's disease), abnormal renal excretion, alcoholism, or treatment with diuretic drugs. It can also be caused by hereditary conditions, for example, acrodermatitis enteropathica [1073].

## The effects of zinc on growth

Zinc deficiency attenuates growth factor signalling, specifically impacting the insulin-like growth factor axis [1074]. Periods of rapid growth (e.g. late pregnancy, infancy, and adolescence) are the most susceptible to the effects of dietary zinc deficiency. In childhood, zinc deficiency is associated with poor growth and delayed sexual development, and the prevalence of low zinc intake correlates with the prevalence of stunting (low height for age) in children under 5 years of age [1070]. Zinc affects appetite, and anorexia is a symptom of deficiency. This can further potentiate the negative effect of inadequate zinc on growth [1075]. Correction of low zinc intake by zinc supplementation (10 mg/day) of growth-stunted infants and children aged 4–36 months in rural Vietnam increased plasma insulin-like growth factor 1 levels and promoted growth (increased weight and height gain), as compared with placebo [1076]. Infants displaying failure-to-thrive also benefitted from supplemental zinc in a placebo-controlled study in the US [1077]. However, effects of zinc supplementation on growth have not been observed in well-nourished children [1078].

## The effects of zinc on immune function

Zinc affects multiple aspects of the immune system. Inadequate zinc intake increases the risk and severity of infection. Likewise, zinc supplements can have beneficial effects in reducing the duration of infectious illness, including the common cold [1079]. In developing countries with widespread zinc deficiency, decreased resistance to infection is common in children. Preventive zinc supplementation has been shown to reduce childhood mortality from diarrhoeal diseases and pneumonia in such settings [1080]

## The effects of zinc on neurological development

Deficiency of zinc in infancy and early childhood can lead to impaired cognitive development, behavioural problems, and neuronal atrophy [1081]. Low maternal zinc can result in neurobehavioural deficits in animals [1082]. There is some evidence that human maternal zinc deficiency or inadequacy affects the neurological development of the fetus, resulting in alterations in attention, activity, motor development, and neuropsychological behaviour [1083]. However, supplementation with 25 mg/day zinc during the second half of pregnancy had no effect on the neurological development of offspring up to 5 years of age [1084]

## Zinc in pregnancy

Daily zinc requirements increase by up to 40 per cent during pregnancy. It has been estimated that non-pregnant women need to absorb approximately 2.0 mg zinc/day; during pregnancy the maternal/fetal unit requires 2.6 mg/day. Because absorption is only partial (estimated 25%), the calculated intake requirement is approximately 10.5 mg zinc/day in late pregnancy (this has been rounded to 11 mg/day for the recommended dietary allowance (RDA)—see 'Zinc sources and bioavailability') [1085, 1086]. Placental zinc transport is bidirectional and does not occur against a concentration gradient [1087], so if maternal zinc levels are inappropriately low, the movement of zinc to the fetus is reduced. Adequate zinc stores should be ensured prior to pregnancy so that the high requirements of the developing fetus can be met. There is an adaptive increase in zinc absorption during pregnancy and lactation to compensate for some of the increased demand [1088, 1089].

Inadequate maternal zinc intake can have adverse effects on a number of outcomes of pregnancy [1090]. Gestational zinc deficiency is known to be teratogenic in animals, causing intrauterine growth restriction and structural abnormalities [1091, 1092]. This teratogenicity appears to be potentiated by other factors such as infection, inflammatory disease, and alcohol intake, all of which are significant risk factors in pregnant women with low zinc status. These triggers increase the expression of the zinc-binding protein metallothionein in the liver, the effect of which is to decrease zinc transfer to the fetus [1086, 1087].

Low maternal zinc levels are generally thought to contribute to the risk of infants being of low birthweight or small for gestational age; however, study results are inconsistent. Most studies show no significant effect of maternal zinc supplementation with infant birthweight [1093–1096]. Two meta-analyses of 20 zinc intervention trials in over 15,000 women and their infants concluded that zinc supplementation in pregnancy had a small but significant effect on the reduction of preterm birth (−14% with zinc), but not on low birthweight or other outcomes [1097, 1098]. Babies who are born premature may miss the critical period of zinc accumulation during late gestation. It is recommended that such infants be supplemented with zinc [1099].

Because of its role in immunity, zinc supplementation has been evaluated in immunocompromised pregnancies. A study of HIV-infected pregnant women in Tanzania found that the addition of zinc (25 mg/day as zinc sulphate) to a supplemental regimen of multivitamins, iron, and folate had no significant beneficial effects on pregnancy outcomes [1100]. Other studies have shown that zinc supplementation in populations at high risk, such as those in developing countries, reduces the incidence of preterm delivery, childhood diarrhoea, and acute lower respiratory tract infections, and increases growth and weight gain in infants and children [1101, 1102]. Data do not support the use of zinc supplementation for reducing gestational hypertension or pre-eclampsia [1097].

## Zinc in lactation and infant feeding

Infants require approximately 2 mg zinc per day for the first 6 months of life [260]. Breast milk from well-nourished mothers supplies all the nutritional zinc required by the infant for first few months. The zinc supply in breast milk is not particularly sensitive to changes in maternal zinc intake; instead, a homeostatic mechanism involving high fractional absorption (twofold higher during lactation) and intestinal retention ensures maintenance of the zinc supply despite potentially low zinc intake and high demands of the nursing infant [1088, 1089]. Nonetheless, malnourished women usually produce milk that lacks sufficient zinc to meet infant demands during lactation, and supplementation of mothers with zinc during lactation does not appear to increase the zinc concentration in their milk [1103].

The stage of lactation affects zinc concentrations in milk, which decline rapidly from 4 mg/L at 2 weeks, to 1.2 mg/L at 6 months postpartum. These levels provide the newborn infant with approximately 2.3 mg zinc/day for the first month, declining to approximately 1 mg/day at 6 months. Impaired growth resulting from zinc deficiency has been observed in some exclusively breastfed infants from 4–6 months of age [1104]. Such a decline in growth velocity can occur despite apparently adequate energy intake and responds to supplemental zinc, implicating zinc as a growth-limiting micronutrient. Maternal zinc supplementation has no significant effect on the decline in breast milk zinc concentration during the course of lactation [1103]. Requirements of older breastfed infants (6+ months) therefore cannot be met without the consumption of complementary foods such as meat or zinc-fortified cereals/infant foods, or by infant supplementation [1105].

Infants with the hereditary zinc deficiency disorder acrodermatitis enteropathica, which is caused by an autosomally recessive mutation in the zinc transporter gene *SLC39A4*, are protected during breastfeeding by the supply of zinc from their mothers' milk but later show signs of deficiency and require zinc supplementation. On the other hand, women with this disorder produce milk that is deficient in zinc, and their infants, if exclusively breastfed, show symptoms similar to acrodermatitis enteropathica if not supplemented with zinc [1106, 1107]. Similarly, mutations in the zinc transporter gene *SLC30A2*, which is expressed in mammary gland epithelial cells, inhibit zinc excretion into breast milk, resulting in transient zinc deficiency in exclusively breastfed infants [1108, 1109].

## Zinc sources and bioavailability

Oysters are very high in zinc; other shellfish (e.g. crab) and red meat (beef) are also rich sources with high zinc bioavailability. Additional food sources include nuts and legumes, poultry, eggs, whole grains, some fruits (e.g. watermelon and blackberries), seeds (e.g. sesame seeds, pumpkin seeds, and sunflower seeds), and dairy products. The typical Western diet is considered adequate to supply zinc for pregnant and lactating women, providing an average intake of ~13 mg/day [1103]. However, in a study of middle- and upper-income pregnant women in the US (n = 63), 30 per cent did not achieve the estimated average requirement of 9.5 mg/day and more failed to meet the RDA (11 mg/day) [369]. Regular consumption of zinc-rich or zinc-fortified foods during pregnancy is necessary to meet the requirement. Fortification of flour with zinc has been recommended in some areas [1110].

The average availability of zinc from the diet is 25 per cent. Intake of phytate, which is present in most plant foods—particularly grains and legumes—has a significant effect on zinc absorption. Zinc absorption is lower in vegetarian diets because of a higher consumption of phytate-containing foods and an avoidance of zinc-rich meats and seafood. Low-income women in developing countries have low zinc intakes [1103], and the bioavailability of zinc from the diet is generally less than that from Western diets, which are higher in red meat. Diets in developing countries are typically high in unrefined, unfermented, and ungerminated cereal grain, and intake of animal protein is often negligible. Zinc bioavailability is especially low when the cereal grains are fortified with inorganic calcium salts.

Iron and calcium supplements also decrease zinc absorption, although intake of iron and calcium from food has little effect [1111, 1112]. Zinc and iron compete for intestinal absorption because they can bind the same transporter. The routine use of iron supplements during pregnancy may therefore interfere with zinc bioavailability at a time when it is in high demand [1113]. Including zinc in supplements with iron may reduce this effect, and this approach may be important in populations at risk for both deficiencies. Populations with high zinc requirements, including pregnant and lactating women, infants, and adolescents, may be more sensitive to iron-zinc interactions [1114]. Zinc interacts with other micronutrients, including copper, folic acid, and vitamin A. As a component of the copper–zinc superoxide dismutase enzyme (in which copper is catalytic and zinc is structural), high zinc intakes ($\geq$ 50 mg/day) interfere with copper absorption.

## Risks of excess zinc

Supplemental doses of zinc from 50–150 mg/day can cause gastrointestinal distress [1115]. Acute toxicity causing abdominal pain, diarrhoea, nausea, and vomiting can occur from consumption of food or beverages contaminated with zinc released from galvanized containers. Long-term excess zinc consumption (50 mg/day as supplements in addition to 10 mg/day from food) causes copper deficiency; the US Institute of Medicine (IOM) therefore recommends a tolerable upper intake level of 40 mg/day [260]. There is no evidence of toxicity from the intake of naturally occurring zinc in food.

## Agency guidelines for zinc intake

The US RDA for zinc for non-pregnant women is 8 mg/day [260]. The UK recommendation for women is 4.0–7.0 mg/day (lower than that from the US), with a total intake of up to 50 mg/day considered safe [1116]. The RDA for pregnant women 14–18 years of age is 12 mg/day and is 11 mg/day for pregnant women 19 and over. During lactation, an additional 1 mg/day is recommended (13 mg/day for 14–18 years; 12 mg/day for 19+). The upper limit set by the IOM for pregnancy and lactation is 34 mg/day for adolescents, and 40 mg/day for women aged 19 years and above [260] (Box 25.1).

There are some groups that require special consideration. Absorption of zinc is lower from vegetarian diets, especially those high in calcium; this combination may result in low zinc status. The zinc requirement for vegetarians may be up to 50 per cent higher [260, 1117]. The UK Food Standards Agency guidelines indicate that persons taking iron supplements of 30 mg or more per day should also take 15 mg zinc, along with 2 mg of copper [1116]. Long-term excessive alcohol consumption leads to impaired zinc absorption, increased zinc excretion, and possibly an increased daily zinc requirement [1118].

The IOM recommendation for infants 0–6 months of age is 2.0 mg/day zinc. This level reflects the average intake of infants fed breast milk only. Absorption of zinc from human milk is higher than from cow's milk, although cow's milk formulas generally contain higher levels of zinc, so formula-fed infants achieve

## Box 25.1  US Institute of Medicine recommended dietary allowances for zinc

Infants 0–6 months (adequate intake) = 2 mg/day
Infants 7–12 months = 3 mg/day
Children 1–3 years = 3 mg/day
Females 14–18 years = 9 mg/day
Females 19+ years = 8 mg/day
Pregnancy 14–18 years = 12 mg/day
Pregnancy 19+ years = 11 mg/day
Lactation 14–18 years = 13 mg/day
Lactation 19+ years = 12 mg/day
Tolerable upper intake level 14–18 years = 34 mg/day
Tolerable upper intake level 19+ years = 40 mg/day

Source: Institute of Medicine, Food and Nutrition Board, *Dietary Reference Intakes for Vitamin A, Vitamin K, Arsenic, Boron, Chromium, Copper, Iodine, Iron, Manganese, Molybdenum, Nickel, Silicon, Vanadium, and Zinc*, The National Academies Press, Washington, DC, copyright © 2001. [260]

similar intakes to those who are breastfed. Older infants require complementary foods to meet zinc intake needs. The RDA for infants 7 months or older (up to 3 years) is 3 mg/day, which cannot be obtained from breast milk alone. Introduction of lean meats (finely minced) and/or zinc-fortified cereals is recommended from 6 months of age [260]. The tolerable upper intake level for infants is 4 mg/day up to 6 months, and 5 mg/day from 7–12 months.

The WHO is developing recommendations for zinc supplementation for susceptible children (10 mg/day for 0–6 months; 20 mg/day) for the prevention and management of diarrhoea and other health issues, which mainly affect developing countries [1119].

## Our recommendations for zinc intake during pregnancy and lactation

Zinc is required for male fertility, and supplementation may improve fertility in subfertile men. Zinc supplementation in pregnancy has not been shown to improve outcomes for mothers or infants, except possibly to reduce the risk of preterm birth. Women consuming diets that are low in bioavailable zinc (i.e. those that are high in unrefined cereal grain and low in animal protein) or who have risk factors for preterm delivery should be advised to take a prenatal multivitamin containing zinc.

Most prenatal multivitamins contain between 12 and 20 mg of elemental zinc, which is at or above the IOM RDA for pregnant women. These amounts have not been found to be harmful, although they can cause stomach upset in some women. Nonetheless, since iron supplementation is widely prescribed to pregnant women and may lower zinc absorption, inclusion of zinc in multivitamins is recommended. Intake from all sources should not exceed 40 mg/day. Breastfed infants should be introduced to zinc-rich complementary foods (e.g. fortified cereals) by 6 months of age to prevent possible zinc deficiency resulting from declining zinc content in breast milk.

Chapter 26

# Manganese in pregnancy and breastfeeding

## Manganese functions

Manganese is both an essential element and a potent neurotoxin. It is involved in cellular metabolic processes and, as a component of antioxidant enzymes such as manganese superoxide dismutase, is protective against lipid peroxidation. Other manganese metalloenzymes include arginase, glutamine synthetase, and phosphoenolpyruvate decarboxylase.

Uptake and efflux of manganese is tightly regulated, as both deficiency and excess can result in disease states. Most manganese is located on erythrocytes [1120] and is taken up from blood by the liver and transported by transferrin. Absorption of manganese is low, and retention is affected by dietary calcium, iron, and phosphorus [1121–1123]. Women usually have lower iron status than men and have been found to absorb more manganese [1124]. Despite its low bioavailability, manganese deficiency is rare in humans, as manganese is found naturally in a number of commonly consumed foods.

Animal studies have shown that manganese is particularly critical during gestation and early infancy. In manganese deficiency, elevated concentrations of serum calcium, phosphorus, and alkaline phosphatase have been observed, suggestive of bone resorption in humans [1125] and animals [1126]. Manganese is directly involved in bone growth as a cofactor of glycosyl transferases [1127] and participates in insulin-like growth factor metabolism [1128]. Manganese deficiency interferes with normal skeletal development in animals because the manganese-dependent enzyme prolidase is needed for collagen formation and wound healing. However, in human pregnancy, manganese levels do not correlate with newborn bone growth parameters [1129].

## Indicators of manganese status/exposure

Serum or plasma manganese concentrations have been reported to respond to dietary intake [1130], as has urinary manganese excretion [1125]. However, there is some disagreement on the use of these measurements as indicators of manganese status [260]. Serum manganese concentrations in combination with lymphocyte manganese superoxide dismutase activity may be the best biomarkers for monitoring manganese intake. Blood arginase activity may also be used. Brain MRI scans and neuro-functional tests are used to assess overexposure to manganese [1122]. The normal blood level of manganese is between 4 and 14 μg/ml, but there is no clear 'normal' range for young children.

## Manganese in pregnancy

Manganese status and metabolism change in pregnancy. Since manganese is primarily found in association with erythrocytes, its concentration would be expected to decrease with haemodilution over the course of pregnancy. However, manganese absorption in inversely correlated with iron status [1131], which tends to decrease in pregnancy. Accordingly, manganese content in blood has been shown to increase in pregnancy [1132, 1133]. The increase is slightly lower in women who receive iron supplements [1132] and may be related to accelerated erythropoiesis. Transfer of manganese to the fetus appears to be limited by the placenta [260].

In the brain, homeostatic mechanisms operate between iron and manganese transporters. Neonatal dietary iron deficiency upregulates manganese transporters in the developing brain and results in elevated brain manganese accumulation [1134]. This has been shown in animals to influence manganese neurotoxicity [1135].

The retention rate for manganese in the neonate is high, and high levels are observed in early infancy [1136]. In infants, both low and high blood manganese levels were associated with lower scores on a standard test of cognitive development at 12 months in a longitudinal study of Mexican children [1137]. The observed U-shaped association between manganese and cognitive development might be explained by effects on oxidative stress at both high and low levels of manganese, with deficiency increasing sensitivity to oxidative injury, and excess causing manganese to act as an oxidant itself [1138].

Approximately 3 μg/day of manganese is secreted in human milk. Although this is a low level compared with other species, it is the recommended adequate intake (AI) level for infants up to 6 months of age. Although the concentration of manganese in human milk is low, infant formulas can vary widely, containing between 30 and 300 μg/L. Infants 7–12 months of age who are fed complementary foods are estimated to consume around 70–80 μg/kg manganese per day. Based on this, the AI for these infants is calculated as 0.6mg/day [260].

## Manganese sources

Manganese is found in high amounts in nuts, seeds, tea, and whole grains, with levels sometimes exceeding 30 mg/kg. Only very small amounts are present in meats, dairy products, and sugary and refined foods [1139]. Manganese is also present in drinking water and may be more bioavailable from water than from food. Many dietary supplements contain manganese at levels between 5 and 20 mg [260]. The average dietary intake for adults is less than 5 mg/day. Heavy tea drinkers, and vegetarians who consume foods rich in manganese such as grains, beans, and nuts may have a higher intake of manganese than the average person [1138].

## Risks of excess manganese

Over-ingestion of manganese from food sources is not likely to cause problems, except in individuals with severe iron deficiency or chronic liver disease. High intake of supplements or exposure to contaminants from occupations such as welding or steel metal work may increase the chance of excessive intake of manganese. The symptoms of manganese toxicity in adults appear slowly over months and years [1138]. The major recognized symptoms of manganese toxicity relate to the CNS. Accumulation of manganese in dopamine-rich brain regions that control muscle movement causes damage to the extrapyramidal system, leading to dyskinesias and neuropsychiatric disturbances [1140]. Liver damage has also been reported [1141].

Several factors, including higher rates of intestinal absorption and brain delivery, potentially predispose the neonate to enhanced manganese accumulation and increased toxicity [1142]. Homeostatic mechanisms control plasma manganese concentrations but can be overwhelmed at high exposure levels [1143]. The developing striatum may be particularly vulnerable to damage from excess manganese in utero and during early neonatal development [1144].

## Agency guidelines for manganese intake

No recommended dietary allowance has been established for manganese intake, although AI recommendations have been made (Box 26.1). The AI for pregnancy and lactation represent an increase based on average intake above that of the non-pregnant state, at 2 mg/day of manganese for pregnant women of all ages and 2.6 mg/day for lactation [260].

Guidelines from Australia and New Zealand for manganese intake by adults differ somewhat from those of the US Institute of Medicine, being 5.0 mg/day for women, regardless of pregnancy or lactation status. The advised intake for non-pregnant adolescents (14–18 years) is 3.0 mg/day, although

## Box 26.1 US Institute of Medicine recommended adequate intake levels for manganese

Infants 0–6 months = 3 μg/day
Infants 7–12 months = 0.6 mg/day
Children 1–3 years = 1.2 mg/day
Females 14–18 years = 1.6 mg/day
Females 19+ = 1.8 mg/day
Pregnancy = 2.0 mg/day
Lactation = 2.6 mg/day
Tolerable upper intake level 14–18 years = 9 mg/day
Tolerable upper intake level 19+ y = 11 mg/day

Source: Institute of Medicine, Food and Nutrition Board, *Dietary Reference Intakes for Vitamin A, Vitamin K, Arsenic, Boron, Chromium, Copper, Iodine, Iron, Manganese, Molybdenum, Nickel, Silicon, Vanadium, and Zinc*, The National Academies Press, Washington, DC, copyright © 2001. [260]

this age group follows the adult recommendation of 5.0 mg/day during pregnancy and lactation [1145].

The WHO evaluated manganese intakes in adult diets and found that the average daily consumption ranged from 2.0–8.8 mg/day, with higher intakes associated with diets high in wholegrain cereals, nuts, green leafy vegetables, and tea. An intake of 2–3 mg manganese per day is therefore considered adequate for adults, and intakes of 8–9 mg/day are deemed safe. Intake from drinking water is considered to make only a minor contribution to manganese intake in general [1146].

Taking into consideration the ubiquity of manganese in foods, and the limited evidence for deficiency in humans, the European Food Safety Authority recommends that exposure to manganese should remain low and should not exceed that found in the diet. Nonetheless, it states that supplemental intakes of 4 mg manganese/day are unlikely to produce adverse effects in the general population. Such supplementation would result in a total intake of 12.2 mg/day, taking into a consideration a dietary intake level of 8.2 mg/day (which may be a high estimate). Specific recommendations have not been made for pregnant and lactating women [1147].

## Our recommendations for manganese intake during pregnancy and lactation

The hazard posed by overexposure to manganese must be weighed against the necessity for some minimum amount of manganese in the diet. Manganese has essential functions in maternal health and fetal development, and in healthy women adequate amounts can be obtained from a mixed diet of grains, cereals, and fruits. Supplements containing manganese should be used with caution, as excess intake can have neurotoxic effects on the developing brain. Newborn infants and young children are the most vulnerable. Maternal intake in pregnancy and lactation is not a cause for concern in most cases, as transfer of manganese to the fetus and into breast milk is limited. However, in situations of iron deficiency or chronic liver disease, excess manganese accumulation can occur and should be monitored.

Chapter 27

# Prebiotics and probiotics in pregnancy and breastfeeding

## Prebiotic and probiotic functions

Probiotics are live, non-pathogenic commensal microorganisms with benefi-cial effects on the host organism; they improve and/or maintain intestinal flora balance by suppressing and displacing harmful bacteria. Prebiotics are nondigestible food components that stimulate growth or activity of these beneficial intestinal bacteria. Probiotics are found in fermented foods such as yoghurt; prebiotics are found in whole grains, soybeans, bananas, onions, gar-lic, honey, and artichokes. It has been claimed that prebiotic and probiotic supplements improve the symptoms of irritable bowel syndrome, diarrhoea, intestinal infections, and vaginal yeast infections and prevent or treat eczema, colds, and flu. When prebiotics and probiotics are combined, they are referred to as synbiotics [1148].

Gut bacteria synthesize some essential vitamins (e.g. vitamin K) and break-down indigestible polysaccharides to short-chain fatty acids. Such microorgan-isms form an integral part of the intestinal mucosal defence system [1149] and are important for the development and maturation of the infant's gastrointes-tinal tract. The infant gut is initially colonized by bacteria that it obtains from the mother during birth, with different patterns of colonization occurring dependent on the mode of delivery: with caesarean delivery, the infant does not come into contact with the mother's intestinal and vaginal microbiota, and the acquisition of some species (e.g. bifidobacteria) is delayed [1150].

Human milk contains functional oligosaccharides with prebiotic effects [1151]. These oligosaccharides modulate bacteria–host interactions and affect the composition of infant gut microbiota. They also serve as decoy receptors that prevent the attachment of pathogenic bacteria to the intestinal lining. In addition to prebiotic compounds, probiotic microbes are present in breast milk and in the gut of breastfed infants, where bifidobacteria and lactobacilli predominate [1148]. These organisms produce antimicrobial compounds and compete with other pathogens for available nutrients. They also strengthen the intestinal barrier against further pathogenic infections

[1152]. Some infant formula is supplemented with factors that mimic the prebiotic effects of human milk and produce similar effects on the gut microbial composition [1153].

## Probiotics and the immune system—the 'hygiene hypothesis'

The basis of the hygiene hypothesis is that increased hygienic standards prevent the neonate from experiencing the immune stimulus of microbial infection that provides a driver for the maturation of the immune system and gut, thereby predisposing the individual to allergies [1154]. Conversely, early microbial exposure promotes B-cell maturation and reduces susceptibility to infections and sensitization to environmental antigens later in life [1155]. Infants in developing countries with poorer hygiene have more rapid colonization than infants in developed countries, where the prevalence of allergic disorders is rising [1156].

Maternal probiotic and prebiotic supplementation has been reported to enhance the development and maturation of the neonatal gastrointestinal tract [1157]. In a randomized, double-blind trial, lactobacillus supplementation to pregnant women for 2–4 weeks ($1 \times 10^{10}$ colony-forming units/day) before expected delivery halved the occurrence of atopic eczema in their offspring at 2 years of age, as compared with placebo [1158]. Probiotics at weaning reduced the risk of developing eczema (early manifestation of allergy) at 13 months in a double-blind, placebo-controlled study [1159]. A higher Th1/Th2 ratio was observed in the probiotic group, suggesting enhanced T cell-mediated immune responses. Feeding infants that were between 4 and 13 months of age (weaning) with cereals containing probiotics also decreased levels of monounsaturated fatty acids, which have been linked to visceral obesity, and raised levels of polyamines that are important for gut maturation and integrity [1160].

## A potential role of probiotics in the prevention of gestational diabetes mellitus

Dietary interventions and lifestyle modifications, as well as medical therapies, have been recommended for the management of insulin resistance during pregnancy. Probiotics have recently been proposed to play a role in prevention of gestational diabetes. Studies in animal models have reported the beneficial effects of probiotics on fasting plasma glucose levels as well as on improved insulin resistance [1161, 1162]. Since probiotics utilize glucose as their primary energy source, they can influence blood glucose and insulin levels through their effects on decreased glucose absorption. Probiotics can also improve insulin resistance through their impact on reduced inflammatory signalling [1162], upregulated expression of proglucagons [1161], and decreased adiposity [1163].

Trials involving probiotic supplementation in pregnancy examining metabolic outcomes are limited. A study involving 256 normal weight pregnant women in Finland demonstrated that women who received probiotic supplementation that consisted of *Lactobacillus rhamnosus* GG and *Bifidobacterium lactis* BB12, along with dietary counselling, had a reduced risk of elevated maternal glucose concentration [1164] and a reduced frequency of gestational diabetes [1165], as well as a reduced frequency of having a maternal waist circumference of 80 cm or more [1166]. Both maternal fasting glucose and insulin levels in the third trimester were significantly lower in mothers who received the probiotic supplement and dietary counselling [1164]. There was no significant difference in the infant weights [1165]. A recent randomized controlled trial [1167] found that pregnant women who consumed 200 g of probiotic yoghurt for 9 weeks were more likely to maintain their insulin levels and avoid the development of insulin resistance compared with women who consumed regular yoghurt for the same period.

## Our recommendations for prebiotic and probiotic intake during pregnancy and lactation

Evidence is accumulating that prebiotics and probiotics ingested during pregnancy and lactation or provided to the weaning infant are beneficial for the infant's developing gastrointestinal and immune systems. We recommend that prebiotics and probiotics be acquired from food sources as the first option, unless other circumstances such as the use of antibiotics suggest that supplementation may be necessary. A diet including yoghurt, whole grains, soybeans, bananas, onions, and garlic should provide sufficient amounts of pre- and probiotics for the health of both mother and nursing infant. Some of these foods can also be introduced to the weaning infant. Further research is needed before prebiotic or probiotic supplements should be routinely considered.

# Section 3

# A healthy lifestyle for a healthy pregnancy

Adopting a healthy lifestyle and reducing behaviours that have adverse effects on health is essential for ensuring the best pregnancy outcomes for both mother and child. This should ideally begin before conception, as many critical embryonic and fetal developmental processes and maternal adaptations to pregnancy occur during the first trimester. This section provides information on aspects of lifestyle that can have significant effects on pregnancy, including safe and unsafe foods, exercise, and exposure to potential toxins, as well as weight guidelines for pregnancy.

# Chapter 28

# Pre-conception maternal body composition and gestational weight gain

## The impact of maternal pre-conception bodyweight

In addition to diet, a woman's body composition at conception is an important factor in her overall health and influences both the amount of weight she gains during pregnancy and infant growth patterns [1168]. It has been known for many years that size at birth is more related to maternal than paternal size [1169, 1170]. Shorter mothers in general give birth to children who are shorter in length, and maternal short stature (height less than 148 cm) is also strongly associated with the risk of low birthweight in term deliveries [1171]. Maternal lean body mass is positively associated with fetal growth [1172, 1173], and both obesity and underweight at the start of pregnancy are associated with birthweight [1174–1176]. Excessive or inadequate weight gain is also detrimental to fetal development.

### Under-nutrition and underweight at conception

Low maternal pre-pregnancy weight, low BMI, and low attained weight throughout pregnancy are associated with impaired fetal growth [1177]. In the developing world there remain many women who have low body mass at conception [1178], although the proportion is decreasing. In developed countries, the prevalence of underweight in pre-pregnant women has also decreased with time [1179], and in the US approximately 5 per cent of women begin pregnancy underweight (BMI <18.5 kg/m²) [1180]. Underweight mothers or those with low BMIs (<19.5 kg/m²) are also at increased risk of both small-for-gestational-age and spontaneous preterm birth [30, 1181], particularly if their gestational weight gain is low [1182]. In studies that considered pre-pregnancy BMI as a continuous variable, an increased preterm delivery risk correlated with a decreasing BMI below 22–26 kg/m² [1181, 1183].

## Pre-pregnancy obesity

Obesity prior to and during pregnancy has been associated with adverse outcomes for both mother and fetus. In 2004–2005, 23 per cent of women in the US began pregnancy as overweight (BMI 25.0–29.9 kg/m$^2$), and 19 per cent began pregnancy as obese (BMI ≥30.0 kg/m$^2$) [1180]. A more recent UK study showed that 50 per cent of women of childbearing age were either overweight (BMI 25.0–29.9 kg/m$^2$) or obese (BMI >30 kg/m$^2$) [1184]. The rates of female overweight and obesity are also rising rapidly in low- and middle-income countries as they become increasingly urbanized and use different food sources [1185–1187].

Overweight and obesity increases the risks of developing gestational diabetes mellitus (GDM) [1174, 1188, 1189], with obese women having up to a fivefold higher risk compared to normal-weight women [1190]. Obese women also have a higher risk of pre-eclampsia compared to their normal-weight counterparts [30, 1191], and this increased risk may be related to an increase in inflammatory factors associated with obesity [1192, 1193]. Obesity in pregnancy also increases the risks of thromboembolism [1194, 1195], infection [1191, 1196], caesarean delivery [1197, 1198], congenital anomalies [404], labour induction [1199], stillbirth [1200, 1201], shoulder dystocia [1191], and preterm delivery [1202]. Being obese at the start of pregnancy is associated with fetal macrosomia [1203], and large-for-gestational-age infants, and the risk increases as the pre-pregnancy BMI increases [1204–1206].

Obesity, both at conception and during pregnancy, can also have long-term effects on the offspring, such as greater risks of adiposity, cardiovascular and metabolic dysfunction, and poor cognitive development [59, 1207–1209]. While these trans-generational effects may in part be cultural, reflecting intrafamilial feeding behaviour, there is growing experimental evidence of the biological effects of maternal obesity leading to obesity in the offspring [1210]. These effects include induced epigenetic changes [1211, 1212]. Additionally, maternal obesity is frequently associated with mild hyperglycaemia, which leads to fetal hyperinsulinaemia and thus greater adipogenesis in utero [1213].

## Gestational weight gain

Gestational weight gain has an impact on both short- and long-term pregnancy outcomes. Low weight gain in pregnant women without diabetes is associated with reduced fetal growth and increased risk of preterm birth [1204], whereas high weight gain is associated with a greater risk of excessive fetal growth [1214]. However there is a paucity of data on which to base good management guidelines. To date only the US Institute of Medicine (IOM) has produced guidelines (see 'Agency guidelines for weight gain during pregnancy'), which are based on US data and opinion and do not extrapolate directly to other societies and across ethnicities where body habitus and healthy BMI ranges may differ. Furthermore, the IOM guidelines are seen as rather broad and in need of revision.

While adopting the IOM recommendations seems to be beneficial for underweight and normal-weight mothers, different guidelines or thresholds might be more appropriate for overweight and obese mothers in order to avoid adverse short-term pregnancy outcomes. In a large German population-based data set, overweight and obese mothers who gained weight within the IOM recommendations for gestational weight gain had a lower incidence of pre-eclampsia and fewer non-elective caesarean deliveries, but higher risks for GDM, small-for-gestational-age birth, preterm delivery, and perinatal mortality [1215]. Unfortunately, overweight and obese women are nearly twice as likely to exceed the recommended guidelines for gestational weight gain compared with normal-weight women, and underweight women are more likely to fall below IOM guidelines.

The issue of whether reducing gestational weight gain affects the risk of pre-eclampsia is controversial, and, if it has any effect, it is likely restricted to obese women [1216–1218]. Nonetheless, in some countries such as Japan, it is still considered preferable to limit weight gain, even in normal- and underweight women. This practice is of considerable concern given the consequences that the resulting lowered birthweight can have for the offspring (see 'Active management of gestational weight gain').

## Gestational weight gain and offspring obesity

There is considerable interest in the relationship between gestational weight gain and the risk of offspring obesity. Maternal obesity and high gestational weight gain are associated with weight gain in childhood and adolescence [1189, 1219–1221]. In a study of ~3,000 singleton births to women without pregnancy complications, weight gain in all trimesters was significantly and independently associated with birthweight, although only first trimester weight gain was associated with child BMI outcomes [1222]. In analyses of 3,600 participants from the Early Childhood Longitudinal Study Birth Cohort, after adjusting for socio-demographics and family lifestyle, there was a significant overall association between gestational weight gain and child adiposity among normal and overweight mothers [1223]. In Germany, a higher risk of both overweight and abdominal adiposity at school entry has been observed in children of mothers who gained weight excessively (as defined by the IOM guidelines) during pregnancies [31].

In a study cohort of ~6,500 mother–child pairs, women who avoided excessive weight gain in the third trimester had children with a 31 per cent lower probability of being overweight [1224]. A similar reduction (27% lower probability) was also observed for women who reversed from excessive weight gain in the first or second trimester to normal weight gain in the third trimester. A meta-analysis [1225] demonstrated that at least a 21 per cent risk for childhood overweight was related to excessive gestational weight gain and that further efforts to design appropriate interventions against excessive weight gain were warranted.

## Agency guidelines for weight gain during pregnancy

To date, the only generally accepted guidelines for weight gain during pregnancy are those developed by the IOM in 1990 and which provide recommendations for women of different BMIs. The guidelines were slightly revised in 2009 [1226] (see Box 28.1) The IOM intended these guidelines to be used for women in the US; however, the IOM committee suggested that these guidelines are potentially 'applicable to women in other developed countries' [1215]. Further research is needed to achieve population specific guidelines because of the very different maternal height and body shape norms between populations.

Maternal height has been considered in the design of two similar charts [1227, 1228]. The latter chart, based on a Chilean population, is now being used in several Latin American countries and could be also adopted in other developing countries where maternal height is shorter than in the US. In this chart, short and tall women are recommended to gain proportionately more and less weight, respectively, than average-height women.

---

### Box 28.1 Gestational weight gain recommendations according to the revised US Institute of Medicine guidelines

Underweight women (BMI <18.5 kg/m$^2$) should gain 12.5–18.0 kg

Normal-weight women (BMI between 18.5 and 25 kg/m$^2$) should gain 11.5–16.0 kg

Overweight women (BMI between 25 and 30 kg/m$^2$) should gain 7.0–11.5 kg

Obese women (BMI ≥30 kg/m$^2$) should gain 5.0–9.0 kg

Source: Yaktine, A.L. and K.M. Rasmussen, eds., *Weight Gain during Pregnancy: Reexamining the Guidelines*, Institute of Medicine, Washington, DC, copyright © 2009. [1226]

## Active management of gestational weight gain

The evidence presented above clearly demonstrates that it is crucial for over-weight and obese mothers to gain weight within population-appropriate guidelines. Advice to restrict energy intake to between 1,800 and 2,000 kcal/day, with an intake of carbohydrates between 150 and 180 g/day, has been shown to reduce gestational weight gain by 50 per cent and to lower fasting insulin concentrations in late pregnancy [1217, 1229]. A behavioural inter-vention programme (including a face-to-face visit, weekly mailed materials that promoted an appropriate weight gain, healthy eating, and exercise, use of individual graphs of weight gain and telephone-based feedback) promot-ed adherence to IOM recommendations in normal-weight women and increased the percentages of normal and overweight/obese women who returned to their pre-conception weights or below by 6 months postpartum [1230]. Another intervention programme, named the Lifestyle in Pregnancy Study, produced significantly lower gestational weight gain by providing dietary guidance, free membership to fitness centres, and physical training, as well as personal coaching, although the obstetric outcomes were similar in both the intervention and control groups [1231]. Weight management interventions in pregnancy have been found to be effective in reducing the incidence of pre-eclampsia and shoulder dystocia and may also reduce the incidence of GDM [1184]. The interventions, however, showed no differ-ences in the incidence of small-for-gestational-age infants between the groups.

It should also be emphasized that these studies involved only minor weight reduction. In contrast, in Japan there has been a tendency toward much more stringent dietary advice, apparently in an attempt to reduce the inci-dence of pre-eclampsia. This has been associated with a much more dramatic fall in gestational weight gain, on the order of 4 kg/pregnancy [1232], accom-panied by a considerable fall in birthweight and a rise in the rate of small-for-gestational-age births [1233]. These very low gestational weight gains fall outside the IOM advisory range. Our own view is that this is a most unwise practice, unlikely to confer additional protection against pre-eclampsia and likely to have long-term adverse effects on the offspring. Maternal under-nutrition is practised in some less developed African societies to reduce the risk of complications at delivery, and we are aware of arguments in some Asian countries to promote a marked reduction in gestational weight gain to reduce the rate of caesarean section. For similar reasons we think this unwise, particularly given that the high rates of caesarean section have a major elec-tive component.

## Our recommendations for pre-conceptional maternal body composition and gestational weight gain

Maternal weight status, lifestyles, and general health during pregnancy play important roles in the offspring's development and can contribute to the risk of non-communicable disease in the offspring in adulthood. Maternal weight in particular seems to have the most dominant effect in influencing the offspring's body composition, which can consequently affect future health outcomes. Women who are underweight at the beginning of pregnancy have a greater risk of having smaller babies and shorter gestational lengths. The offspring may have long-term sequelae of this peri-conceptual under-nutrition. Women who are overweight prior to pregnancy and those who gain more weight than the recommended guidelines during pregnancy may develop GDM and maternal obesity, both of which can have adverse effects on the fetus and child.

Currently the IOM guidelines are the only ones available for developed countries, where mean maternal height is similar to that in the US. We would recommend that attention be given to body composition before pregnancy and that the IOM guidelines be followed, but that simple measures of habitus such as maternal height are taken into account in applying them. Alternatives that include the influence of maternal height to proportionally guide weight gain may be considered for developing countries.

# Chapter 29

# Exercise and physical activity in pregnancy

## Exercise and physiological changes in pregnancy

Regular physical exercise is known to reduce cardiovascular disease risk factors such as blood pressure and plasma lipid levels and can improve insulin sensitivity, increase lean body mass, and reduce fat mass [40]. As these factors have important consequences for pregnancy, there is an increasing focus on the role of exercise in maintaining a healthy pregnancy. At the same time, there is a need to consider whether extreme exercise or excessive physical exertion might have adverse effects on pregnant women.

Various mechanisms beyond straightforward changes in energy homeostasis have been proposed to explain how exercise can alter the physiology of pregnancy, including promotion of placental growth and vascularization, reducing oxidative stress, and improving maternal vascular endothelial function and immune and inflammatory responses [1234]. Trophoblastic, endothelial, and stromal cell proliferation is increased in active pregnant women [1235], as is functional tissue volume in the placenta [1236], resulting in an improved surface area for gas and nutrient exchange [1237]. Exercise in pregnant women has been shown to increase the circulation of pro-angiogenic factors while reducing anti-angiogenic factors [1238]. Likewise, exercise training has been shown to increase circulating anti-inflammatory cytokines such as interleukin-10 and reduce pro-inflammatory factors such as interleukin-1 beta, interleukin-6, and tumour necrosis factor alpha [1234]. An elevation in the levels of anti-angiogenic and pro-inflammatory factors may contribute to the pathophysiology of pre-eclampsia [1234, 1239].

## Cultural factors influencing exercise during pregnancy

There are wide cultural and population differences in the energy expenditure of pregnant women. In many low-income countries, pregnant women continue with hard physical exertion, such as carrying heavy loads of water over long distances, well into pregnancy [1240, 1241]. Coupled with poor nutrition, this high-energy expenditure can impair fetal growth and maternal health [1242], Conversely, modern sedentary lifestyles have contributed to a greatly increased prevalence of obesity and type 2 diabetes in both developed and developing countries, where, in many areas, women of reproductive age are more likely than not to be overweight.

## The benefits of exercise for expecting mothers

Compared with sedentary pregnant women, those who exercise moderately at least once a week are less likely to have low back pain and depression. In addition, more frequent exercise can help reduce pelvic girdle pain [1243]. Women who exercise in accordance with the 2002 American Congress of Obstetricians and Gynecologists (ACOG) guidelines [1244] (see 'Agency guidelines on exercise for pregnant women') exhibit significantly improved fitness levels and muscular strength, and recover faster post-delivery [1243].

### The effects of exercise on gestational weight gain

Regular physical activity is important for maintaining optimal maternal body-weight during pregnancy. Both excessive and inadequate gestational weight gain are associated with adverse maternal and infant outcomes (see chapter 28). Many studies have shown that intervention programmes that include leisure time physical activity/exercise can be successful in preventing excessive gestational weight gain. Such activities include aqua-aerobics, supervised walking/biking, a progressive walking programme, and unsupervised free gym membership with personal coaching [1231, 1246–1248].

### The effects of exercise on gestational diabetes and pre-eclampsia

Because of its potential effects on insulin resistance, angiogenesis, and blood pressure, exercise has been suggested as a means to reduce the risks of gestational diabetes mellitus (GDM) and pre-eclampsia. However, evidence for an effect of physical activity on these outcomes has been mixed [1247, 1249–1256]. Most studies that examined the impact of physical activity before conception reported a significant impact in reducing the risk of pre-eclampsia [1254, 1257], but some reported no benefit [1258]. A recent Cochrane systematic review reported no significant differences in the incidence of GDM in women who received exercise interventions compared with those who received routine antenatal care [1259]. Based on these outcomes, there was not enough conclusive evidence to recommend a prescriptive exercise programme and establish a standard guideline and practice.

## The effect of exercise on preterm birth

Physical activity throughout pregnancy has been reported to have a protective effect against delivery before 37 weeks gestation [1260–1262]. In a population-based cohort study of >61,000 singleton pregnancies in Norway, women who exercised 3 to 5 times a week in mid-pregnancy had a longer gestation than those who did not exercise [1263]. Frequent vigorous recreational activity (e.g. jogging, swimming, and brisk walking) in the first trimester was associated with longer gestation and a reduced risk of preterm birth [1264].

## Stress management during pregnancy through yoga

Maternal stress and anxiety can have negative consequences for the growth and development of the fetus [1265–1267]. Stress increases fetal exposure to gluco-corticoids and has been suggested as a risk factor for the development of atten-tion deficit hyperactivity disorder or lowered performance on executive function tests in the offspring [1268, 1269]. More detail on the effects of pre-natal stress on pregnancy outcomes is provided in chapter 33.

Yoga has gained popularity as a method of reducing stress, anxiety, depres-sion, and chronic pain syndromes in adults. In high-risk women, yoga per-formed 3 times per week from the 12th to the 28th week of gestation significantly reduced the risk of pregnancy-induced hypertension, pre-eclampsia, GDM, and intrauterine growth restriction [1270]. In addition, women who practised yoga were significantly less likely to have a baby that was small for gestational age or had a low Apgar score at birth. Two recent reviews of both controlled and observational trials reached similar conclusions regarding a reduction in the rates of preterm labour, intrauterine growth restriction, low birthweight, sleep disturbance, and stress [1271, 1272].

## The effects of moderate maternal exercise on the offspring

In general, non-extreme exercise is reported to have minimal risk and potential indirect (i.e. via mother's health) benefits to the fetus [1273, 1274]. Regular aerobic exercise during pregnancy is associated with lower fetal heart rate and higher heart rate variability at rest [1275, 1276]. The exact mechanisms by which maternal exercise may affect fetal heart rate control are uncertain, but a dose-response relationship has been demonstrated [1277].

Maternal physical activity before and during pregnancy may have a beneficial impact on the timing of delivery, birthweight, and offspring health [1278]. In a study of >79,000 pregnant women from the Danish National Birth Cohort, women who exercised during pregnancy had a reduced risk of giving birth to small-for-gestational-age or large-for-gestational-age infants compared with those who did not exercise [1279]. Data from >9,000 women who were involved in the National Maternal and Infant Health Survey also demonstrated a protective effect of leisure physical activity during pregnancy against low birthweight outcomes [1280].

## The long-term effects of maternal exercise on the offspring

Little is known of the long-term effects of maternal exercise on offspring health. In general, the apparent reduction in preterm delivery and the associated improvements in maternal health might be expected to improve offspring health. Whether the physiological effects on the fetus of moderate maternal exercise provide long-term benefit is not clear.

Children of mothers who exercised during pregnancy had a leaner body mass and better neurodevelopmental outcome at 5 years of age [1281]. The mechanisms of this long-term protective effect are unknown. A confounder on such studies is that the social environment of families where mothers were committed to regular exercise may be sufficiently different to impact on the child's development independently of the woman's exercise pattern.

# The potential risks of exercise during pregnancy

## The potential risks of exercise in swimming pools during pregnancy

It has been suggested that swimming in pools during pregnancy might be harmful for pregnant women because the chlorine disinfection by-products may be toxic to the fetus [1282]. Although several studies have suggested that exposure to such by-products may increase the risk of low birthweight, the evidence is inconclusive [1283]. There are few studies of swimming exposure per se, but these are reassuring. The Avon Longitudinal Study of Parents and Children birth cohort of >11,000 pregnant women found no apparent association between swimming and birthweight [1284]. Similarly, a more recent study in nearly 75,000 singleton pregnancies from the Danish National Birth Cohort reported that swimming in pool water was not associated with adverse reproductive outcomes [1282], and in fact women who swam in early/mid-pregnancy had a slightly reduced risk of having preterm birth. Based on the limited studies that have been conducted and reported so far, the current practice of swimming in pools for pregnant women should be safe.

## Extreme exercise in pregnancy

While there is strong evidence for the benefit of moderate and regular exercise in well-nourished pregnancies, there is more debate about the wisdom of severe exercise in pregnancy, particularly in late pregnancy, because of its effects on birthweight. Studies suggest that women who perform vigorous exercise (e.g. running, aerobic dance, and cross-country skiing) throughout pregnancy give birth to infants with reduced birthweight (~300–500 g lighter), compared with those who do not exercise or exercise moderately [1241, 1279, 1286–1288]. A randomized controlled trial in healthy women in the second half of pregnancy showed that vigorous aerobic exercise was associated with lower birthweight and BMI, as well as lowered cord serum insulin-like growth factor 1 and insulin-like growth factor 2 [1289].

Because of this association with reduced birthweight, caution is indicated with respect to extreme exercise in late pregnancy. Whether such reduction in birthweight has long-term consequences for the offspring is not certain but, given that the mechanism of the reduction in birthweight is likely to be analogous to the effects of poor late gestational maternal nutrition, we would suspect that the offspring of mothers undertaking extreme exercise may be at greater risk for the development of obesity, insulin resistance, and other noncommunicable diseases. Further studies are needed to address this question.

## Agency guidelines on exercise for pregnant women

The ACOG recommends that healthy pregnant women should engage in 30 minutes or more of moderate physical activity per day on most, if not all, days of the week. ACOG also states that physically active woman with a history of or risk for preterm labour or fetal growth restriction should reduce their activity in the second and third trimesters [1244]. The Canadian guidelines [1290] recommend that healthy pregnant women should perform aerobic exercise regularly for at least 15 minutes, 3 days per week at the target intensity. The exercise duration can be increased from a minimum of 3 days per week to 4 or 5 days per week over time. Healthy pregnant women who were previously inactive can gradually increase the duration of exercise from 15 to 30 minutes per session during the second trimester. In addition, women should avoid exercising in the supine position after the fourth month as well as performing the Valsalva manoeuvre during resistance exercise (which is easy to do without being aware of it in activities such as weightlifting).

The Royal College of Obstetricians and Gynaecologists suggests that all women be encouraged to participate in aerobic and strength-conditioning exercise as part of a healthy lifestyle during their pregnancy [1291]. Reasonable goals of aerobic conditioning in pregnancy should be to maintain a good fitness level throughout pregnancy without trying to reach peak fitness level or train for athletic competition. Women should choose activities that will minimize the risk of loss of balance and fetal trauma.

## Our recommendations on exercise for pregnant women

Moderate and regular exercise and/or physical activity benefits both mothers and offspring. Although some studies have reported the benefits of exercise in reducing the risks of GDM, pre-eclampsia, and caesarean delivery, others have not been able to demonstrate these benefits. Exercise/physical activity also been reported to reduce the risks of large-for-gestational-age/small-for-gestational-age babies and of preterm birth.

Although there are various exercise guidelines for women during pregnancy, the consensus is that 30 minutes or more of moderate physical activity per day on most, if not all, days of the week is desirable. However extreme exercise in late gestation is associated with lower birthweight and the possibility of long-term adverse consequences on the offspring. We therefore would counsel, at this stage of our knowledge, against such extreme forms exercise during the later stages of pregnancy and suggest a more moderate approach.

Chapter 30

# Foods, exposures, and lifestyle risk factors in pregnancy and breastfeeding

## Deciphering the messages about foods and exposures to avoid during pregnancy

Pregnant women can feel bombarded with messages from various sources regarding foods and exposures to avoid during pregnancy. Some of this guidance is sound and should be followed. However, other commonly propagated advice is not based on scientific evidence and may in fact be disadvantageous in some situations. For example, despite common belief, avoidance of certain foods in pregnancy has not been shown to reduce the risk of childhood allergies. In a large population-based UK birth cohort, some dietary patterns were associated with eczema, IgE, lung function, and asthma; however, none had any effect after allowing for other environmental confounders [1292].

Previous advice on food avoidance has included peanut consumption in pregnancy as a potential risk factor for development of peanut allergy in the offspring of women with familial risk factors. A study of the effect of this advice in the UK found that the prevalence of peanut sensitization more than doubled in the ten-year period after the advice on peanut avoidance was publicized [1293]. A recent systematic review of available evidence concluded allergen avoidance in the maternal diet during pregnancy is unlikely to reduce offspring susceptibility to atopic disease, even in high-risk women [1294]. In fact, recent studies have shown that in utero allergen exposure (peanuts and tree nuts) may increase offspring tolerance and reduce the risk of childhood food allergy [1295, 1296]. Hence, avoidance diets in pregnancy, including peanut avoidance, are no longer advocated for the prevention of allergy.

There are, however, various natural substances and toxic contaminants present in our environment and in common foods and drinks that may be harmful to the developing fetus, and consumption of or contact with these substances should be restricted or avoided during pregnancy. There are also a number of known occupational, behavioural, or environmental factors that can affect pregnancy outcomes. Women need to know the possible impact of these so that precautions can be taken and harmful contacts can be minimized.

## Foods to avoid during pregnancy and lactation

Teratogens are substances that have been found to interfere with fetal development and cause birth defects, either in animal studies or from reports of human exposure. Some foods and drinks have been identified as containing teratogens, usually when consumed in high amounts early in pregnancy. There are specific vulnerable periods at different stages of fetal development.

Organogenesis begins around day 16 and continues up to the 8th week post conception. Major malformation of the brain, eyes, ears, limbs, lungs, heart, and kidneys can be caused by the ingestion of teratogens during this critical period. Neural tube defects and some craniofacial malformations stem from disruptions or toxic insults during this window of fetal development. Cleft palate, micro-opthalmia, and hydrocephalus can occur as a result of exposures between days 40 and 60 of gestation. Sexual differentiation starts in this period, and from that point on, exposure to endocrine disruptors can affect male genital development. From the 8th to the 15th week, interference with neuronal proliferation, differentiation, and migration can occur, disrupting brain growth and cognitive development. CNS maturation is also vulnerable throughout the remainder of pregnancy [1297].

### Liver consumption during pregnancy and the risk of excess vitamin A

High maternal exposure to vitamin A or retinoic acid early in pregnancy has been shown to be teratogenic in rodents and humans [229, 1298], causing craniofacial, CNS, thymic, and heart defects. Avoidance of foods and supplements containing high concentrations of preformed vitamin A is strongly recommended (see chapter 6). As vitamin A is stored in the liver of animals, eating liver, especially during early pregnancy, should be avoided.

### Herbal tea consumption during pregnancy and potential risks from polyphenols and phytotoxins

Herbal teas are widely consumed around the world and are rich in polyphenolic compounds with antioxidant and anti-inflammatory properties [1299, 1300]. While these may seem beneficial for pregnant women, overconsumption may have adverse effects. Oral administration of polyphenols extracted from green tea can inhibit the activity of cyclo-oxygenase 2, which mediates the transformation of arachidonic acid into prostaglandins. Substances with the capacity to inhibit maternal circulating prostaglandins in pregnancy can have a constricting effect on the fetal ductus arteriosus, altering fetal haemodynamics and potentially resulting in neonatal pulmonary hypertension. Indeed, maternal consumption of large quantities of polyphenol-rich foods in late pregnancy is reported to be associated with fetal arterial ductal constriction [708]. Among other types of herbal teas, chamomile tea consumption in pregnancy has been associated with constriction of the ductus arteriosus in case reports [1301].

Pyrrolizidine alkaloids are phytotoxins found in plants used in Chinese and Indian (Ayurvedic) herbal remedies and teas, and are contraindicated in pregnancy as they are potentially teratogenic. Comfrey tea preparations can contain pyrrolizidine alkaloids, and cases of fetal hepatic veno-occlusive disease have been reported from high maternal consumption [1302]. This fatal birth defect was also observed following daily consumption of an herbal cooking mixture containing pyrrolizidine alkaloids [1303]. Honey made from plants of genera that produce pyrrolizidine alkaloids, particularly *Senecio*, *Borago*, and *Echium* spp., is another source of ingestion. These plants are significant contributors to honey production in many countries [1304, 1305]. However, most women would not consume enough honey for this to be a problem, and honey is not currently contraindicated in pregnancy.

## Avoidance of contaminated grains during pregnancy and lactation

Mycotoxins are produced by fungi that can contaminate grains such as rice, corn, and wheat. Peanuts, almonds, walnuts, sunflower seeds, and spices, including black pepper and coriander, are also potential sources of contamination. Food can be contaminated during processing, storage, or transport in conditions favourable for mould growth.

Aflatoxins are the most prevalent of the mycotoxin food contaminants, and exposure is common in sub-Saharan Africa and East and South East Asia [1306], where aflatoxins are known to contribute to increased risk of hepatocellular carcinoma [1307, 1308]. Aflatoxin exposure in utero can occur via placental transfer following maternal intake of contaminated foods [1309] or during lactation via contaminated breast milk and has been shown to increase the risk for growth faltering [1310]. Exposure to aflatoxins can cause growth impairment in children [44].

## The consumption of predatory fish during pregnancy

Several toxicants that can negatively affect fetal development have been identified in predatory fish from some regions. These include PCBs, hexachlorobenzene, and mercury. PCBs and hexachlorobenzene are banned industrial organochlorine chemicals that were used extensively in North America and Europe and appear as persistent environmental contaminants in fish and marine mammals living in surrounding waters [1311]. In seafood-eating populations such as Inuit Indians, in utero exposure to moderately high levels of organochlorines and mercury is associated with shortened gestational length and consequent lower birthweight and reduced length and head circumference [1312]. PCBs also interfere with thyroid function during development, resulting in learning and behavioural problems in childhood [1313].

Mercury in the aquatic environment is methylated by bacteria to methylmercury, which is accumulated through the food chain such that the bodies of predatory fish including swordfish, tuna, and shark can acquire high concentrations. All fish contain some level of methylmercury, which may act as a neurotoxicant even at low levels of exposure. The fetus is particularly vulnerable, as many developmental processes are susceptible to disruption by mercury. There are examples of congenital poisoning, for example, following environmental contamination in Japan [1314] and Iraq [1315], resulting in neurological abnormalities and severe developmental delays in children even when mothers showed little or no overt signs of toxicity. The American Pregnancy Association advises that fish containing modest levels of mercury (e.g. bass, carp, Alaskan cod, halibut, Mahi Mahi, freshwater perch, monkfish, sea trout, snapper, and canned tuna) be limited to 1–2 meals per week [216].

The beneficial effects of omega-3 long-chain polyunsaturated fatty acids from a diet high in fish may partially mask the adverse effects of prenatal methylmercury exposure [1316]. Longitudinal studies in a population of high fish consumers have shown no long-term neurological consequences in prenatally exposed offspring at 9 years of age [1317], suggesting that the beneficial influence of fish-derived polyunsaturated fatty acids may counteract the possible adverse effects of prenatal methylmercury exposure. Fish consumption is still recommended during pregnancy, but high consumption of predatory fish and marine mammals should be avoided.

## Sources of foodborne infections during pregnancy

During pregnancy, hormonal changes occur that down-regulate cell-mediated immune function to accommodate the semi-allogenic fetus [1318]. A consequence of these changes is that pregnant women may be more susceptible to some types of infections, or at risk for more severe disease [1319]. For example, *Listeria monocytogenes* infection (listeriosis) occurs most frequently in people whose cellular immunity has been suppressed by drugs, disease, or pregnancy. In healthy adults, including pregnant women, listeriosis causes only minor (usually gastrointestinal) illness but can have profound effects on the developing fetus. *L. monocytogenes* is a gram-positive bacterium that can grow in aerobic or anaerobic conditions. It is a particular concern with regard to food contamination because it can grow at refrigerator temperature and is not killed by freezing [1320]. Ready-to-eat foods such as cold cuts or deli meats and cheeses or other dairy products are likely sources of contamination. In particular, it is advisable that pregnant women avoid mould-ripened soft cheeses (e.g. Camembert, Brie, and blue-veined cheese), unpasteurized milk (or products containing it), pâté (any kind, including vegetable), and uncooked or undercooked ready-prepared meals and meats.

Toxoplasmosis, caused by infection by the protozoan parasite *Toxoplasma gondii*, is another foodborne illness of significant concern for pregnant women. *T. gondii* infection is very common worldwide. Pregnant women who were previously unexposed to the parasite and who become infected during pregnancy usually transmit the infection to their fetus, with potentially serious and lasting consequences, including intellectual disability, blindness, and epilepsy [1321]. Toxoplasmosis can be acquired from eating undercooked meat (mainly pork), or salad vegetables contaminated with soil. *T. gondii* is also present in cat faeces and litter, and pregnant women are advised to avoid coming into contact with cat litter trays. There are some concerns that the increasing use of free-range farming increases the risk of exposure of pigs to grass, soil, feed, and water potentially contaminated with *T. gondii*, possibly increasing the risk of toxoplasmosis from the consumption of organically raised pork [1322]. More studies are needed before advice can be provided on organic vs traditionally farmed meat products for pregnant women at this stage.

In any case, pork and other meats should be cooked thoroughly and eaten soon after cooking to avoid the potential for infection with this parasite during pregnancy. Rare-cooked lamb is also a potential source of infection. It is advisable to cook whole cuts of lamb, pork, veal, or beef to at least 65.6°C (150°F) as measured by a food thermometer [1323]. Fruits and vegetables should be peeled or thoroughly washed before eating. Cutting boards and utensils should be washed with hot soapy water after they have been in contact with raw meat, poultry, seafood, or unwashed fruits or vegetables [1324].

The gram-negative bacteria *Salmonella enterica* can contaminate raw or partially cooked eggs (or foods that may contain them, e.g. mayonnaise and home-made Caesar salad dressing), raw or partially cooked meat (especially poultry), and raw sprouts [1324]. Although pregnant women are at no greater risk of salmonellosis than the general population, if infection occurs in pregnancy it can be transmitted to the fetus, possibly leading to preterm delivery or intrauterine death. As a general precaution, pregnant women are advised not to eat raw or partially cooked meat or eggs. Eggs should be cooked until the yolk and white are firm.

To avoid possible infection with pathogens that may cause fetal harm, all pregnant women, regardless of their diet, are advised to be vigilant about the washing, cooking, and storage of foods. The opinion of researchers from the Motherisk programme in Canada is that improved hygiene standards and surveillance have substantially lowered the risk of infection from deli meats and soft cheeses, such that these no longer need to be avoided if acquired from reputable establishments [1325]. However, most agencies continue to recommend against consumption of these foods. Foods that should be avoided in pregnancy are listed in Table 30.1

**Table 30.1** Forbidden foods

| Food | Risk in pregnancy | Comment/advice |
|---|---|---|
| Liver | Excess vitamin A—teratogenic | Best to avoid, particularly in early pregnancy. |
| Fish with mercury[a] | Fetal brain damage/developmental delay | Avoid large predatory fish. |
| Fish exposed to pollutants (PCBs)[b] | Birth defects | Check with local health authorities whether locally caught fish is safe to eat. |
| Cold deli meat | Listeriosis | Reheat cold meats until steaming hot. |
| Cold smoked seafood[c] | Listeriosis | Reheat until steaming hot. |
| Soft cheeses[d] | Listeriosis | Avoid unless made from pasteurized milk. |
| Pâté (including vegetable) | Listeriosis | Avoid all refrigerated pâtés. Canned or shelf-safe pâtés can be eaten. |
| Unwashed fruits and vegetables | Toxoplasmosis | Peel or wash fruits and vegetables thoroughly before eating. |
| Undercooked or raw meat, poultry or seafood | Toxoplasmosis, salmonella | Cook food thoroughly and eat while hot. |
| Raw eggs[e] | Salmonella | Avoid . |

[a] Predatory fish: swordfish, marlin, tuna, shark, orange roughy, king mackerel, bigeye or Ahi tuna, and tilefish

[b] From contaminated rivers and lakes (locally caught, not from supermarket): bluefish, striped bass, salmon, pike, trout, and walleye

[c] Deli or cold packaged. Canned or shelf-safe smoked seafood is safe to eat

[d] Cheeses made from unpasteurized milk: Brie, Camembert, Roquefort, feta, Gorgonzola, Mexican style cheeses (queso blanco and queso fresco)

[e] Includes homemade dressings made with raw eggs, e.g. Caesar and Hollandaise; also homemade ice creams or custards. Commercially available dressings, custards, and ice creams are made with pasteurized eggs and are considered safe to eat

Source: American Pregnancy Association, *Food to avoid during pregnancy*, copyright © 2014 American Pregnancy Association. <http://americanpregnancy.org/pregnancyhealth/foodstoavoid.html>; US Department of Health and Human Services, *Checklist of foods to avoid during pregnancy*. 2014, <http://www.foodsafety.gov/poisoning/risk/pregnant/chklist_pregnancy.html>; NSW Food Authority, *Foods to eat or avoid when pregnant*, copyright © State of New South Wales through the NSW Food Authority. 2014, <http://www.foodauthority.nsw.gov.au>.

## Caffeine consumption during pregnancy

Approximately 70 per cent of pregnant women in the US report consumption of coffee, soft drinks, and/or tea during pregnancy, at average caffeine intakes of around 150 mg/day [1326]. The methylxanthines theophylline and caffeine found in tea and coffee, and theobromine (an active derivative of caffeine) found in chocolate, are subject to uninhibited transport through the placenta to the fetus [1327]. Caffeine also passes into milk during lactation. Metabolism of methylxanthines is impaired in pregnant women, fetuses, and neonates, allowing accumulation of these substances [1328].

Caffeine increases the levels of catecholamines, which can induce placental vasoconstriction [1329]. High maternal caffeine consumption (>300 mg/day) is mainly associated with an increased risk of fetal growth restriction [1330–1333], although there are also reports of increased risks of spontaneous abortion [1334, 1335], or stillbirth [1336]. Even in the intake range of 200–299 mg/day (3 single espressos or 4–6 cups of tea), caffeine consumption was found to be associated with a statistically significant increased risk of fetal growth restriction, with the strongest effect in women who were rapid metabolizers of caffeine [41].

A longitudinal study demonstrated that exposure to caffeine was related to poorer neuromuscular development and significant increases in breech presentation of fetuses; breech presentation was doubled with caffeine use above 444 mg/day from coffee, tea, and/or chocolate [1337]. The Food Standards Agency in the UK now recommends that women be aware of all the sources of caffeine in the diet that will contribute to their daily intake, including chocolate, energy drinks, and colas in addition to tea and coffee, and to limit their intake of caffeine to 200 mg/day [1338]. In a study in which caffeine consumption was recorded by interview, the level of intake during pregnancy did not have an effect on the sleep patterns of infants up to 3 months of age, although night-time waking was most frequent in infants of mothers with the highest intakes (≥300 mg/day) throughout pregnancy and breastfeeding [1339].

In addition to the possible risks of high caffeine intake during pregnancy, pre-pregnancy caffeine consumption may affect a couple's ability to conceive. Caffeine metabolism varies during the menstrual cycle, with reduced clearance during the luteal phase. This results in caffeine accumulation during the period of implantation and early embryonic development [1340]. High caffeine intake has been shown to reduce conception rates [1341], with a similar decline in fertility in both females and males, the latter effect possibly resulting from an impact of caffeine on semen quality.

Despite numerous reports in the literature, the risks associated with caffeine consumption are still a matter of debate. A recent comprehensive review of 17 epidemiological studies since 2000 concluded that it is not possible to verify a causal relationship between outcomes and caffeine consumption because of confounding issues such as imprecise calculation of caffeine consumption, recall bias, etc. [1342]. Common advice is to limit caffeine intake to 200 mg/day (~2 medium cups of filtered coffee) during pregnancy and breastfeeding, a recommendation that continues to be justified based on the available data.

## Effects of exposure to environmental toxicants during pregnancy and lactation

Prenatal exposures to some relatively low-level environmental contaminants may have significant effects on later development. For example, prenatal lead exposure affects behavioural and cognitive development in children. Endocrine disruptors, a classification of substances that interfere with hormone action, can alter fetal hormone signalling, inappropriately modulating fetal growth and organ development. Indeed the same phenomenon of altered developmental programming that increases susceptibility to diseases later in life as a result of altered maternal nutrition can also be shown for many cases of chemicals with endocrine-disrupting activity. Some commonly encountered toxins that pregnant and lactating women should be aware of are discussed below. This is by no means comprehensive, and there is growing interest in a broader range of potential exposures [1343].

## Lead exposure during pregnancy and lactation

Lead exposure remains a concern for pregnant and lactating women, despite improved policies in many countries to reduce environmental and workplace sources of exposure [1344]. Lead is non-biodegradable and accumulates in soil and dust near industries that utilize lead in manufacturing, and near electronic waste dumps, in addition to its presence in lead paints in old houses, some ceramic glazes, and even common foods and home remedies in some countries [1345, 1346]. Lead accumulates in the skeleton over time, and the increased bone demineralization that occurs during pregnancy causes the release of lead from bone into blood. This results in fetal exposure, as lead readily crosses the placenta via diffusion.

In utero lead exposure can affect the developing nervous system, and in extreme cases leads to spontaneous abortion or fetal death. Prenatal exposure of low levels of lead (less than 10 µg/dL in maternal blood) has been shown to affect indices of infant cognition at 7 months of age [1347]. Paternal employment in the lead industry or other occupations that are associated with exposure to lead (e.g. automotive painting and/or radiator repair, scrap handling, house renovation/paint stripping, demolition of ships or old buildings, etc.) is regarded as an indirect risk to the fetus, as lead dust can be brought into the home on clothing, skin, and hair [1348].

The intellectual functioning of children is affected by lead exposure from an early age, and the effects are long-lasting and irreversible. Therefore, prevention is critical. Recent studies indicate that even low lead exposure can have subtle negative effects on cognitive, behavioural, and neuropsychological development and that every 10 μg/dL increase in blood lead level in children correlates with a drop of 4.6 IQ points [1348].

There are nutritional influences on lead toxicity. Calcium, iron, and vitamin C help protect the developing fetus from the harmful effects of lead exposure. Increased intake of calcium in the diet is known to decrease the gastrointestinal absorption of lead. Women with inadequate calcium intake during pregnancy are more likely to have elevated blood lead levels [1349]. High calcium intake also reduces blood lead exposure in pregnancy by minimizing bone demineralization and the consequent release of lead from bone [1350]. A randomized trial in pregnant women who received 1.2 g calcium/day or placebo starting in the first trimester demonstrated a modest reduction in blood lead levels (with the highest reduction seen in the most compliant group) [1351]. When given during lactation, calcium supplementation (1.2 g/day) has been shown to reduce lead levels in maternal blood (by 15–20%) and breast milk (by 5–10%) [1352, 1353]. Supplementation with 1 g calcium per day during pregnancy and 6 months postpartum delayed the increase in blood lead levels until later in the postpartum period [1354].

Vitamin C has a chelating effect: higher serum ascorbic acid levels correlate with significantly lower blood lead levels [1355, 1356]. The mechanism of the interaction of iron and lead is less well understood, but it is known that iron deficiency increases susceptibility to lead toxicity. Both iron and lead affect the haem biosynthetic process; in particular, lead inhibits the enzyme ferrochelatase, which catalyses the insertion of ferrous iron into protoporphyrin, forming haem. When iron deficiency is present, ferrochelatase is more sensitive to lead effects. Because iron deficiency is common in pregnancy (see chapter 20), it serves as an additional risk factor for lead toxicity. The precautionary advice for pregnant women provided by the US CDC [1357] is outlined in Box 30.1.

Recognition and removal of lead sources is important for the prevention of maternal and neonatal morbidity. Universal screening for maternal lead exposure is recommended in some areas [1345].

## Box 30.1 Advice of the US CDC: precautions for pregnant women regarding lead exposure

◆ Avoid dust from the renovation of older homes—paint peeling or cracking in older homes may release dangerous lead dust.

◆ Stay out of the house if a room with lead paint is being cleaned, painted, or remodelled.

◆ Discuss the use of any home remedies or supplements, some of which may contain lead, with a doctor.

◆ Cravings to eat dirt or clay should also be made known to the doctor.

◆ Avoid work that may involve lead exposure, such as auto refinishing, construction, and plumbing.

◆ Note that indirect maternal exposure can occur when a worker brings home lead dust on clothing.

◆ Household members involved in such occupations should change to clean clothing before entering the home.

◆ Eat foods high in calcium, iron, and vitamin C.

◆ Avoid candies, spices, and non-commercial food products from foreign countries, which sometimes contain lead.

◆ Store food properly—avoid lead-glazed pottery and pewter.

Source: CDC, *Lead: pregnant women*. <http://www.cdc.gov/nceh/lead/tips/pregnant.htm> accessed 7 May 2013. [1357]

## Pesticide exposure during pregnancy and lactation

Pesticides can have neurotoxic and endocrine-disrupting effects in humans and can be harmful to the developing fetus. Several studies have suggested that maternal occupational exposure to agricultural pesticides during pregnancy is associated with increased risk of impaired reproductive development in male offspring [1358–1360]. Among these pesticides is vinclozolin, a fungicide that has been shown to alter epigenetic programming of the male germ line in animals (rats) [1361]. The principal toxic effects induced by vinclozolin and/or its metabolites are related to its anti-androgenic activity.

The organochlorine pesticide dichloro-diphenyl-trichloroethane (DDT) is an effective and relatively inexpensive means of mosquito (malarial vector) control that is still used in some regions, despite being banned in the US in 1972 and its use curtailed around the world in 2001. DDT persists as an environmental contaminant worldwide and accumulates in fatty tissues of animals and humans. Prenatal exposure to DDT was associated with neurodevelopmental delays during early childhood in a highly exposed population working on farms in California [1362]. Other studies have shown that in utero exposure to low-level, background concentrations of DDT may also decrease cognitive function, particularly in girls [1363]. Notably, there was a beneficial effect of breastfeeding, even in highly exposed women.

A longitudinal study of children born to women who were occupationally exposed to pesticides during pregnancy showed immediate and long-term effects on body composition. The exposed children had thicker skin folds and higher body fat percentage at school age than their non-exposed counterparts, with higher exposure correlating with higher adiposity [1364]. The effect was amplified if the children had also been exposed to cigarette smoke in utero. In addition, organophosphate insecticides inhibit acetylcholinesterase, thereby prolonging the action of acetylcholine. A study of an agricultural community with relatively high exposure to these chemicals indicated that in utero exposure has a detrimental impact on neurobehavioural functioning in newborns [1365].

Aside from occupational exposure, substantial exposure to pesticides that may affect the developing fetus can occur in and around the home and garden. Metabolites of indoor pesticides are frequently found in blood samples of pregnant women. Moreover, these substances are able to cross the placental barrier and are detectable in newborn blood [1366].

It is advisable to be aware of and limit occupational exposure to pesticides during pregnancy, including paternal exposure that may be tracked into the household on clothing and skin. Within the home, pesticides should be used with caution and under conditions of adequate ventilation. Protective clothing or gloves should be worn if handling is necessary.

## Herbicide exposure during pregnancy

Atrazine is the herbicide most commonly used in the US and around the world for weed control and is a potent endocrine disruptor. Although monitored by the US EPA [1367], significant concentrations are occasionally found in drinking water in some areas, as a result of run-off from crops sprayed with the chemical. The use of atrazine in plant protection products was banned by the European Commission in 2003 [1368].

Gastroschisis, an increasingly common birth defect involving incomplete closure of the abdominal wall, has been attributed in part to in utero exposure to agricultural chemicals, including atrazine [1369]. A seasonal variation in incidence has been observed, relating to exposure during the peri-conceptional period [1369, 1370]. The mechanism is thought to involve oestrogen disruption. A recent study has shown that the effect is specific to offspring of women ≥25 years of age, as compared with those from younger mothers, possibly relating to the fact that older women have lower first trimester oestrogen levels than younger women, making them more sensitive to oestrogen disruption [1371].

Increased risk for intrauterine growth restriction has also been observed in communities where the municipal drinking water contained higher atrazine concentrations (2.2 µg/L vs 0.6 µg/L) [1372]. Dermal and inhalation exposure of atrazine in farming communities has also been associated with increased incidence of preterm delivery and spontaneous abortion [1373, 1374]. The latter studies involved farming couples where in most cases the fathers had direct exposure to the chemical, and mothers were mainly indirectly exposed through contact with contaminated clothing or by consuming contaminated drinking water. This emphasizes the often overlooked influence of paternal factors, in particular the contribution to potentially damaging exposures, on birth outcomes (see chapter 35 for more detail).

## Exposure to polycyclic aromatic hydrocarbons during pregnancy

Polycyclic aromatic hydrocarbons (PAHs) are formed from incomplete burning of coal, oil, gas, wood, and other organic substances such as tobacco or chargrilled meat. PAHs are found throughout the environment; exposure is mainly as vapours (e.g. cigarette smoke, exhaust fumes, and wood fires) or attached to dust particles. Food grown in contaminated soils may also contain PAHs. Some PAHs, such as benzopyrene, are known to cause tumours in laboratory animals [1375] and DNA damage in humans [1376].

Cigarette smoke exposure increases PAH metabolism in human placental tissue [1377]. However, PAHs do not readily cross the placental barrier, so maternal and placental levels are higher than fetal levels [1378]. In epidemiological studies, prenatal PAH exposure was associated with impaired fetal growth, resulting in reduced birthweight, smaller head circumference, and/or small size for gestational age [1379]. as well as diminished cognitive development [1380, 1381].

The fetus has a heightened susceptibility to PAH-associated DNA damage in early development because of high cell proliferation rates. A critical window of vulnerability to exposure in the first gestational month has been identified [1382], although pre-conception parental exposure is also a factor. Paternal pre-conceptional exposure to PAHs from cigarette smoke or occupational exposure (e.g. oil and gas production, coal-fired and other power plants, and restaurants) has been reported to increase the risk of childhood brain tumours in their offspring [1383], although this assumption remains unconfirmed. Maternal occupational exposure has been linked with an increased risk of gastroschisis [1384]. Occupational exposure to PAHs should be limited if possible, particularly maternally during the first month of pregnancy. Exposure (both first-hand and second-hand) to cigarette smoke should be avoided throughout pregnancy.

## Exposure to bisphenol A during pregnancy

Bisphenol A (BPA) is an endocrine-disrupting chemical present in polycarbonate plastic and epoxy resins and is ubiquitous in the environment. It is classified as a xenoestrogen, meaning it has estrogenic properties. Very small amounts of BPA (below the no-observed-adverse-effect level typical of environmental exposure) alter the development of reproductive organs in mice [1385]. In utero exposure to BPA in sheep increased the fetal expression of CYP19, which is involved in the conversion of androgens to oestrogens, and disrupts the expression of microRNAs involved in regulating oestrogen signalling and insulin homeostasis [1386]. Consequent to such exposure, puberty is accelerated and body weight is increased [1387].

Animal studies suggest that BPA might augment the allergic immune response [1388, 1389], and that prenatal exposure has more profound effects than exposure in adulthood [1390]. A recent study of allergic/asthmatic outcomes relating to prenatal and postnatal BPA exposure measured urinary BPA concentrations in pregnant women (n = 568) and their children at ages 3, 5, and 7 years and found an inverse correlation between prenatal urinary BPA levels and wheeze in children at 5 years of age but a positive association between childhood urinary levels and wheeze or asthma [1391].

BPA is detectable in urine in most people, including pregnant women, and fetal tissues accumulate BPA [1392]. BPA is used in linings of food cans, and has been shown to leach into the food products. Women who regularly eat canned vegetables had higher urinary BPA levels than those who did not. BPA is also found in cigarette filters, and women exposed to cigarette smoke had levels of BPA that were 20 per cent higher than unexposed women. Leaching of BPA from plastic products is increased with heating (microwave) or with repeated use [1393]. Exposure was found to affect childhood behaviour, with higher exposure linked to increased aggression [1394].

Research towards improved understanding of the effect of BPA on humans is ongoing, although preliminary data suggest that caution concerning BPA exposure is warranted, especially for pregnant women and infants. Recommendations for avoiding excess BPA exposure include reducing the amount of canned foods (including beverages) that are consumed, rinsing canned fruits and vegetables before eating them, decreasing the use of plastic food-storage containers, and avoiding heating foods in plastic containers in the microwave. There has been a move away from BPA-containing plasticware used for infant feeding.

## Exposure to arsenic during pregnancy

Arsenic is at the top of the US Agency for Toxic Substances and Disease Registry Priority List of Hazardous Substances [1395]. Its presence in variable amounts in drinking water and some foods is a worldwide health concern. Arsenic readily crosses the placenta, and animal studies suggest it may have growth inhibiting and possibly teratogenic effects, even at low doses that are equivalent to common human exposure in drinking water [1396]. There has been widespread arsenic poisoning in Bangladesh due to groundwater contamination in the Ganges basin [1397], and a prospective cohort study of 1,578 mother–infant pairs in this region showed that arsenic exposure in utero was associated with smaller size at birth [1398]. Other studies have implicated arsenic exposure in increased stillbirth and preterm birth rates [1399].

Grape and apple juices have been reported to contain arsenic, and rice, particularly brown rice grown in the US, is also a potential source. A study found that consumption of one half-cup cooked rice provided the same arsenic exposure as drinking one litre of tap water containing arsenic at the US Environmental Protection Agency's highest allowable level [1400]. A concern has been raised that daily consumption of rice, as in some Asian cultures, may result in elevated exposure to arsenic at levels that may be of concern for the developing fetus.

## Exposure to cadmium during pregnancy

Like arsenic, cadmium is a toxic metal with potential adverse effects for the developing fetus, and is among the top ten substances on the most recent Agency for Toxic Substances and Disease Registry Priority List of Hazardous Substances (2011) [1395]. Cadmium is embryotoxic and teratogenic in animals [1401], although the impact of in utero exposure in humans is not well documented. A negative correlation between maternal and cord blood cadmium levels and infant birth size has been noted [1402]. The mechanism of cadmium teratogenicity may relate to the substitution of cadmium for zinc or calcium in biological processes, and these minerals may be important in lowering the toxicity of cadmium exposure, although human data are minimal [1401]. Individuals with iron, calcium, or zinc deficiency or with protein malnutrition may absorb cadmium at an increased rate [1403].

Inhalation of tobacco smoke is a major source of human exposure to cadmium. Cadmium is used in batteries, pigments, coatings, and platings, as well as stabilizers for plastics, and can enter the food chain, resulting in exposure through foods such as cereals and seafood [1404]. Pregnant women can be exposed to cadmium through their own or their partners' work in cadmium-emitting industries such as smelting and electroplating, wherein the main route of exposure is inhalation of dust and fumes. Exposure can be controlled through the use of protective equipment and good hygiene practices such that cadmium dust is not transferred to the home from the workplace [1405].

## Maternal behaviours that affect pregnancy outcomes

### Alcohol consumption during pregnancy and lactation

Alcohol is considered a dietary teratogen when consumed in large quantities. Acute exposure to ethanol in early gestation compromises development of the cerebral cortex [1406]. In an Australian study of approximately 4,700 women who gave birth between 1995 and 1997, those classified as 'heavy' drinkers in the first trimester were four times more likely to have a baby with a birth defect than those who did not drink [1407]. Chronic or frequent heavy alcohol use during pregnancy confers significant risk of fetal alcohol spectrum disorders, manifestations of which include facial abnormalities, growth deficiency, and nervous system defects. Yet alcohol consumption remains common among pregnant women: a report from Australia found that around 30 per cent of women consumed some alcohol during their pregnancies [1408], and the issue of mild alcohol consumption during pregnancy remains controversial.

In 2001, the Australian National Health and Medical Research Council changed their recommendation from abstinence during pregnancy to advising that women should consume less than seven standard drinks per week, and no more than two standard drinks on any one day [1409]. This message was reversed in 2009 to advise that alcohol avoidance is the safest option for pregnant and breastfeeding women [1410]. The UK Royal College of Obstetricians and Gynaecologists (RCOG) concurs with this opinion, advising that the safest approach in pregnancy is to choose not to drink at all [1411]. Various studies have reported no effect of 'light' alcohol consumption in pregnancy with negative childhood outcomes [1412, 1413], although this is potentially confounded by the fact that light alcohol drinkers tend to be socially advantaged, which may account for some of the favourable development of their offspring.

It is important to note that women are more likely to avoid eating foods that can potentially be contaminated with *Listeria* than to avoid alcoholic beverages, even although the rate of fetal harm from infections is lower than the risk from prenatal alcohol exposure [1414]. Health care professionals need to be more proactive in informing women about the possible harm of alcohol consumption on the fetus. It remains the opinion of most researchers that avoidance of alcohol is the safest choice, as there remains no known safe level of consumption during pregnancy.

## Smoking during pregnancy

Numerous studies have addressed the impact of maternal smoking during pregnancy on infant outcomes (for a review, see [1414]). Although environmental and genetic confounders may limit the interpretation of studies of maternal smoking behaviour in pregnancy and offspring outcome, maternal smoking is clearly a fetal stressor, with multiple potential toxic exposures to the fetus including nicotine, carbon monoxide, and heavy metals. There are also indirect effects resulting from alteration of placental function and umbilical artery blood flow that may impair oxygen exchange across the placenta [1415].

Infants of mothers who smoke during pregnancy are at increased risk of low birthweight and smaller head circumference [1416–1418]. Maternal smoking has also been linked to preterm birth. In an analysis of over 150,000 births in Germany [1419], the risks of preterm delivery and premature rupture of membranes were directly related to the number of cigarettes smoked per day. The incidence of intrauterine growth restriction increased from 5.7 per cent in non-smokers to 15.8 per cent in patients who smoked >10 cigarettes per day. Smoking is associated with an increased risk of intrapartum stillbirth, which is accentuated in adolescent mothers [1420].

Maternal smoking has also been linked to offspring obesity in later life. Women who were exposed to cigarette smoke in utero were at a significantly higher risk of obesity in adulthood, and gestational diabetes in their own pregnancies [1421]. A recent study of >1,600 births reported an increased risk of overweight, specifically in boys at 5 years of age [1422].

Smoking and exposure to second-hand smoke are among the most important preventable risk factors for adverse pregnancy outcomes. Smoking cessation interventions have been shown in numerous studies to reduce the risks associated with maternal smoking [1423]. Efforts should be made by health care professionals to encourage and implement cessation strategies for their patients who are pregnant or planning a pregnancy. According to National Institute for Clinical Excellence guidelines issued in 2008 [266], nicotine replacement therapy should be offered to pregnant women, with instruction that nicotine patches should be removed at night.

## Pica during pregnancy

Pica is a compulsive dietary aberration that occurs worldwide and is prevalent among pregnant women. It is defined as the pathological/persistent craving and consumption of non-food matter such as clay or dirt (geophagia), purified starch (amylophagia), or other substances, including charcoal, ash, paper, chalk, coffee grounds, or egg shells. In a form of pica known as pagophagia, pregnant women consume large quantities of ice (averaging 700 g daily).

Pica is most common in, but not limited to, low socio-economic and under-developed populations and may have strong cultural implications. Among a group of pregnant women studied in rural Kenya in 1999, 73 per cent ate soil (mainly from the walls of houses) on a regular basis. Soil eating was considered to be related to fertility and reproduction, and although not entirely endorsed, was regarded as acceptable behaviour in pregnancy in this society [1424]. Among a US cohort of 553 African American women in an urban environment, 8.3 per cent of women said that they consumed non-food substances before they became pregnant. A larger proportion of this group (28.2%) said that they had seen other family members eat non-foods; the women themselves were most likely to practice pica if the person they had observed doing this was their mother, although the substances they consumed were often different [1425]. Pica was more common among rural, socio-economically disadvantaged African American women; 38 per cent reported pagophagia during pregnancy in a multicentre prospective study [1426].

The primary hypothesis to explain this enigmatic behaviour is that it is associated with specific nutrient deficiencies, particularly of iron, zinc, and calcium. Other proposed explanations for pica suggest that it may be motivated by hunger, psychological stress, or gastrointestinal distress [1427]. However, despite decades of study, the causes of pica remain poorly understood.

Iron supplementation has been evaluated for the treatment of pica, with mixed results [1428]. Pagophagia appears to respond most consistently to supplemental iron treatment. Zinc treatment has also been used with some success in children and mentally handicapped adults [1429], but controlled studies are lacking. Although iron deficiency is thought to be a possible cause of pica, it also appears to be a consequence in some cases, either as a result of decreased consumption of nutritional, iron-containing foods, or because the ingested substances bind (and thereby sequester) elemental iron [1430].

In pregnancy, amylophagia may be involved in precipitating gestational diabetes [1430] or pre-eclampsia [1431]. Potential complications of geophagia include helminth infection [1432] or lead toxicity [1433]. High maternal blood lead levels have been observed in women with geophagia in pregnancy [1434], and fetal lead poisoning can occur as a result of maternal ingestion of plaster [1435]. In the urban African American population described above, women with pica (mainly amylophagia and pagophagia) gave birth to infants with smaller head circumference, compared with nonpica women [1425]. In addition to traces of lead, some soils that are consumed in geophagia may contain *Bacillus* and *Clostridium* spores and should be considered harmful in pregnancy, despite providing a proportion of recommended daily intakes of iron and zinc, as well as traces of magnesium and calcium [1436].

Pica in pregnancy may be under-reported. Anecdotal evidence suggests that few health care professionals question women about pica, despite its apparently widespread prevalence. Women are unlikely to volunteer information about pica, but should be asked, in a non-judgemental manner, if they have any unusual cravings during pregnancy.

## The use of over-the-counter drugs during pregnancy

The use of pain relieving/anti-inflammatory drugs is common in pregnancy. Some of these drugs are available over-the-counter, such as paracetamol (acetaminophen) and the nonsteroidal anti-inflammatory drugs (NSAIDs) ibuprofen, diclofenac, naproxen, and aspirin. Data are conflicting regarding the effect of prescribed or over-the-counter NSAIDs on pregnancy outcomes, with some studies linking use in early pregnancy with spontaneous abortion [1437, 1438], but others finding no such association. Most studies were not able to find associations with specific NSAIDs. A study looking specifically at over-the-counter NSAIDs found no evidence that non-prescription drugs such as ibuprofen are linked to an increased risk of spontaneous abortion [1439].

Other studies have suggested that NSAID use in late pregnancy is associated with persistent pulmonary hypertension in the newborn, a serious and sometimes fatal disorder caused by a maladaptive pulmonary vascular response during the transition at birth from fetal to neonatal circulation [1440, 1441]. This association is biologically plausible, given the inhibitory effect of NSAIDs on prostaglandin synthesis, which are involved in the regulation of pulmonary vasculature and maintenance of ductal patency [1442]. However, a recent large multicentre epidemiological study did not find evidence to support the hypothesis that NSAID use in pregnancy increases the risk of persistent pulmonary hypertension [1443].

Regular or frequent paracetamol use in late pregnancy was associated with an increased risk of childhood asthma and wheeze in a population-based longitudinal study in the UK [1444]. The increased risk was observed in the offspring followed up to 7 years of age [1445] and is supported by a recent meta-analysis of additional studies [1446]. The effect of paracetamol on asthma risk may be related to increased oxidative stress, brought on by a reduction in glutathione [1447, 1448].

The link between paracetamol use and asthma is also supported by a number of epidemiological studies in adults, and exposures in young children (for reviews and meta-analysis see [1449, 1450]). It is therefore advisable for pregnant women to limit their use of paracetamol, especially during late gestation. A recent study has also suggested that prolonged paracetamol use (≥28 days) during pregnancy may increase the risk of poor gross motor functioning and other adverse developmental outcomes, including externalizing behaviour and negative emotionality in children. There was a trend towards stronger effects following exposure during the third trimester [1451].

## Skipping breakfast or maintaining a low-carbohydrate diet during pregnancy

Skipping breakfast or maintaining a very low-carbohydrate diet during pregnancy can result in amplification of maternal ketosis. Ketones are produced as by-products of fatty acid metabolism. Conditions that amplify maternal ketosis, such as diabetes and malnutrition, are associated with a less favourable fetal outcome. Hyperketonaemia can cause increased circulating levels of pro-inflammatory cytokines and markers of oxidative stress [1452]. Ketones readily cross the placenta and may impair fetal neuropsychological development if present in excess [1453].

Ketone levels rise threefold in pregnant women when breakfast is omitted, a condition that has been referred to as 'accelerated starvation' [1454]. Accelerated starvation is a mechanism occurring in pregnancy whereby carbohydrate depletion causes a rapid adaptation to metabolize fat as energy, so that less expendable fuels, such as glucose and amino acids, are spared for the growth of the fetus. It is associated with hypoglycaemia, elevated plasma levels of free fatty acids, and increased urinary excretion of nitrogen and ketones. As glucose is transferred for fetal consumption, the resulting fall in maternal circulating glucose suppresses insulin secretion, enhancing lipolysis and conversion of fatty acids to ketones. Fetal blood glucose levels also fall and ketone levels rise in response to prolonged maternal fasting [1455].

Non-diabetic pregnant women are vulnerable to enhanced ketosis during brief periods of fasting in the third trimester. Falls in insulin and glucose coincident with increased free fatty acids and ketones are factors in widespread metabolic changes [1456]. Because such conditions partially mimic the diabetic state, this is thought to be harmful in pregnancy, both for the mother and the fetus. However, several studies indicate no adverse effect of gestational Ramadan fasting in healthy pregnant women on maternal oxidative stress, fetal development, or birthweight [1457–1459], despite a higher incidence of ketonuria observed in fasting women [1460] (see also chapter 31).

The increasing popularity of low-carbohydrate diets, including the 'Palaeolithic' diet (which is known to be ketogenic), has raised questions about the effect of enhanced ketosis on pregnancy outcomes. Although there are examples of healthy women and their offspring coping with fasting and enhanced ketosis during gestation, thorough studies on the effect of this metabolic shift on fetal outcomes are lacking. Results from prospective cohort studies such as the Southampton Women's Survey and other studies show that unbalanced diets (especially a low-carbohydrate, high-protein diet) in early pregnancy are associated with alterations in cardiovascular structure, blood pressure, cortisol levels, and adiposity in the children [88, 1461–1463]. In general, such diets and fasting are currently not recommended during pregnancy. Women who choose to follow these practices should be closely monitored, although it should be recognized that educational and other socio-economic factors often contribute to the consumption of such diets, so they are not always a matter of choice.

## The use of hair dyes and skincare products during pregnancy and lactation

A recent report released by the RCOG [1464] has suggested that pregnant women might wish to consider minimizing the use of various personal care products, including moisturizers, cosmetics, shower gels, and fragrances, because of the potential for harmful exposure to their fetuses. However, a review of multiple studies on the level of exposure from such products concluded that use of cosmetics and other personal care products confers minimal exposure risk [1465]. This is consistent with data from other sources as reviewed in 2005 by the Cosmetic Ingredient Review Expert Panel in the US [1466].

In general, skincare products act locally and have little systemic effect and therefore most are safe to use during pregnancy. However there are notable exceptions, including the skin-bleaching agent hydroquinone and the acne medication tretinoin/isotretinoin, both of which can cause birth defects [1467]. Acne creams containing benzoyl peroxide or salicylic acid are considered safe to use during pregnancy. Topical preparations containing glycolic acid (an alpha-hydroxy acid) are also assumed to be safe to use, as very little is expected to be absorbed systemically. Similarly, topical hair removal agents containing thioglycolic acid (<5%), and hair bleaching creams containing hydrogen peroxide are not expected to cause problems if not used excessively [1467].

Various claims have been made about the safety of hair dyes, which contain N-nitroso compounds that have been shown to be mutagenic and carcinogenic in animals. As with most other topical cosmetic products, ingredients in hair dyes exhibit only minimal penetration of skin. Nonetheless, there is some concern that use of hair dyes could increase the likelihood of cancers in the offspring, despite inconsistent data.

For example, although a possible connection between maternal hair dye use in pregnancy and childhood brain tumours was not confirmed [1468], one study found some association with increased risk of neuroblastoma, and, specifically, more risk with temporary dyes than with permanent dyes [1469]. The effect was seen with exposure one month before and/or during pregnancy. An increased risk of childhood germ cell tumours was also observed with exposure to hair dyes one month prior to conception [1470]. Interestingly, this effect was sex-specific, with an increased risk for male offspring. The same study noted an increased risk for germ cell tumours in female offspring of mothers exposed to hair dyes while breastfeeding [1470]. Thus, although the risk may be low, we would advise women to delay the use of hair dyes until at least the end of the first trimester, if not throughout pregnancy and breastfeeding. Occupational exposure to hair dyes does not appear to pose a risk [1471].

## Our recommendations concerning foods, exposures, and lifestyle risk factors during pregnancy and lactation

The lists of food, lifestyle, and environmental risk factors to be avoided may seem dauntingly long to newly pregnant women. New advice, often based on minimal evidence, is publicized in the news media or online on a near daily basis. This can cause undue stress during a time when stress should be minimized for the wellbeing of both mother and fetus (see chapter 33 for more on maternal stress).

While certain chemical exposures can cause serious adverse effects in the developing fetus, a report from the United Nations Environment Program and the WHO concluded that most effects of endocrine-disrupting chemicals have been observed in areas where chemical contamination was high [1472]. However, occupational exposures should be minimized, and, where possible, reduction of exposures in the home is advisable. Although evidence is still accumulating, it also appears prudent to try to minimize exposure to BPA during pregnancy.

With regard to food and lifestyle factors, women with reasonably healthy lifestyles prior to pregnancy should not find the recommendations above too onerous. The most important modifiable risk factors discussed here include smoking and exposure to second-hand smoke, alcohol consumption, and avoidance of foodborne illness. Excess consumption of caffeine and herbal teas should also be avoided, along with seafood that is high in mercury. Unusual cravings (pica) should be discussed, and measures taken to curb consumption of non-food items if this occurs. We recommend that alcohol, tobacco, and illicit drugs be avoided completely during pregnancy, and we would suggest that where practical, both parents should abstain from the use of these substances in the weeks prior to conception.

# Chapter 31

# Cultural and traditional food practices in pregnancy and breastfeeding

## Pregnancy-related diet, food practices, and 'taboos'

A woman's dietary intake before and during pregnancy and through lactation is influenced by her sociocultural environment. Some traditional health care beliefs and food practices favoured in different cultures appear to result from efforts to address specific environmental challenges. For instance, Native American populations incorporated lye, ash, or lime (which were all alkaline) into their maize cooking procedures in a manner that balances the essential amino acids and frees the otherwise unavailable niacin [1473]. Without these practices, they would face widespread malnutrition, including niacin deficiency (pellagra) and a lack of certain essential amino acids [1473]. Other examples include intricate processing techniques which would protect foraging and horticultural populations from the toxins present in otherwise valuable food sources such as acorns, cycads, and cassava [1474–1476]. The use of pathogen-killing spices in meat preparations are believed to protect people in warmer climates from foodborne illnesses [1477]. This chapter discusses the implications of some common food practices, as well as cultural practices that are specific to pregnancy and lactation, on maternal and infant health.

Cultural beliefs and practices can markedly influence a woman's pregnancy and childbirth experiences, and may shape her mothering behaviour. Immigrants to a new country often attempt to balance the values of their cultural heritage with those of the host society, which can create tension for pregnant women. Their traditional beliefs and practices may not always follow the biomedical norms of maternal nutrition for optimal fetal growth and obstetric outcomes [1478]. Yet it is important to recognize and respect these beliefs while guiding women towards optimum nutrition and away from harmful practices or prohibitions.

Food taboos exist in virtually all human societies. What may be considered unsuitable by one group may be perfectly acceptable to another. Even when

**Table 31.1** 'Hot' and 'cold' foods according to Indian custom[a] [1481]

| Hot foods—prohibited in pregnancy[b] | Cold foods—encouraged in pregnancy |
| --- | --- |
| Meat, chicken | Milk, yoghurt[a], buttermilk[a] |
| Eggs | Butter, ghee[a] |
| Fish | Coconut |
| Ghee[c] | Green leafy vegetables |
| Pulses/lentils | Wheat[a] |
| Aubergine (eggplant) | Rice[a] |
| Onion, garlic | Bananas[a] |
| Dates | |
| Jaggery[d], sugar | |
| Alcohol | |
| Coffee, tea | |
| Most spices, including ginger and chilies | |
| Papaya | |
| Banana | |
| Pumpkin | |
| Wheat | |
| Rice | |
| Yoghurt[a], buttermilk[a] | |

[a] The perception of these foods as hot or cold varies from region to region in India

[b] Hot foods are encouraged in late pregnancy to facilitate labour

[c] Clarified butter

[d] Course, dark brown sugar

Source: Choudhry, U.K., Traditional practices of women from India: pregnancy, childbirth, and newborn care, *Journal of Obstetric, Gynecologic, and Neonatal Nursing*, Volume 26, Issue 5, pp. 533–9, copyright © 2007 John Wiley & Sons, Inc.

based on myths and misconceptions, they can serve bring a society together, maintain its identity, and create a sense of belonging for the group. In many cases the 'taboo' food is not something that would be considered essential for pregnant women, unless it is among few other sources of essential nutrients in their normal diet. Several cultures adhere to a practice of restricting certain fishes from the pregnancy diet (e.g. some populations in West Malaysia, Papua New Guinea [1479], and Fiji [1480]). If the woman has no other significant source of omega-3 fatty acids in pregnancy, this restriction may be of concern but otherwise may not be harmful. In some cases, these food taboos may even have a utilitarian origin because they selectively target the most toxic marine species, effectively reducing a woman's chances of poisoning during pregnancy and breastfeeding [1480].

In India, and for many immigrant women of Indian descent, there is a belief that pregnancy generates a 'hot' state, and foods that are considered 'cold' are desirable in order to achieve a balance. 'Hot' foods should be avoided to reduce the risk of miscarriage but are given in the last stages of pregnancy to facilitate labour. These terms do not relate to the temperature or spiciness of the food but rather to its perceived nature, although most spices are considered hot (see Table 31.1). Some of these perceptions of 'hot' and 'cold' foods vary by region in India, such that foods considered hot in one region are viewed as cold in another [1481].

Koreans have a long history of food beliefs influenced by centuries-old practices of shamanism (animism), Buddhism, Taoism, and Confucianism. Ancient cures often included the use of garlic and ginseng, among other herbs [1482]. Foods such as seaweed soup, beef, and rice are considered to have qualities that will strengthen the body during the difficult time of pregnancy [1482].

## Fasting and dieting during pregnancy

In some societies in Africa and Asia, small women practice 'eating down' in pregnancy [1188, 1481, 1483, 1484]. This practice is based on the idea that a small baby is less likely to hurt or kill the mother in childbirth, and its origin is understandable in places where midwifery is non-existent. It is concerning that proposals for the promotion of 'eating down' are currently being considered in some Asian cities to reduce the rates of caesarean section, without consideration of the long-term potential harm of such behaviours for the offspring. The outcome of famine restricted to the last trimester has been well documented in the Dutch famine and includes a greater risk of obesity, glucose intolerance, and hypertension [32, 1485]. These findings are supported by studies of the Chinese famine of the Great Leap Forward era [34, 1486] and of the Biafra civil war famine [33].

Ramadan is the one-month obligatory fasting period in Islamic religion, during which no food or drink (including water) can be consumed from dawn to sunset. Although pregnant women are allowed to defer fasting until after pregnancy, many pregnant women prefer to fast in order to share the spiritual and social experiences of Ramadan with their families. Pregnant women who fast during Ramadan are reported to have symptoms of 'accelerated starvation' (as characterized by low serum levels of glucose and alanine and high levels of free fatty acids—see chapter 30, 'Maternal behaviours to limit during pregnancy and lactation') [1487, 1488]. While there have been conflicting reports, more robust studies suggest that Ramadan fasting is associated with reduced birth size and possibly placental size [1488–1490]. In general, dieting prior to and in pregnancy is not recommended except in the management of gestational diabetes and significant obesity; fad diets and diets for cosmetic reasons should be avoided.

## Postpartum food practices and beliefs

In certain cultures and societies, women practice postpartum food restriction (also known as confinement diets) and behaviour following delivery. Women in several Asian countries such as China, Korea, Thailand, and Singapore are known to perform a traditional postpartum practice called 'doing the month' or 'sitting month' [1491–1493]. During this month, women lie in bed continually, with doors and windows closed [1494–1496]. These women are advised to consume plenty of eggs, meat, chicken soup, brown sugar water, and millet every day, often with large amounts of ginger and garlic, while simultaneously avoiding any raw and cold foods such as fruits and vegetables, which are believed to be unfavourable for postpartum recovery [1494–1496]. Many Chinese women who have immigrated to Western countries still believe in the importance of this traditional postpartum practice [1497–1500].

The Indian belief that the state of 'hotness' generated by pregnancy is balanced by the consumption of 'cold' foods has a postpartum counterpart. It is believed that delivery of the baby upsets the balance achieved during pregnancy and brings about weakness; so, to return a new mother to a state of balance, it is desirable to include milk, ghee, nuts, and jagerry in the diet, and to avoid consuming cold food and water. Dried ginger is eaten in the belief that it helps control postpartum bleeding and acts as a uterine cleansing agent [1481].

Many cultures, particularly the lower educated segments of the populations, maintain a practice of withholding colostrum and giving newborns prelacteal feeds that often include honey or sugar water. These practices have been reported in Africa [1501, 1502], India [1481], China, and other Asian societies [1503]. This practice continues today, for instance in Ethiopia [1492], where colostrum is considered either non-nutritive or harmful to infant health. Prelacteal feeding behaviours continue and in most cases are maladaptive, as they do not provide the immunological benefits of colostrum and may contain harmful contaminants. A 2009 study in Turkey found that newborn infants are commonly fed sugar water [1504]. Many postnatal practices which are considered harmful have been identified in Turkey [1505].

## Summary and recommendations concerning cultural and traditional food practices during pregnancy and lactation

Cultural beliefs and practices play a role in the distribution of nutrition messages to the community, and those adopted by pregnant women can affect their birth outcomes. Many of these beliefs and practices have been passed down for generations without any scientific or validated health reasons behind them. Postpartum food restrictions and practices may also affect the mother's and infant's health following delivery.

It is important to examine different contributing and constraining factors (e.g. pregnancy experience, food habits, and related beliefs and practices) not only for effective health care and awareness about traditional food beliefs and habits but also to make subsequent improvements in overall health and pregnancy outcomes of women globally. Interventions and educational support are also needed in order to improve the quality of maternal diet, in particular for those who are still practising cultural traditions that may be harmful to the mother's and their offspring's health outcomes.

Chapter 32

# Traditional and herbal remedies in pregnancy and breastfeeding

## The use of complementary medicine during pregnancy and lactation

Women are the highest consumers of complementary and alternative medicine [1506], and the use of herbal medicine during pregnancy has become very common worldwide. Those who use these therapies tend to believe they offer safe alternatives to pharmaceuticals, allow greater choice and control over the childbearing experiences, and are compatible with their holistic health beliefs. Regarding herbal products, pregnant women tend to rely on advice from family and friends and often do not disclose their use of herbal medicine to their health care providers [1501]. However, it is important for health care providers to be aware of the effects of and precautions associated with the use of herbal medicine, bearing in mind the weak evidence base to support claims for efficacy and the lack of standards of quality and potency for many of the available products.

Herbs that are frequently used by pregnant women include ginger, chamomile, liquorice, fennel, aloe, valerian, echinacea, almond oil, propolis, and cranberry [1507]. Among Chinese populations, traditional Chinese medicine is officially recognized as a medical profession and remains an important form of medical care, including that for pregnant and breastfeeding women [1508, 1509]. In a study of ~21,000 women from the Taiwan Birth Cohort Study, at least one Chinese herbal medicine was used by 33.6 per cent and 87.7 per cent of the participants during pregnancy and the postpartum period, respectively [1510].

## Indications for the use of herbal remedies during pregnancy

### The use of herbal remedies for pregnancy-induced nausea and vomiting

Ginger root (*Zingiber officinale*) has been used worldwide for morning sickness, and some efficacy has been shown in a few small randomized trials [1511–1513].

However, the use of ginger during pregnancy is not without precautions. Ginger is known for its anticoagulant effect [1514], and women taking anticoagulant therapy such as heparin or warfarin, nonsteroidal anti-inflammatories, aspirin, or other drugs or herbs which have a similar action are recommended to avoid ginger completely. In addition, women prone to dizziness, which affects some expectant mothers, as well as those on anti-hypertensive medication, are recommended not to take ginger [1514].

Although there is no real evidence of adverse effects of ginger on the developing fetus, the German E Commission on herbal medicines recommends that ginger should be avoided during pregnancy [1514]. Finland has placed a warning on the labels of all ginger medicinal products as being unsafe for use in pregnancy due to the possibility of the impairment of fetal development [1515]. Denmark has also issued warnings to pregnant women about the high levels of ginger in a particular product, GraviFrisk™, which was banned in 2008 [1516].

### The use of herbal remedies for urinary tract infections during pregnancy

Unsweetened cranberry juice or cranberry pills have been used as a complementary support for the treatment of urinary tract infections (UTIs) during pregnancy. Cranberries are claimed to help prevent and inhibit infections by preventing *E. coli* bacteria from sticking to the bladder wall [1517, 1518]. Daily consumption of cranberry juice in multiple doses has been reported to have a trend in reducing UTIs, with no effects on either obstetric or neonatal outcomes [1519].

Among women receiving cranberry juice, there was a reduction in the frequency of both asymptomatic bacteriuria (57%) and the prevalence of UTIs (41%) [1519]. The 2012 Cochrane review on the use of cranberry for the prevention and treatment of UTIs reported a small benefit for women with recurrent UTIs; however, there were no statistically significant differences when the results of a much larger study were included [1520]. Since UTIs can also be a precursor to preterm labour [1521], the use of herbal medicine should not be used solely in the treatment of UTIs, and it should always be monitored by the physician.

### The use of herbal remedies to treat mild depression during pregnancy

St John's wort (*Hypericum perforatum*) is commonly used in both the US and Europe to treat mild depression. St John's Wort contains hypericin and hyperforin, which play a significant role in this herb's pharmacological effect in the treatment of depression [1522, 1523]. However, safety concerns regarding the use of this herb have been raised, as studies indicated that its use may potentiate other antidepressant drugs and decrease the effectiveness of oral contraceptives and the protease inhibitors used to treat HIV [1517]. Its safety in pregnancy is not known.

## The use of herbal remedies to treat skin conditions during pregnancy

Aloe vera gel is one of the ten most commonly used herbs but should be used externally only. Topical use is considered safe in pregnancy. The gel is effective for the quick healing of burns [1517].

## The use of herbal remedies as labour aids

Raspberry, castor oil, and blue cohosh have been administered to pregnant women for labour aid [1507]. Evidence is thus far insufficient to support claims of efficacy for raspberry leaf, in the form of tea, tablets, or tincture [1524, 1525]. The most common adverse effect is lowered blood pressure. Because of the lack of efficacy and safety data, the use of raspberry leaf extracts in pregnancy is questionable [1526].

Castor oil has also been used to initiate labour. In a prospective cohort study of 103 singleton pregnancies with intact membranes at 40 to 42 weeks gestation, participants were alternately assigned to receive either a single oral dose of castor oil (60 mL) or no treatment [1527]. The study revealed that women who received castor oil had an increased likelihood of initiation of labour within 24 hours compared to women who received no treatment. Specifically, following treatment with castor oil, 30 of 52 women (57.7%) began active labour compared to 2 of 48 (4.2%) receiving no treatment. In addition, 83.3 per cent (25/30) of the women who received castor oil delivered vaginally.

Blue cohosh however, should be avoided for labour aid. Jones and Lawson [1528] reported that a newborn infant whose mother ingested an herbal medication containing blue cohosh to promote uterine contractions experienced acute myocardial infarction associated with profound congestive heart failure and shock. Severe cases of multi-organ hypoxic injury and perinatal stroke have also been reported in neonates whose mothers consumed blue cohosh [1529, 1530].

# Summary and recommendations for the use of traditional and herbal remedies during pregnancy and lactation

Women commonly look towards herbal remedies as 'natural' alternatives to promote and maintain health during pregnancy and breastfeeding. Some pregnant women believe that herbal remedies are more effective and that they have fewer side effects than prescription medications. Although the use of these products has been widely promoted by television, magazines, and the internet, the evidence for efficacy of most of the products is extremely limited.

There is some government regulation of herbal medicine in Europe. However, in the US, herbs are classified as dietary supplements. Therefore, manufacturers are not required to conduct studies of the efficacy or safety of herbs before selling them to the public, and, overall, too few studies have been conducted to permit clinical guidance. With the exception of ginger, there is currently not enough data to support the use of any other herbal supplements during pregnancy. Therefore, it is recommended that women who are interested in using herbal remedies should discuss their symptoms and wishes with their doctors. Pregnant women should not use over-the-counter herbs and supplements in pregnancy without prior consultation with their health care providers.

Chapter 33

# Maternal stress in pregnancy and breastfeeding

## The stress response during pregnancy

There are a number of reasons for women to avoid stress as much as possible in pregnancy. Acute stress can trigger maternal vasoconstriction, decreasing uterine blood flow [1531] and possibly resulting in the restriction of oxygen and vital nutrients to the fetus, as evidenced in studies in primates [1532, 1533]. Chronic stress can lead to chronic hypercortisolaemia, with metabolic consequences for mother and fetus. There is also growing evidence to suggest that a parent's adverse experience both pre-conceptionally and during pregnancy can affect the ability of their offspring to cope with adverse life events.

Acute stress triggers an autonomic response involving release of the catecholamines epinephrine and norepinephrine [1534]. Chronic stress is associated with increased reactivity of the hypothalamic–pituitary–adrenal axis, which mediates a sustained neuro-endocrine response. In this stress response, corticotropin-releasing hormone is synthesized in the hypothalamus, promoting the release of adrenocorticotropic hormone into the bloodstream. This hormone stimulates the adrenal cortex to release glucocorticoids, mainly cortisol, which acts both centrally and peripherally through ubiquitously distributed intracellular receptors. Glucocorticoids normally play a role in energy metabolism, growth processes, and in the functioning of the immune system and the brain. During exposure to stressful stimuli, they govern the intensity of the stress response and are key to its termination via negative feedback control [1535, 1536].

The placenta provides a barrier to natural glucocorticoids, buffering the fetus from minor changes in maternal cortisol levels. The enzyme 11-beta-hydroxysteroid dehydrogenase type 2 inactivates cortisol into the relatively inactive cortisone. However, this barrier can be saturated by high maternal levels of cortisol, and, under conditions of maternal under-nutrition and where there is placental compromise, levels of the enzyme are reduced [1537, 1538]. The consequent higher levels of cortisol in the fetal circulation may play some role in accelerating fetal maturation to make a premature birth more viable, but they are also strongly implicated in the longer term consequences as reflected in the cluster of phenomena related to the developmental origins of health and disease [1539–1541].

## Stress and conception

Stressors prior to pregnancy may impact the ability to conceive, as physiological stress responses could affect ovulation, implantation, or other aspects of successful conception. A relatively high degree of anxiety and depression has been noted among infertile couples (both idiopathic and non-idiopathic), although dissecting the cause from the effect of stress in these situations is difficult [1542]. A recent meta-analysis of 14 prospective studies conveyed an assurance to women that emotional distress, which is often associated with unintended childlessness, should not significantly reduce the chances of successful conception via IVF [1543].

## Stress and pregnancy outcomes

### The effect of stress on preterm birth and low birthweight

High maternal antenatal stress or anxiety is predictive of poorer obstetric outcomes, most commonly preterm delivery and/or low birthweight [1544]. In a large Danish epidemiological study (n = 5,873), the experience of life events during pregnancy that were perceived by the mother as highly stressful was associated with a greater risk of preterm delivery [1545]. The effect appears to be stronger in more socio-economically deprived groups.

In poor African American and Hispanic groups, women experiencing high levels of stress (a combination of life events, anxiety, and perceived stress), were several-fold more likely to deliver preterm [1546]. Unfortunately, studies of interventions designed to provide psychosocial support for such high-risk women were not found to reduce the incidence of low birthweight among infants [1547, 1548]. A recent study showed that infants born in New York to women who were pregnant at the time of the September 11, 2001 terrorist attacks on the World Trade Center and the Pentagon were more likely to be born preterm, or to be small for gestational age or of low birthweight. It was hypothesized that environmental pollution and stress in New York at that time contributed to this trend [1549].

### The effect of stress on offspring behavioural outcomes

Increases in maternal glucocorticoid levels can provide hormonal cues to the fetus about its future environment, potentially resulting in profound changes in offspring phenotype [1550]. There is growing evidence that exposure to stressful influences in prenatal life can permanently alter the biological response to stress later in life [1551]. In a controlled study, young adults whose mothers had experienced extreme social stress during pregnancy had higher corticotropin-releasing hormone neuronal activity when exposed to psychosocial stress in the Trier Social Stress Test. When exposed to this test, the prenatally stressed subjects also showed a higher increase in cortisol than control subjects, despite having lower cortisol levels prior to the test [1552].

Numerous studies have shown consistent associations between maternal stress during pregnancy and an increased risk of emotional and behavioural problems and impaired cognitive development in their offspring [1553, 1554]. Some have suggested a direct effect of maternal anxiety on fetal brain development [1555], with specific influences on the amygdala, which is involved in the generation of anxiety responses [1556]. The amygdala is activated in the presence of fear-provoking stimuli in humans, and a larger amygdala has been noted in children with generalized anxiety disorder [1557]. A recent study has linked maternal stress hormone levels in human pregnancy with subsequent volume of the amygdala and affective problems in childhood [1558]. Some large cohort studies have found an elevated incidence of autism or attention deficit hyperactivity disorder in children born to women exposed to stressful situations during pregnancy, particularly during the third trimester [1559–1561]. Other studies, however, have not found support for this association [1562].

## The effect of stress on the risk of congenital malformations

There is very limited evidence that offspring of women exposed to emotional stress from severe life events (e.g. death of a child) during the first trimester are at higher risk of congenital abnormalities. The defects were predominantly cleft lip and/or palate and congenital heart malformations. The tissues involved in such abnormalities originate from the cranial neural crest and are vulnerable to disruption during early pregnancy [1563].

## Stress hormones and lactation

Transmission of abnormally high levels of glucocorticoids through breast milk has been shown in animal models to modify brain development. Animals exposed to elevated levels of glucocorticoids in milk during infancy display stably altered hypothalamic–pituitary–adrenal axis regulation and altered behavioural responses to stress [1564]. In humans, glucocorticoids in breast milk, which rise in relation to stress, have been shown to influence infant behaviour and temperament, particularly among female offspring [1565, 1566].

## Stress and the offspring sex ratio

The secondary sex ratio refers to the proportion of male births in a population and is usually around 0.51 (i.e. a slight excess of males). A prominent hypothesis is that the sex ratio is partially controlled by the hormone levels of both parents at the time of conception, girls being favoured by high levels of gonadotropins and low levels of testosterone [1567]. The sex ratio may also be affected by maternal stress, as it has been reported to decline after environmental or natural disasters [1568, 1569], war [1570, 1571], and periods of economic instability [1572, 1573]. In general, male fetuses appear to be more susceptible to maternal stress than female fetuses. For example, women who were pregnant during times of social stress such as the 1995 Kobe earthquake in Japan [1569] and the September 11 World Trade Center attacks [1574] produced significantly fewer male offspring than female offspring. Paternal stress could also contribute to this effect, as reduced sperm motility was observed among stressed males after the Kobe earthquake [1575].

## Summary and recommendations for managing maternal stress during pregnancy and lactation

Multiple threads of evidence suggest that severe stress is detrimental to both the mother and her fetus during pregnancy, with effects that can be long-lasting for the offspring. Unfortunately this type of stress is not always easily avoided. The effects of day-to-day stress on pregnancy outcomes are difficult to measure and have not been adequately studied.

Pregnancy itself can be stressful for women in many ways. The ever-growing list of what prospective mothers should and should not do, and the potential to blame oneself for failing to do or avoid those things, are not insignificant factors in this. Yet being stressed is itself counted among the prohibited behaviours that a pregnant woman may feel guilty about—continuing the cycle of stress [1576].

We recommend that women be cautious about behaviours that are known to carry significant potential risks to their unborn child (e.g. smoking, heavy drinking, eating risky foods, and exposure to known toxins/teratogens) but not to worry too much about unknown risks or factors that cannot be controlled. Anxiety in pregnancy is a predictor of postpartum depression [1577]; for this and the other reasons outlined above, caregivers should do what they can to reduce the anxiety levels in their patients by providing sound advice that is not overly burdensome for pregnant women to follow.

Chapter 34

# Effects of maternal age on pregnancy outcomes

## Advanced maternal age in pregnancy and breastfeeding

Maternal age on both ends of the reproductive spectrum (teenage and 35+) is associated with increased risk of adverse pregnancy outcomes compared with the 20–34 year old age range. Pregnancy in women in their late 30s to mid -40s is becoming increasingly more common. However, advanced maternal age (≥44 years) is associated with significantly higher odds of medical complications during pregnancy and more interventions during delivery [1578].

Analysis of a large data set from the US National Center for Health Statistics (the Birth Cohort Linked Birth and Infant Death Data, 1995–2000; n > 8 million singleton pregnancies) showed a decrease in mean birthweight and an increase in the proportion of low-birthweight babies and preterm births among older mothers [1579]. Maternal age ≥45 years was associated with an increase in the risk of hypertension, diabetes, and infant death, including death due to congenital abnormalities. Older women were at higher risk for excessive bleeding and breech presentation and were more likely to have prolonged, dysfunctional labour. These factors contributed increased frequencies of labour induction, use of forceps or vacuum, and caesarean delivery with advancing maternal age [1579].

Diminishing cardiovascular reserve and a reduced ability to adapt to physical stress, both of which accompany the normal ageing process, may contribute to some of these outcomes. Additional factors such as the higher prevalence of overweight and obesity [1580] and uterine fibroids among older mothers [1581] are also likely to influence the poorer pregnancy outcomes in this group. The risk of adverse pregnancy outcomes is elevated in women who receive treatment for infertility, the majority of whom are over 30 years of age, although some of this increased risk may be related to the cause of the infertility itself.

## The effects of advanced maternal age on maternal morbidity and mortality

Some of the increase in pregnancy complications in older mothers is caused by underlying age-related health issues such as hypertension and diabetes, which increase linearly with increasing age [1582]. Related diseases can also develop during pregnancy, including gestational diabetes, severe pre-eclampsia, and pregnancy-induced hypertension, for which older mothers are at increased risk, as underlying factors are exacerbated by the physiological effects of pregnancy. Among other reports, these increased risks have been confirmed by analysis of the Swedish Medical Birth Registry data on >31,000 women aged 40–45 years, and >1,200 women >45 years of age [1583].

The overall maternal mortality rate increases with increasing maternal age. Thromboembolic complications during pregnancy, labour, and puerperium together with intrapartum and postpartum haemorrhage account for a large proportion of maternal deaths and are also the strongest determinants of the age-related obstetric risk to mothers [1584]. Maternal deaths remote from the time of birth but possibly related to aggravation of thromboembolic risk factors are likely to be under-reported.

## The effects of advanced maternal age on birth defects and neonatal mortality

A 7-year prospective study of over 100,000 pregnancies in the US observed increasing risk for specific non-chromosomal fetal malformations, including cardiac defects, club foot, and diaphragmatic hernia, with advancing maternal age [1585]. These data included stillborn fetuses and terminated pregnancies and therefore were at variance with some earlier studies that did not find a relationship between maternal age and congenital malformations [1586, 1587]. Maternal age 40 years and older at delivery was reported as an independent risk factor for perinatal mortality in a study cohort of over 36,000 women in the First and Second Trimester Evaluation of Risk trial, a prospective multicentre investigation of singleton pregnancies from an unselected obstetric population [1588].

Other studies have also found an increase in perinatal and neonatal death with increasing maternal age. Data from the National Infant Mortality Surveillance Project in the US in 1980 (n = 1,579,854 births and 14,591 deaths) indicated that infants born to mothers 35–39 years of age were at a slightly elevated (18% higher) risk of perinatal and neonatal death compared to those born to mothers 25–24 years of age, and those born to mothers 40–49 years of age were at a much more elevated (69% higher) risk [1589].

Trisomy 21 is a common chromosomal non-disjunction error resulting in Down's syndrome, the risk for which increases with maternal age [1590–1592]. There may be an added effect of paternal age on Down's syndrome risk, but this is yet to be definitively proven, and the relative contribution is likely to be small (see chapter 35).

## The effects of advanced maternal age on lactation

Older mothers tend to experience more difficulty in establishing breastfeeding and maintaining lactation, in part because breast milk yield decreases with advancing maternal age [1593]. Colostrum of older mothers is higher in fat content, possibly because of decreased water content [1594]. However, once breastfeeding is established, the composition of milk is not significantly different between older and younger mothers.

# Pregnancy and lactation during adolescence

Young maternal age also comes with risks. Pregnant adolescents are more likely than adults to consume micronutrient-poor, energy-dense diets. They are also more likely to have inadequate prenatal care, often as a result of less favourable social and economic circumstances. Statistically, teenage pregnancy is associated with increased risk of maternal complications from pregnancy and delivery, and anaemia is highly prevalent [1595].

## Infant birthweight and preterm birth in adolescent pregnancy

Compared with pregnant adults, young women who are still growing more often give birth prematurely or have low-birthweight infants. In a study of >15,000 adolescent pregnancies (age 13–17 years) and >90,000 pregnancies in women aged 20–24 years, young age was found to be a significant intrinsic risk factor for low birthweight and prematurity, independent of socio-demographic factors that may also predispose adolescent mothers to poorer outcomes [1596]. The poorer fetal growth associated with adolescent pregnancy possibly results from a competition for nutrients, as the adolescent mother may still be growing herself [1597, 1598].

Pregnant adolescents are prone to having abnormal weight gain in pregnancy. In addition, teenage mothers are more likely than older, non-growing mothers to retain more weight postpartum [1598]. However, the Camden Study, which prospectively evaluated nutrition and pregnancy in teenage girls vs older mothers in one of the poorest cities in the US, found that, despite a larger total weight gain in growing teenage mothers, their infants weighed significantly less at birth than those of older, non-growing mothers [1598].

## Birth defects in adolescent pregnancy

The effect of young maternal age on the incidence of birth defects was assessed in a California population of over a million births, which included 29,848 malformations. Risks were substantially increased for mothers younger than 20 years for some types of birth defects, with the highest risks observed for nervous system and abdominal wall anomalies [1599]. The risk elevation in young mothers was comparable to the oldest group (women over 40 years of age; i.e. risk showed a U-shaped pattern).

## Breastfeeding in adolescence

A prospective study of breastfeeding behaviours among adolescent mothers in the US found that, while the percentage of adolescent mothers who initiated breastfeeding was high (71%), breastfeeding duration was very short as compared to that observed with older mothers [1600]. In addition, obese adolescents had significantly lower odds of breastfeeding compared with their normal weight peers. This may relate to body image issues, which may prevent them from breastfeeding outside the home.

## Bone loss in adolescent pregnancy

Maternal bone loss following pregnancy and lactation is an important issue in women with low calcium and vitamin D status and intake. This is of particular concern in adolescents, whose bones are still growing and whose diets are often low in calcium [1601–1603]. Some studies have suggested that an increase in calcium intake during pregnancy and lactation may help reduce postpartum bone loss in adolescent mothers [1604]. In a recent placebo-controlled study, supplementation with 600 mg/day calcium and 200 IU/day vitamin D from 26 weeks gestation in adolescents whose normal dietary intake of calcium was below 600 mg/day resulted in higher maternal bone mass and reduced bone loss in the first 20 weeks of lactation [1605].

# Summary and recommendations concerning maternal age during pregnancy and lactation

Because pregnancy at both extremes of the reproductive age spectrum comes with risks to both mother and fetus, both adolescents and older women should be closely monitored during pregnancy. Adolescents, especially those who are still growing, will often benefit from dietary advice and monitoring of nutritional status. Although calcium supplementation is not generally required for pregnant women who consume a healthy diet, young women whose bones are still growing do benefit from additional calcium in the form of supplements.

Adolescent mothers are less likely to have consumed folic acid supplements pre-conceptionally but should be encouraged to do so as soon as possible in early pregnancy. They should be made aware of the impact of excessive gestational weight gain from high-fat diets and be encouraged to select a variety of foods specifically including fruits and vegetables.

Older mothers [35–40 years] who do not have underlying risk factors for diabetes and hypertension should receive advice similar to younger mothers. However, those who are overweight, obese, or who already have hypertension or diabetes should be encouraged to reduce their risk of aggravating these disorders during pregnancy. This can include dietary improvement and moderate exercise, and gestational weight gain within recommended ranges (see chapters 28 and 29).

# Chapter 35

# Paternal factors that affect conception and pregnancy

## Paternal pre-conception nutrition and lifestyle

The father's nutrition and lifestyle can influence pregnancy outcomes in a number of ways. In the pre-conception period, several modifiable factors can influence sperm count and quality and consequently affect fertility. For example, sperm count and quality is affected by alcohol, recreational drugs, prescription drugs, infections, tobacco, and environmental toxins. In addition, a father's BMI and metabolic status may have some impact on the metabolic trajectory of his offspring. Other aspects of a father's behaviour can indirectly affect the developing fetus through environmental exposures.

## The effects of paternal obesity, BMI, and diabetes on conception and fertility

Obese males or those with poorly controlled diabetes may have difficulty conceiving. Diabetes affects the endocrine control of spermatogenesis and can lead to structural and genetic abnormalities in spermatozoa [1606, 1607]. In addition, poor glycemic control can affect sperm quality and testicular function [1608]. A prospective observational study in the Netherlands (n = 450 men) found that BMI and waist circumference had an effect on sperm quality in men of subfertile couples, independent of other lifestyle factors. Ejaculation volume, sperm concentration, and motility were reduced with increasing BMI and central adiposity [1609]. In a study of >1,500 young men in Denmark, BMI was related to sperm count, which decreased with both high and low BMI [1610].

A systematic review of 31 studies did not find evidence for a disadvantage of high BMI on sperm parameters but did note strong evidence of a negative relationship between BMI and testosterone levels. However, the heterogeneous nature of the studies meant that confounding factors could not be accounted for [1611]. A recent prospective cohort study observed a significant (84%) decrease in the odds of a live birth following the use of the assisted reproduction technique of intracytoplasmic sperm injection with sperm from an obese male partner. However, male BMI was unrelated to other IVF outcomes [1612].

## Nutritional factors and male fertility

A healthy and nutritionally balanced diet is as important for male fertility as it is for females. Diets lacking sufficient quantities of certain micronutrients may affect a man's sperm count and quality, lowering his chance of conceiving a healthy infant. There is also some evidence to suggest that men who consume obesogenic diets may pass on poor metabolic attributes to their offspring.

Folate, for instance, is an important pre-conception micronutrient for men as well as women. Potential fathers require adequate folate in their diets, as low folate concentrations in seminal plasma may be detrimental to the stability of sperm DNA [1613]. Associations have also been found between folate deficiency and sperm aneuploidy [1614] and low sperm count [1615]. A recent study also links paternal folate levels with adverse pregnancy outcomes [1616].

Zinc also has a significant impact on male fertility, as it is involved in DNA synthesis and is required for spermatogenesis. Zinc levels in semen correlate positively with sperm count [1617], and poor zinc nutrition is a risk factor for low sperm quality and male infertility [1618]. An early sign of zinc deficiency in males is an arrest of spermatogenesis, manifested in a lack of elongated spermatozoa [1619].

Supplementation of subfertile men with a combination of folic acid (5 mg/day) and zinc sulphate (66 mg/day) for 26 weeks increased sperm count by 74 per cent in a randomized, placebo-controlled trial (n = 108 subfertile men and 107 fertile men). Zinc alone also increased sperm count but not to a statistically significant level [1620]. In its antioxidant capacity, zinc may protect cells, including sperm, from the negative effects of alcohol consumption and cigarette smoking. In rats, tobacco smoke-induced changes in spermatozoa were prevented by zinc treatment [1621].

Several selenium-dependent proteins are important in male fertility. The selenoprotein glutathione peroxidase 4 is essential for sperm structure and function. In addition, the sperm mitochondrial capsule selenoprotein has both structural and enzymatic roles in sperm tail motility and integrity. A study in Glasgow (an area with low selenium intakes) found enhanced sperm motility in men receiving selenium supplements (100 µg selenium or selenium plus vitamins A, C, and E daily), compared with a placebo control group [1032]. A more recent randomized, controlled trial in Iran found that supplementation of infertile men with selenium (200 µg/day) and/or N-acetyl cysteine increased sperm count and sperm motility after 26 weeks of treatment [1033].

The influence of reactive oxygen species (ROS) on fertility, and the possible benefits of antioxidant nutrients, has been the subject of investigation with particular emphasis on the possible role of ROS in idiopathic male infertility. Human sperm produce ROS and are susceptible to ROS-mediated peroxidative damage. Elevated production of ROS and increased sperm membrane damage has been observed in men with reduced sperm motility (asthenozospermia) [1622]. Because of this, protective agents against ROS, including vitamins C and E, have been postulated as useful agents in the treatment of male infertility. However, an 8-week placebo-controlled trial of daily high-dose vitamin C and E (1,000 mg vitamin C and 800 mg vitamin E) did not improve semen parameters or sperm survival in men with asthenozospermia [1623]. Several systematic reviews have confirmed that while dietary antioxidants may be beneficial for sperm health, there is currently no established role for supplemental antioxidants, including high-dose vitamin C and E, in the treatment of male infertility [1624–1626].

Overall dietary patterns may impact semen quality. A typical 'Western' diet characterized by high intake of red and/or processed meat, refined grains, snacks, high-energy drinks, and sweets has been associated with lower sperm motility as compared to a diet including high intakes of fish, chicken, fruit, vegetables, legumes, and whole grains [1627, 1628]. A recent cross-sectional study found an inverse association between intake of full-fat dairy products and semen quality (sperm motility and morphology) [1629]. This result needs confirmation in prospective longitudinal studies but may suggest that high intake of full-fat dairy foods such as cheese be reduced in men trying to conceive a pregnancy. There was no correlation between reduced-fat dairy foods and semen quality. In addition, high caffeine intake has been shown to reduce conception rates [1341], with a similar decline in fertility in both females and males, the latter effect possibly resulting from an impact of caffeine on semen quality.

## Paternal environmental and occupational exposures that can affect conception and pregnancy

Substances that induce mutations or epimutations in spermatic DNA have the potential to cause birth defects or cancers in offspring. Such mutagens include ionizing radiation, pesticides, ethylene dichloride, and vinyl chloride. Exposure to some of these agents may be occupational [1630].

Xenobiotic agents, including polycyclic aromatic hydrocarbons, PCBs, dioxins, and phthlates, have been shown to cause oxidative stress and DNA damage to the sperm and can therefore decrease fertility or result in birth defects, childhood cancers, or miscarriage of defected fetuses [1631]. Occupations that involve exposure to metals, combustion products, solvents, and pesticides (e.g. welding, painting, auto mechanics, firefighting, and agriculture) have been implicated, although various studies have failed to replicate such findings. Paternal exposure to paints, hydrocarbons or exhaust fumes, and to a lesser extent pesticides, has been consistently shown to increase risks of childhood cancers [1632]. These agents are discussed in chapter 30 with respect to their impact on the fetus. Development of immature sperm to mature sperm takes approximately 72 days and is a continual process; therefore a 3-month period of freedom from exposure is desirable to improve sperm quality prior to a planned pregnancy.

## The effects of paternal cigarette smoking on conception and pregnancy

Tobacco smoke contains a large number of agents with mutagenic, aneugenic, and/or carcinogenic properties that can damage sperm. Cigarette smoking is associated with an increased concentration of leukocytes in seminal fluid, considered to be a marker of low semen quality [1633]. Among subfertile men, smokers had reduced sperm motility, poorer sperm morphology, and a higher leukocyte count in seminal fluid than non-smokers [1634]. Leukocytes are the major source of ROS in the ejaculate, and elevations in their concentration are thought to increase oxidative DNA damage in sperm and thus reduce fertility [1635]. The sperm antioxidant defence system is sensitive to disruption by cigarette smoking [1636], and there are reports of tobacco-induced oxidative damage to sperm DNA [1637, 1638].

## The effects of paternal drug and alcohol use on conception and pregnancy

Most drugs to which the male has been exposed can be found in seminal fluid and transmitted to the female in the ejaculate. Some of these, such as the cancer drug cyclophosphamide, have demonstrated the potential to confer pre-implantation loss or embryopathy. There is also an increase in sperm aneuploidy during chemotherapy, and men should be advised not attempt to conceive pregnancy during such exposure or in the first cycle of spermatogenesis following termination of therapy [1639]. Toxins such as cocaine may also bind to sperm and be transported to the ovum at fertilization [1640], as has also been demonstrated with sperm exposed to viruses [1641]. In addition, the use of anabolic steroids for increasing muscle mass has been shown to decrease sperm count and alter sperm morphology, in some cases resulting in azoospermia [1642].

The effect of alcohol on sperm parameters is not yet fully understood. Although some studies have not observed significant effects of alcohol on sperm parameters [1643–1645], the balance of evidence suggests that alcohol contributes to developmental defects of sperm morphology and sperm production (reduced sperm count), the incidence of which increases with increasing alcohol consumption [1646–1650]. Alcohol withdrawal improves semen quality and has been shown to completely and rapidly reverse alcohol-associated azospermia [1651, 1652]. The use of alcohol or marijuana is associated with elevated leukocyte levels in seminal fluid and thus with low semen quality [1653]. Marijuana also interferes with spermatogenesis, resulting in lower sperm density and motility and increased numbers of sperm with morphologic abnormalities [1653].

## Paternal factors and pregnancy outcomes

The impact of paternal nutrition and lifestyle does not end at conception, although pre-conception behaviours can result in germline mutations or epigenetic changes that can be passed on to their progeny. Cigarette smoking, for example, has been linked to genetic damage in sperm, with the potential to cause developmental defects in the offspring. An epidemiological study in China found a paternally mediated effect of smoking on the risk of birth defects, including a more than twofold increased risk of anencephalus and spina bifida. Infants of fathers who smoked were also more likely to have a diaphragmatic hernia and were more than three times more likely to have skin pigmentary anomalies than infants of non-smokers [1654].

### Paternal factors influencing infant birthweight and metabolic health

A father's metabolic status can have an influence on development of the fetus, as well as possible long-term effects on the offspring's metabolic development. In the international SCOPE Study cohort, paternal obesity and central adiposity were both associated with a 60 per cent increase in risk of fathering a small-for-gestational-age infant [1655]. In addition, when analysed for the influence of parental BMI on childhood obesity, the Avon Longitudinal Study of Parents and Children data revealed an equivalent relationship between either maternal or paternal BMI and the BMI of the offspring at age 7, arguing against a significant effect of the intrauterine environment [1656]. However, paternally derived epigenetic influences could be a factor that enhances paternal effects. This hypothesis has been suggested to explain the trans-generational influence of paternal smoking on offspring BMI, a pattern seen in cohorts from both the Avon study and the Swedish Överkalix study [1657].

Fathers consuming high-fat diets pre-conceptionally may be at increased risk of having offspring with diabetes. Evidence from a rodent model suggests that obese fathers are likely to have offspring with diabetes [1658]. Another recent study found that a high-fat diet causing paternal obesity and impaired glucose tolerance in the offspring also induced paternal sperm microRNA profile alterations that were transmitted to a second generation, indicating transgenerational paternal effects of obesity on glucose tolerance [1659].

## The effects of paternal age on pregnancy and child outcomes

There have been a number of recent studies on the effect of advanced paternal age on pregnancy and child outcomes. Paternal age is thought to influence the accumulation of de novo germline mutations and/or methylation of paternally imprinted genes. Advanced paternal age is also associated with a reduced capacity for DNA repair, and increased mutagenesis. A recent study demonstrated an exponential increase in germline point mutations as men age, beginning at a rate of approximately 2 mutations per year and doubling every 16.5 years [1660]. This study also found that men transmit a higher number of mutations to their children than women, despite a higher rate of recombination in females, which also increases with maternal age.

Down's syndrome, which results from the non-disjunction of chromosome 21 during meiosis, is known to be influenced by the advancing age of the female gametes [1590–1592]. Whether there is an effect of paternal age on the incidence of trisomy 21 has been the subject of debate [1661], but studies in specific populations (e.g. Norway) have reported an increased risk, independent of maternal age, with paternal age >50 years [1662]. Other studies also suggest some influence of paternal age [1663, 1664], but more recent reanalyses suggest that the effect is small and unlikely to influence family-planning decisions [1661].

Epidemiological studies have shown that the risk of schizophrenia in the offspring increases significantly with increasing paternal age [1665], possibly involving a mutational hotspot in a schizophrenia-related gene, or impaired imprinting [1666]. Additionally, over 20 genetic disorders have been associated with older paternal age, including achondroplasia, cardiomyopathy, multiple endocrine neoplasia, osteogenesis imperfecta, and craniosynostosis syndromes (causing craniofacial anomalies) [1667]. On the other hand, offspring of very young fathers have an elevated risk for de novo genetic disorders—possibly because spermatids are immature and DNA repair and antioxidant activities are low [1668].

Such a U-shaped relationship between paternal age and adverse offspring outcomes has also been observed in regard to cognitive development. A significant U-shaped relationship was observed between paternal age and offspring IQ scores in a study of >44,000 births in an Israeli cohort [1669]. A similar U-shaped relationship between paternal age and the risk of type 1 diabetes was also observed in a small Taiwanese study [1670].

## Paternal occupational exposures and offspring outcomes

Paternal occupation can affect birth outcomes in two ways. Occupational exposure to harmful substances can cause genetic alterations in the male germ cell line, as discussed in 'Paternal pre-conception nutrition and lifestyle'. Alternatively, such exposure can lead to exposure of the mother (through contaminated clothing or skin).

Paternal employment in the lead industry or other occupations that are associated with exposure to lead (e.g. automotive painting and/or radiator repair, scrap handling, house renovation/paint stripping of old buildings, demolition of ships or old buildings, etc.) is regarded as an indirect risk to the fetus, as lead dust can be brought into the home on clothing, skin, and hair [1345]. High or prolonged paternal occupational lead exposures (including the period from 6 months before conception to the end of pregnancy) were associated with a higher risk of low birthweight and preterm birth [1671]. In addition, the offspring of workers exposed to benzene, chromium, and other minerals have a higher risk of being small for gestational age, and offspring of men exposed to X-rays have a higher risk of preterm birth [1672].

Between 1980 and 2002, flour mill workers exposed to various fumigants in Washington State fathered fewer male offspring, and male infants had significantly reduced birthweight [1673]. The results suggest that the workers' exposure had an effect on testicular function, as seen with the now-banned fumigant dibromochlorpropane (a nematocide for worm control), which causes oligospermia or azoospermia [1674]. This chemical was used extensively in the US between 1955 and 1977 for controlling crop-damaging parasitic worms and is still found in groundwater in areas of past high use.

# Our recommendations concerning paternal factors in pregnancy

Prospective fathers need to be conscious of their personal health and nutrition, as well as of environmental factors that may influence both their ability to conceive and the health of their future offspring. Poor dietary habits that contribute to obesity and type 2 diabetes have a negative impact on male fertility and, potentially, on the metabolic health of their children. Eating habits are learned and perpetuated within families, but biology also suggests that metabolic trajectories are established to some extent in utero, with the paternal status contributing to this outcome.

Nutrients including zinc and selenium are important for male fertility, but in most cases can be obtained from a balanced diet. However, subfertile men may benefit from supplementation with these minerals. Antioxidant therapy with vitamins C and/or E is not recommended to improve male fertility.

Smoking is detrimental not only to sperm and reproductive health but also to the fetus via maternal exposure to second-hand smoke. Men should be encouraged to quit smoking before trying to conceive, or, at a minimum, to restrict their smoking behaviours so that the mother (and the infant after birth) is not exposed. In addition, although evidence is still accumulating, it is prudent to advise men to limit alcohol consumption and curtail recreational drug use, as both may cause sperm damage and lead to birth defects. Men should also be made aware of the potential impact of various occupational exposures that can cause genetic damage to sperm or be transmitted to the mother and fetus through dust on clothing brought into the home.

# A management guide— from before conception to weaning

In practice, health care providers do not deal with individual nutrients or behaviours but must take a holistic approach to providing advice at each stage of pregnancy, from preconception through birth and breastfeeding. In this section, we provide a summary checklist of points to consider in interacting with parents at each pregnancy stage. The justification and sources of the recommendations made in this chapter are encompassed in sections 2 and 3 of this book and will not be again referenced here.

Chapter 36

# Guidelines for the pre-conception period

## Advice for a healthy pre-pregnancy state

An increasing number of parents seek pre-pregnancy counselling. That creates an opportunity to address issues of lifestyle and nutrition as well as addressing any specific medical problems. We would suggest similar advice be given where possible to both prospective parents. The central effort should be to encourage and inform about a healthy diet, install healthy exercise behaviour, and promote abstinence from harmful substances such as tobacco, alcohol, and non-medically indicated drugs.

The evidence suggests that attention to the potential mother's BMI is important; both low and high BMIs are associated with poorer pregnancy outcomes, and there is growing evidence that this may also be true for the paternal BMI. The issue becomes more complex when the mother has a very high BMI as, based on animal experiments, severe dieting at conception may have adverse epigenetic effects on the embryo. It is therefore best to try to address these issues ahead of the proposed pregnancy.

Establishing and/or maintaining optimal nutritional intakes prior to conception will help minimize adverse outcomes for both mothers and offspring. Pre-conception nutrition remains a challenge worldwide, with under-nutrition still a concerning issue in low-and middle-income countries, and poor/unbalanced diet or over-nutrition predominating in developed countries. Poor nutrition around the time of conception can influence the fetal growth trajectory and weight at birth and has been documented to increase the risk of preterm birth. A well-balanced diet consisting of fruits, vegetables, iron, and calcium-rich foods, as well as protein-containing food, should be consumed. Health care professionals should address optimal weight gain, healthy diet, eating guidelines, and the use of dietary supplements as part of pre-conception care and counselling.

# Recommended nutrition and supplementation prior to conception

Ideally most aspects of nutrition can be addressed by a balanced diet, particularly one containing adequate amounts of oily fish to provide omega-3 fatty acids. Supplementation is usually only required for a few nutrients, except in certain cases as outlined below. Folic acid supplementation has been shown to have protective effects against birth defects, in particular neural tube defects (NTDs), and all women of reproductive age, especially those who are planning a pregnancy, are recommended to consume 0.4 mg (400 μg) of synthetic folic acid daily, obtained from supplements and/or fortified foods. Where possible, this should be associated with a blood test for vitamin $B_{12}$ and folate status, and in some circumstances this will lead to different dose requirements. Vitamin D status also needs to be considered; covert deficiency is far more common that generally recognized, and low-dose supplementation (400 IU/day) may be necessary. Women residing in areas with a high prevalence of vitamin A deficiency may need pre-conception supplementation, but otherwise vitamin A should be obtained from food sources.

Depending on the context, the health care professional may need to consider other forms of supplementation, including iodine, zinc, iron, and some B group vitamins. In strict vegetarians, the status of vitamin $B_{12}$ and iron needs particular consideration. Vegetarian diets contain low levels of alpha-linolenic acid and are devoid of omega-3 fatty acids. Zinc absorption is lower in vegetarian diets because of a higher consumption of phytate-containing foods and the avoidance of zinc-rich meats and seafood. Choline may also be low in vegetarians. A summary of daily requirements for non-pregnant women prior to conception is given in Table 36.1, along with increases for pregnancy and lactation. Details of those nutrients for which supplementation may be considered are provided in the sections that follow.

## Folic acid supplementation prior to conception

Folic acid is a B-complex vitamin that is recognized to have protective effects against NTDs. Dietary sources that are rich in folic acid include legumes, green leafy vegetables, citrus fruits and juices, and breads and cereals that contain flour enriched with folic acid. Women of reproductive age are advised to consume 0.4 mg (400 μg) of synthetic folic acid daily, obtained from fortified foods and/or supplements.

Women with a prior history of NTD-affected pregnancy are advised to take a dosage of 4–5 mg folic acid per day, under the guidance of a physician, for at

**Table 36.1** Recommended dietary allowances (or adequate intake levels) in the pre-conception, pregnancy, and lactation periods

| Nutrient | Maternal status | | |
|---|---|---|---|
| | Pre-pregnancy | Pregnancy | Lactation |
| Protein (g/day) | 46 | 71 | 71 |
| Fibre (g/day) | 25 | 28 | 29 |
| Carbohydrate (g/day) | 130 | 175 | 210 |
| n-6 PUFAs[a] (g/day)** | 11–12 | 13 | 13 |
| n-3 PUFAs[a] (g/day)** | 1.1 | 1.4 | 1.3 |
| Vitamin A (µg/day)[b] | | | |
| 14–18 yrs | 700 | 750 | 1200 |
| 19+ yrs | 700 | 770 | 1300 |
| Vitamin $B_1$ (thiamine; mg/day) | 1.0 | 1.4 | 1.4 |
| 14–18 yrs | 1.1 | 1.4 | 1.4 |
| 19+ yrs | | | |
| Vitamin $B_2$ (riboflavin; mg/day) | | | |
| 14–18 yrs | 1.0 | 1.4 | 1.6 |
| 19+ yrs | 1.1 | 1.4 | 1.6 |
| Vitamin $B_3$ (niacin; mg/day)[c] | 14 | 18 | 17 |
| Vitamin $B_6$ (pyridoxine; mg/day) | | | |
| 14–18 yrs | 1.2 | 1.9 | 2.0 |
| 19+ yrs | 1.3 | 1.9 | 2.0 |
| Folate (µg/day)[d] | 400 | 600 | 500 |
| Vitamin $B_{12}$ (cobalamin; µg/day) | 2.4 | 2.6 | 2.8 |
| Vitamin C (mg/day) | | | |
| 14–18 yrs | 65 | 80 | 115 |
| 19+ yrs | 75 | 85 | 120 |
| Vitamin D (µg/day)[e] | 15 | 15 | 15 |
| Vitamin E (mg/day)[f] | 15 | 15 | 19 |
| Biotin (µg/day)** | | | |
| 14–18 yrs | 25 | 30 | 35 |
| 19+ yrs | 30 | 30 | 35 |
| Calcium (mg/day) | | | |
| 14–18 yrs | 1300 | 1300 | 1300 |
| 19+ yrs | 1000 | 1000 | 1000 |

**Table 36.1** (continued) Recommended dietary allowances (or adequate intake levels) in the pre-conception, pregnancy, and lactation periods

| Nutrient | Maternal status | | |
|---|---|---|---|
| | Pre-pregnancy | Pregnancy | Lactation |
| Choline (mg/day)**\*\*g** | | | |
| 14–18 yrs | 400 | 450 | 550 |
| 19+ yrs | 425 | 450 | 550 |
| Copper (µg/day) | | | |
| 14–18 yrs | 890 | 1000 | 1000 |
| 19+ yrs | 900 | 1300 | 1300 |
| Fluoride (mg/day)\*\* | 3 | 3 | 3 |
| Iodine (µg/day) | 150 | 220 | 290 |
| Iron (mg/day) | | | |
| 14–18 yrs | 15 | 27 | 10 |
| 19+ yrs | 18 | 27 | 9 |
| Magnesium (mg/day) | | | |
| 14–18 yrs | 360 | 400 | 360 |
| 19–30 yrs | 310 | 350 | 310 |
| 31–50 yrs | 320 | 360 | 320 |
| Manganese (mg/day)\*\* | | | |
| 14–18 yrs | 1.6 | 2.0 | 2.6 |
| 19+ yrs | 1.8 | 2.0 | 2.6 |
| Phosphorus (mg/day) | | | |
| 14–18 yrs | 1250 | 1250 | 1250 |
| 19+ yrs | 700 | 700 | 700 |
| Selenium (µg/day) | 55 | 60 | 70 |
| Zinc (mg/day) | | | |
| 14–18 yrs | 9 | 12 | 13 |
| 19+ yrs | 8 | 11 | 12 |

\*\* Adequate intake recommendations (insufficient data to establish a recommended dietary allowance)

[a] n-6 PUFAs = omega-6 polyunsaturated fatty acids (e.g. linoleic acid); n-3 PUFAs = omega-3 polyunsaturated fatty acids (e.g. alpha-linolenic acid)

[b] As retinol activity equivalents (RAEs); 1 RAE = 1 µg retinol, 12 µg beta-carotene, 24 µg alpha-carotene, or 24 µg beta-cryptoxanthin. The RAE for dietary provitamin A carotenoids is twofold greater than the retinol equivalent, whereas the RAE for preformed vitamin A is the same as the retinol equivalent

[c] As niacin equivalents; 1 mg of niacin = 60 mg of tryptophan; 0–6 months = preformed niacin (not niacin equivalent)

**Table 36.1** (continued) Recommended dietary allowances (or adequate intake levels) in the pre-conception, pregnancy, and lactation periods

d As dietary folate equivalents; 1 dietary folate equivalent = 1 μg food folate = 0.6 μg of folic acid from fortified food or as a supplement consumed with food = 0.5 μg of a supplement taken on an empty stomach. In view of evidence linking folate intake with the prevention of NTDs in the fetus, it is recommended that all women capable of becoming pregnant consume 400 μg from supplements or fortified foods in addition to intake of food folate from a varied diet

e As cholecalciferol. 1 μg cholecalciferol = 40 IU vitamin D. Recommendations assume minimal exposure to sunlight

f As alpha-tocopherol

g Although adequate intake levels have been set for choline, there are few data to assess whether a dietary supply of choline is needed at all stages of the life cycle, and it may be that the choline requirement can be met by endogenous synthesis at some of these stages

Source: Institute of Medicine, Food and Nutrition Board, *Dietary reference intakes (DRIs): estimated average requirements*, National Academies, Washington, DC, copyright © 2014. <http://www.iom.edu/Activities/Nutrition/SummaryDRIs/~/media/Files/Activity%20Files/Nutrition/DRIs/5_Summary%20Table%20Tables%201-4.pdf>.

least 1 month prior to conception. The risk of NTDs is significantly elevated in overweight and obese women. Thus, those with BMIs ≥30 should be also be advised to take folic acid supplements in the higher dose range.

## Vitamin A intake prior to conception

Vitamin A is crucial for proper visual, fetal growth, reproduction, immunity, and epithelial tissue integrity. However, excess vitamin A can result in miscarriage and birth defects that affect CNS, craniofacial, cardiovascular, and thymus development. The recommended dietary allowance of preformed vitamin A for women is 770 μg RAEs (retinol activity equivalents) per day, with a tolerable upper intake level for pregnancy of 3,000 RAEs/day or 10,000 IU/day. Supplementation is generally advised against prior to conception and in early pregnancy, though women from areas with high prevalence of vitamin A deficiency are recommended supplementation in later pregnancy. For women at low risk, vitamin A should be obtained from food sources.

## Vitamin B$_{12}$ intake prior to conception

Vitamin B$_{12}$ is critical for neurological function. Women who follow strict vegetarian diets are at risk of vitamin B$_{12}$ deficiency, as are their infants, who often have very limited reserves of vitamin B$_{12}$ at birth. Pre-conceptional supplementation with vitamin B$_{12}$ is highly recommended for vegetarian and vegan women, and others who may be at risk of low vitamin B$_{12}$ status. Prenatal multivitamins generally contain vitamin B$_{12}$ in varying doses; it is recommended that such multivitamins, if used, contain at least 6 μg of vitamin B$_{12}$.

## Vitamin D supplementation prior to conception

Vitamin D can be synthesized endogenously in skin exposed to sunlight, or obtained from dietary sources that include milk, orange juice, fatty fish, egg yolks, beef liver, and cheese. A minimum of 400 IU/day is recommended by the US Institute of Medicine for women prior to conception. We would advise that intakes of between 1,000 and 2,000 IU/day, which are in line with the Endocrine Society and American Congress of Obstetricians and Gynecologists recommendations, are likely to be beneficial and not harmful, particularly for women who are at high risk of deficiency (e.g. dark-skinned or veiled individuals, vegetarians, and people living at high or low latitudes with minimal/no sun exposure).

## Calcium intake prior to conception

Calcium is important for pre-conception health; inadequate calcium stores can result in some maternal bone loss during pregnancy, as the fetus draws calcium from the maternal circulation to meet its needs. If intake is adequate, no adjustment will need to be made after conception, as homeostatic mechanisms ensure that levels are appropriate for both mother and fetus. All women should be encouraged to achieve or maintain a dietary calcium intake between 1,000 and 1,300 mg/day prior to conception, by increasing their intake of calcium-rich foods such as dairy products, leafy green vegetables, sardines/anchovies, soy products, and fortified cereals. Supplements are not required in most women, although calcium is included in most prenatal vitamins. Young women (under the age of 25) may benefit from supplementation with 1.0–1.5 g calcium per day if their dietary calcium intake is low.

## Iron intake prior to conception

Many women in the pre-conception period have low iron stores as a result of menstrual blood losses and/or poor diet. Aside from the fact that conception itself is compromised by iron deficiency, building iron stores prior to pregnancy is important to prepare for the high fetal requirement for iron, and the increase in maternal blood volume that occurs during gestation. It is difficult to restore a normal iron level during pregnancy if pre-conception iron status is low, let alone meet the increased fetal demands. It is recommended that, during the pre-conception visit, screening should be conducted for women with risk factors for iron deficiency for the purposes of identifying and treating anaemia. Women who consume little or no animal source foods are likely to benefit from supplementation with low-dose iron (30 mg ferrous iron per day) taken at bedtime or between meals.

## Iodine intake prior to conception

Salt iodization is the recommended, preferred strategy to control and eliminate iodine deficiency. Women of reproductive age should be counselled on the risks of iodine deficiency on pregnancy outcomes, and the importance of maintaining an adequate daily dietary iodine intake of 150 µg prior to conception (increasing to at least 220 µg/day when pregnant). Maintaining this level of intake is necessary to avoid abnormal thyroid gland stimulation during pregnancy, which has negative consequences for both mother and fetus. Women whose diets may be low in iodine, either because they reside in iodine-deficient regions (e.g. inland, mountainous terrain) or because they follow salt-restriction diets or do not consume iodine-fortified bread products, should be advised to take oral iodine supplements of 150 µg/day while trying to conceive. Supplementation with seaweed or kelp tablets is not recommended, as the iodine content of such products is highly variable, and the safe range of iodine intake is narrow. Excess iodine can inhibit thyroid function.

## Zinc intake prior to conception

Zinc is important in the pre-conception period for optimal reproductive health in both males and females. In women who are taking supplemental iron, zinc supplements may be required, because iron interferes with zinc absorption. Most prenatal vitamins contain zinc, though diets that include regular consumption of shellfish and red meat are likely to provide adequate levels of bio-available zinc.

## Biotin intake prior to conception

Marginal or subclinical biotin deficiency may go undetected in many women. Because of the possibility of teratogenicity (mainly cleft lip and palate) it is prudent to ensure that women are not at risk of biotin deficiency in the pre-conception period. Women who regularly consume large amounts of egg whites (without yolk) may risk deficiency, as avidin in egg whites binds biotin (present in excess in egg yolk) and renders it nutritionally unavailable. Women should be encouraged to consume whole eggs rather than egg whites, and when choosing a prenatal vitamin, to choose one containing biotin.

## Essential fatty acid intake prior to conception

During the pre-conception period, women are recommended to consume a diet rich in omega-3 and omega-6 fatty acids, the major source of which is oily fish. However, there is growing concern over levels of mercury in some fish species, including swordfish, king mackerel, shark, and tilefish, and consumption of these species should be limited by women who are attempting to conceive. Consumption of canned albacore tuna should also be limited to 2 meals per week (85 g/meal). Essential fatty acids are available through other dietary sources, including nuts and vegetable oils. More studies are required in order to endorse supplementation for women prior to pregnancy.

## Weight status and exercise prior to conception

Fertility in both females and males is decreased by being either overweight or underweight. Weight loss in non-pregnant overweight and obese women is associated with positive health outcomes and can also improve both fertility and pregnancy outcomes. The pre-conception period is a critical window of opportunity to establish good eating and exercise habits that will set the stage for a healthy pregnancy. Because weight loss is generally not recommended during pregnancy, it is best to have overweight women lose their excess weight prior to conception.

However, advice in this regard is often inadequate and, given that many women do not seek pre-pregnancy health checks, it is also often unheard. Many women with BMIs in the obese range do not consider themselves obese or even overweight. In some communities, obesity is now so common that it is perceived as normal. Adding to this conundrum is the fact that even when advised to lose weight prior to pregnancy, a large proportion of overweight and obese women fail to do so [1675].

Women who require modification in body weight, either loss or gain, should be advised to undertake this gradually prior to pregnancy. Regardless of BMI, women should also be encouraged to engage in regular aerobic exercise (walking, jogging, swimming, etc.) in order to achieve and maintain an acceptable level of fitness, not only for their own general health and well-being, but also to maximize their ability to cope with the demands of pregnancy, and allow the best chance of an optimal outcome for their offspring.

## Pre-conception exposures

Medications and supplements that are not prescribed or approved by a physician should be discouraged in women planning a pregnancy. Some plants used in Chinese and Indian (Ayurvedic) herbal remedies and teas contain phytotoxins that are potentially teratogenic. In addition, some ethnic home remedies have been found to contain hazardous contaminants such as lead and mercury; therefore all supplement consumption should be scrutinized, and unnecessary intake should be avoided.

As mentioned in 'Vitamin A supplementation prior to conception', avoidance of supplements and foods (e.g. liver) containing high concentrations of pre-formed vitamin A is recommended prior to conception, as vitamin A can be teratogenic in early pregnancy if present at high levels. Fish containing high levels of methylmercury, including shark, swordfish, king mackerel, and tilefish should also be limited in women planning a pregnancy. In addition, caffeine should be limited in the pre-conception period, as excess consumption may affect a couple's ability to conceive and contribute to fetal growth restriction during pregnancy. The current advice is to limit the consumption of caffeine from all sources, including chocolate, energy drinks, and colas as well as tea and coffee, to 200 mg/day prior to conception and throughout pregnancy. Tobacco, alcohol, and illegal drugs should also be strongly discouraged in the pre-conception period, as harm from these substances can occur early, before a woman realizes that she is pregnant.

Certain occupations may expose women to relatively high levels of toxi-cants, including heavy metals (e.g. lead, cadmium, and arsenic) that have reproductive and developmental effects. Both the dose and duration will affect the extent of risk, and for many substances, the critical period for harm has not been clearly determined. Some types of factory work that exposed fathers pre-conceptionally to mercury vapour were found to increase the risk of spontaneous abortion in the workers' female partners [1676]. Similarly, peri-conceptional exposure of females to mercury can induce early spontane-ous abortion.

With regard to congenital malformations or childhood cancers, pre-conception occupational exposures of either parent can possibly contribute to increasing the risks. Parental pre-conception exposure to low-level ionizing radiation, for exam-ple, has shown an association with NTDs in the offspring. Exposure to high con-centrations of herbicides, fungicides, pesticides, and other hydrocarbons such as solvents and oil and coal products during the pre-conception period may also contribute to the development of birth defects or cancers. Factory workers, farm-ers, and horticulturalists are among those potentially at risk. Occupational expo-sures of both parents should be queried and, where possible, minimized prior to attempting to achieve a pregnancy. In addition, contact with solvents used in the home, such as paint-stripping and furniture-stripping solvents, metal cleaners, and non-latex-based paints, should be minimized.

## Diabetes control prior to conception

For women with pre-existing diabetes, pre-conception care should focus on achieving and maintaining good glycemic control, which has been shown to reduce the incidence of spontaneous abortions, preterm deliveries, malformations, stillbirths, and neonatal deaths associated with poorly controlled maternal type 1 diabetes [1677]. The target for metabolic control in women with diabetes is to lower glycated haemoglobin levels to near the normal range before conception (43 mmol/mol (6.1%) or lower, according to UK National Institute for Health and Care Excellence guidelines), in order to reduce the risk of abnormal development of fetal organs in early pregnancy [1678].

## Recommendations for a pre-conception diet

A woman's pre-conception diet can affect her chances of conceiving a pregnancy and will also influence the early stages of pregnancy, when the embryo is particularly sensitive to poor intrauterine conditions. A diet high in vegetables, vegetable oils, legumes, and fish and low in saturated fats, meats, and refined carbohydrates (the 'Mediterranean diet') is recommended. The diet should be low in fat, saturated fat, and cholesterol. Components of a healthy pre-conception diet are shown in Table 36.2.

**Table 36.2** Dietary components of a healthy pre-conception diet

| Dietary component | Number of servings/day | Serving size example |
|---|---|---|
| Fruit | 2 | 1 apple, orange, banana, pear, 2 small plums, apricots |
| Vegetables | 3 | 1 cup leafy vegetables |
| Grains* | 6–11 | ½ cup rice, 1 slice bread |
| Lean meat, fish, poultry, legumes | 2 | ½ chicken breast, ¾ cup flaked fish, ½ cup dry beans (1 cup cooked), 2 tbsp peanut butter |
| Low-fat dairy products | 2–3 | 1 cup milk, ⅔ cup yogurt, ⅓ cup shredded cheese |
| Vegetable oils* | 1–2 | 1 tsp olive oil used in cooking or salad dressing |

* Choose whole grains whenever possible

* Choose olive oil, rapeseed oil; avocado oil

# Chapter 37

# Guidelines for pregnancy

## Guidelines for early pregnancy

Once pregnancy is diagnosed, the health care provider has the responsibility to ensure that parents have a clear understanding of the benefit of a good parental lifestyle. This should include advice as to healthy and unhealthy eating, weight gain goals in pregnancy, and a list of unsafe foods (see Table 30.1 in chapter 30). In addition, there should be advice on healthy exercise behaviours, and the effects of alcohol and drugs.

### Diet composition and micronutrient requirements in early pregnancy

If the mother has not had pre-conceptional counselling, it is important to ensure that she understands the importance of a balanced diet and what that means. Women should be advised that their energy intake needs in early pregnancy do not increase from pre-pregnancy levels; they should focus on eating well for pregnancy, and not eating more. Depending on the context, folate, vitamin $B_{12}$, iron (haemoglobin), and vitamin D status may need to be measured.

All women should receive vitamin D and folate supplementation; this is increasingly done in the form of multivitamin supplements that provide other micronutrients that should be present in a balanced diet in any event. Most of the required nutrients should be obtainable from food sources if, for example, women follow a diet similar to the Mediterranean diet, which is replete with fresh fruits and vegetables, fish (aside from large predatory species), legumes, and olive oil as the fat source. The recommended dietary allowances (RDAs) for micronutrients in pregnancy, as compared with the pre-conception requirements, are shown in Table 36.1 in chapter 36. In this section, we provide advice regarding specific micronutrient needs in the early pregnancy period.

### Vitamin A intake in early pregnancy

Vitamin A deficiency in pregnancy confers increased risks of growth failure, depressed immunity, and increased morbidity and mortality due to infectious disease. However, high intakes of preformed vitamin A in early pregnancy are associated with an increased risk of birth defects. Most women can meet their early pregnancy needs for vitamin A from food sources of beta-carotene by consuming at least five servings of darkly coloured fruits and vegetables, or animal sources of retinol, although foods that are very high in vitamin A, such as liver, should be avoided. Supplementation with vitamin A is not recommended in early pregnancy, and even in areas of endemic vitamin A deficiency, supplements containing >10,000 IU of retinol (>700 μg)/day or >25,000 IU weekly should be avoided.

### Folic acid supplementation in early pregnancy

Women should be advised to continue taking folic acid at their pre-conception recommended level (at least 400 μg/day), through the first 12 weeks of pregnancy. Low maternal folate is associated with low birthweight, small-for-gestational-age infants, and maternal pre-eclampsia, as well as an increased risk for neural tube defects. However, women taking high dosages of folic acid should ensure that their vitamin $B_{12}$ intake is also sufficient.

### Vitamin $B_{12}$ intake in early pregnancy

Vitamin $B_{12}$ requirements do not change drastically during pregnancy, but women at risk for deficiency, such as vegans and vegetarians, require supplementation to ensure adequate nutritional status. The requirement for vitamin $B_{12}$ in early pregnancy is 2.6 μg/day. As noted above, vitamin $B_{12}$ status is interlinked with folate status, and both need to be adequate in early pregnancy to ensure optimal pregnancy outcomes and to avoid maternal adverse health effects associated with deficiency for these nutrients.

### Vitamin D supplementation in early pregnancy

Deficient maternal vitamin D status (<30 nmol/L) in early pregnancy is associated with reduced birthweight followed by accelerated growth after birth. This growth pattern may increase the risk of obesity, cardiovascular disease, and insulin resistance in the offspring. Supplementation with vitamin D should be continued through pregnancy, especially in high-risk women. The dose of the vitamin D supplement should be at least 400 IU/day, and the total intake should be in the range of 1,000–2,000 IU/day from dietary and supplemental sources.

### Iron intake in early pregnancy

Maintaining or building optimal maternal body stores of iron in early pregnancy is important in order to prepare for the increased demands of late gestation. Iron status should be monitored, and supplementation is recommended in women with low iron stores or anaemia (haemoglobin <110 g/L in the first trimester), starting in early pregnancy if not prior to conception. All women should be given dietary advice to maximize iron intake and absorption, and should consume ~27 mg iron/day during pregnancy.

## Iodine intake in early pregnancy

Adequate iodine intake should be ensured in early pregnancy. Intake should be increased from the pre-pregnancy recommended level of 150 µg/day, to around 250 µg/day in early pregnancy. In many countries it is difficult to obtain iodine in sufficient quantity purely from dietary sources and, if iodized salt is not used or is used minimally, pregnant women should be encouraged to take iodine supplements (150 µg/day) as early as possible in pregnancy.

# Guidelines for middle and late pregnancy

## Weight gain, exercise, and glucose monitoring in middle and late pregnancy

The rate of weight gain accelerates from mid-pregnancy, and it should be plotted against the US Institute of Medicine norms, taking into account measured or estimated pre-pregnancy BMI. Energy requirements increase from early pregnancy, with an average requirement for an additional 340 calories (~1,422 kilojoules) during the second trimester and an additional ~450 calories during the third trimester. Dieting, except under medical advice to address gestational diabetes or other conditions, should not occur unless weight gain is excessive. It should *not* be used to manage social concerns regarding the ease of labour.

Moderate exercise regimens should be maintained throughout pregnancy. As well as providing maternal health benefits in terms of cardiovascular fitness, moderate to vigorous exercise in the second trimester may reduce the risk of preterm birth by improving placental functional capacity and thus nutrient delivery to the fetus. In addition, all women should have their glucose status measured in mid-pregnancy. While there remains debate as to whether a fasting glucose or a non-fasting polycose test is sufficient unless there are clinical risk factors present, at least in Asia, where the incidence of gestational diabetes is very high, we would recommend an oral glucose tolerance test at 24–28 weeks for all women.

## Diet composition and micronutrient requirements in middle and late pregnancy

Energy requirements increase in general in mid to late pregnancy, but the specific macronutrient composition of the diet may also be important. In particular, there is some evidence that adequate intakes of protein, preferably animal protein, in late pregnancy are important to protect against low birthweight. The intake of vegetable and fruit fibre should be maintained or increased in order to control fasting glucose levels and insulin resistance. Particular attention should be given to ensuring an adequate supply of polyunsaturated fatty acids and, if the diet is low in oily fish, supplementation should be considered.

The RDAs for micronutrients do not change between early and late pregnancy, despite greater energy requirements. Where supplements have been advised starting in early pregnancy, their intake should be continued. Some micronutrients are required in greater amounts in this period (e.g. iron), but the recommendation is that intakes are increased from early pregnancy in order to maintain and/or build adequate stores. Specific requirements to be aware of are discussed below.

### Vitamin A intake in middle and late pregnancy

The growing fetus requires ~100 µg/day of vitamin A in the third trimester. If women have been following appropriate dietary advice for early pregnancy, consuming five or more servings per day of darkly coloured fruits and vegetables, and animal sources, including fish, eggs, and dairy products, their liver stores should be adequate to cope with the increased fetal demand in late pregnancy. In areas of endemic vitamin A deficiency (e.g. sub-Saharan Africa and southern India), supplementation is advisable beginning after day 60 of gestation and continuing for at least 12 weeks to delivery. Supplements should contain up to 10,000 IU vitamin A daily or up to 25,000 IU vitamin A weekly as an oral liquid, oil-based preparation of retinyl palmitate or retinyl acetate.

### Vitamin D intake in middle and late pregnancy

Women in mid to late pregnancy should continue to take vitamin D supplements of *at least* 400 IU/day. The level of supplementation should be higher if they fall into the risk groups for deficiency (e.g. women who are dark-skinned or veiled, avoid the sun or regularly use sunscreens and/or protective clothing, live at high or low latitudes, eat vegan or vegetarian diets, or are obese). The intake should be in the range of 1,000–2,000 IU/day from diet, supplements, and/or sensible sun exposure.

### Calcium intake in middle and late pregnancy

Bone turnover doubles in late pregnancy. Thus, dietary calcium intake in middle and late pregnancy should be maintained to support this. However, women with habitual low intakes of calcium should not increase their consumption markedly, as the maternal adaptive processes may be disrupted, potentially leading to worse outcomes for both mother and infant.

## Iron status in middle and late pregnancy

Requirements for iron increase in the third trimester, but it is preferable that iron stores be built up from pre-conception and through gestation in order to meet the late pregnancy fetal demand. Women should be encouraged to maintain an adequate intake (two servings per day) of a mix of dietary iron sources such as meat, fish, poultry, legumes, nuts, green leafy vegetables, and iron-enriched breakfast cereals. Eating foods rich in vitamin C in the same meal as the iron source will increase the amount of iron that is absorbed. Women consuming a Western diet are likely to have iron intakes of only 12–18 mg/day and therefore may require supplementation in mid to late pregnancy to meet the RDA of 27 mg/day. Because both the intake and absorption of iron tends to be lower in vegetarian women, they are advised to take iron supplements at a dosage of 30 mg/day. Women in developing countries are recommended a supplementation dosage of 60 mg/day from 16 weeks gestation, with larger doses (~100 mg/day) advised in cases of anaemia.

## Zinc intake in middle and late pregnancy

Zinc is required for the rapid fetal growth that occurs in late pregnancy to protect against low birthweight and impaired immune function. For the most part, requirements for zinc can be met through dietary sources such as seafood, red meat, poultry, leafy green vegetables, nuts, and legumes. However, the zinc content of plant-based foods tends to reflect the local soil zinc levels, and in some regions including sub-Saharan Africa and South Asia, the zinc content in the food supply may be inadequate to meet nutritional needs. In addition, diets high in phytate are associated with poor bioavailability of dietary zinc, because phytate forms insoluble complexes with zinc in the gastrointestinal tract. Iron supplementation also reduces zinc absorption, so women taking iron supplements or consuming diets low in bioavailable zinc should be advised to take a daily multivitamin containing zinc.

## Exposures to avoid in middle and late pregnancy

Some substances should be specifically avoided in late pregnancy in order to reduce the potential risk of poor infant outcomes. During the third trimester, women should avoid high intakes of herbal teas and polyphenol-rich foods, which have been associated with the development of fetal ductus arteriosus brought on by inhibition of prostaglandin synthesis. For the same reasons of prostaglandin inhibition, nonsteroidal anti-inflammatory drugs should not be taken in late pregnancy. In addition, paracetamol (acetaminophen) should be avoided late in gestation, as there is some evidence to suggest that its use may increase the risk of childhood asthma. Recent data also suggest that prolonged paracetamol use in pregnancy, particularly during the third trimester, increases the risk for adverse psychomotor outcomes in children.

# Chapter 38

# Guidelines for breastfeeding and weaning

## Benefits of breastfeeding

In the first 4–6 months of life, the infant will double its birthweight from that accumulated during its 9-month gestation. Nonetheless, provided that maternal nutrition is good, the infant requires little other than breast milk during this period. Breastfeeding is regarded as the optimal and most natural form of infant feeding. Milk from well-nourished mothers provides almost all of the nutrient requirements for the growing infant to the age of 6 months.

In developing countries with poor hygiene, breastfeeding is the safest feeding option, preventing infection both by avoiding contaminated water or foods and by provision of protective components, including secretory IgA antibodies and lactoferrin, in breast milk [1679]. Even in developed countries, breastfeeding is associated with a significant reduction of infections, including acute otitis media and gastrointestinal infection [1680]. Observational evidence suggests other positive health benefits for the breastfed infant later in life, including a reduced risk of hypertension and lower total cholesterol in adulthood [1681]. The latter may reflect long-term effects of adjustments in cholesterol metabolism in response to the higher cholesterol content of breast milk compared with infant formulas. In addition, the pattern of infant growth is quite different for breastfed and formula-fed infants [1682, 1683]. Although there are conflicting data, it is generally accepted that exclusive breastfeeding for >4 months is associated with a reduction in the risk of later obesity [1684, 1685].

In addition to its documented benefits for the growing infant, breastfeeding is also beneficial for the mother, reducing postpartum weight retention [1686] and lowering the risk of premenopausal breast cancer, particularly with extended breastfeeding [1687]. Other potential benefits include improved mother–infant bonding and maternal bone health, as well as reduced risks of postpartum depression and endometrial, ovarian, and postmenopausal breast cancer [1688, 1689]. If exclusive breastfeeding for the first 6 months is not accomplished, partial breastfeeding and/or breastfeeding for a shorter time period is also valuable and should be encouraged. Breastfeeding is contraindicated in only a few circumstances, which include cases of maternal HIV-1 or human T-cell lymphotropic virus type I or type II infection, or herpes simplex lesions on the breast [1690]. Yet in resource-poor settings, continued breastfeeding by HIV-infected women is recommended because the risk of morbidity and mortality from other infections or malnutrition outweighs the risk of HIV transmission to the infant.

Nutritional and lifestyle guidance for women during the highly demanding period of lactation is as important as that given before and during pregnancy. Although exclusive breastfeeding for the first 6 months is a desirable goal, we also acknowledge that some women either cannot or choose not to breastfeed their infants. For these women, guidance is required in terms of the optimal infant formulas for their newborns. The weaning period is equally important, and advice on complementary foods should be provided to all women, whether formula feeding or breastfeeding.

## Nutrition for lactation

The need to maintain healthy eating habits into lactation is obvious. This may create some challenges, as in some cultures quite distinct confinement diets are the norm during the first month after birth (see chapter 31). In general, the nutritional needs of women during breastfeeding exceed those of pregnancy, and the micronutrient recommended dietary allowances (RDAs) for lactation are accordingly different to those of pregnancy (see Table 36.1 in chapter 36). Lactating women may need supplementation with a multivitamin.

### Energy and macronutrient requirements during breastfeeding

Breastfeeding women have increased energy requirements to meet both the energy cost of milk production and the energy content of the milk they produce. On average, women who are exclusively breastfeeding their infants produce ~780 mL of milk per day during the first 6 months and ~600 mL/day between 7 and 12 months, and the average energy density of the milk is 0.67 kcal/mL [131]. Part of this energy demand can met by the mobilization of fat stores laid down during pregnancy, and this mobilization occurs at a rate of ~170 kcal/day in well-nourished women [1691].

Weight loss varies during lactation but is most steady in women who exclusively breast feed. Women who are underweight or who had low gestational weight gain require some additional caloric intake above that consumed during pregnancy in order to meet the energy demands of exclusive breastfeeding. The recommended intake is an additional 500 kcal/day during the first 6 months of lactation, in addition to the energy mobilized from fat stores. This extra intake is reduced to 400 kcal/day after 6 months because milk output is reduced as infants begin complementary feeding.

Overweight or obese women do not require additional energy during breast-feeding. On the contrary, they can safely restrict their energy intake at this time, in order to encourage weight loss. This can be accomplished without affecting the growth of their infants by reducing their overall energy consumption by 500 kcal/day [1692]. The proportions of macronutrients required in the lactation diet do not differ from those during non-lactating states [1693]. However, the breast milk composition of some macronutrients is influenced by the amount, proportion, and types of nutrients consumed by the mother.

## Fatty acid requirements during breastfeeding

The type and amount of fat in the maternal diet strongly influences the compos-ition of fatty acids present in breast milk. For example, the trans-fatty acid con-tent of human milk correlates directly with the maternal intake of partially hydrogenated fats and oils [1694]. Long-chain polyunsaturated fatty acids such as docosahexaenoic acid (DHA) are important for infant brain and visual development, and their presence in breast milk is largely determined by the maternal diet.

In addition to its effect on the infant, a decline in maternal DHA status in lac-tation is associated with postpartum depression in the mother [1695]. Supple-mentation with 200–220 mg/day DHA from mid-pregnancy through lactation has been shown to improve maternal DHA status and the amount of DHA pres-ent in breast milk [1696, 1697]. Very premature infants miss out on third tri-mester accretion of DHA and may benefit from maternal supplementation to increase breast milk supply [1698]. Neurological development in preterm, low-birthweight infants is also enhanced by feeding them DHA-enriched formula to match the level of accretion missed in utero [1699].

## Protein requirements during breastfeeding

The RDA for protein intake during lactation is 1.1 g per kg of body weight per day, which is the same as for pregnancy but is an additional 25 g/day above the requirement for non-pregnant, non-lactating women [131]. Body composition does not influence the amount of protein present in breast milk, but increasing dietary protein intake does modify the total amount of protein in milk [1700]. The recommended percentage of energy derived from protein in the lactation diet is 10–35 per cent, which does not differ from that for the general popula-tion. High-quality protein sources such as meat, fish, eggs, and milk provide all the essential amino acids required for lactating women. Vegetarian women need to ensure that their diet contains adequate combinations of plant proteins (legumes, nuts, fruits, starchy root vegetables, cereals) to provide all essential amino acids.

## Carbohydrate requirements during breastfeeding

The carbohydrate content of human milk is mainly lactose, which at 70 g/L makes up the second largest component of milk, after water. The lactose content of milk does not appear to be influenced by the maternal diet. Lactose and oligosaccharides facilitate growth in the gut of *Bifidus* spp., which helps to protect the breastfed infant from gastrointestinal infection. Oligosaccharides differ in composition and quantity in human vs cow's milk [1695]. Infant formulas are quite heterogeneous in their oligosaccharide makeup but in general are more similar to cow's milk than human milk, despite efforts to mimic the human milk composition [1701].

## Micronutrient requirements during breastfeeding

Nutrients are prioritized to breast milk during lactation, often at the expense of maternal reserves. Differences in milk composition, especially with regard to vitamins, can occur as a result of varying dietary intake. The concentrations of vitamins $B_6$, $B_{12}$, A, and D in breast milk are particularly sensitive to maternal intake [1702]. In well-nourished women, most micronutrients will be in adequate supply in their milk, with the exception of vitamins D and K. A number of other micronutrients, including folate, calcium, iodine, and zinc, may also be in short supply in lactating women if their own body stores were low at the end of gestation.

### Vitamin D requirements for breastfeeding mothers and newborns

Vitamin D is one micronutrient that is likely to be present in insufficient quantity in the breast milk of lactating women. Its activity in breast milk is directly related to the vitamin D status of the mother, and recent data suggest that a large percentage of women have less than optimal vitamin D stores during pregnancy. If mothers are deficient in the nutrient, vitamin D will not be detectable in their milk.

The US Institute of Medicine (IOM) RDA for vitamin D during lactation is 600 IU (15 μg/day), the same as for pregnancy. However, as dietary sources of vitamin D are minimal and UV-avoidance behaviour is common, a large proportion of the population requires supplementation in order to obtain adequate vitamin D. The recommended supplementation level of 400 IU/day, generally taken in the form of a multivitamin, has only a modest effect on maternal blood 25-hydroxyvitamin D levels [1702]. The Endocrine Society suggests that lactating women should take a vitamin D supplement of ≥1,000 IU daily *in addition* to the 400 IU/day provided in multivitamins [582].

However, despite such results and advice, maternal high-dose supplementation remains controversial. Supplementation of infants with 400 IU/day orally is therefore increasingly recommended, because provision of adequate vitamin D through breast milk cannot be consistently assured in the absence of high-dose maternal supplementation. Recent recommendations of the European Society of Paediatric Gastroenterology, Hepatology and Nutrition support this advice in order to achieve a 25-hydroxyvitamin D serum concentration in infants of >50 nmol/L (indicating vitamin D sufficiency according to their criteria) [1703].

## Vitamin K requirements for newborns

Regardless of maternal intake or status, vitamin K is generally not deposited in sufficient quantities in breast milk to support the needs of the newborn infant in the first few days of life. Therefore infant supplementation with an initial vitamin K dose shortly after birth is recommended to prevent vitamin K deficiency bleeding. The American Academy of Pediatrics recommendation is intramuscular administration of 0.5 mg vitamin K for infants ≤1,500 g, and 1 mg for infants >1,500 g [677]. Mothers should continue to consume 90 μg/day, obtainable from green leafy vegetables such as kale, spinach, beet greens, and herbs, as well as broccoli, Brussels sprouts, and spring onions.

## Vitamin A requirements during breastfeeding

Breast milk is rich in vitamin A, derived mainly from maternal fat stores and transported in the lipid fraction of milk as retinyl ester. Breast milk vitamin A content is also sensitive to maternal dietary intake, and women with low intakes may be at risk of vitamin A deficiency resulting from further depletion of their body stores, as postnatal uptake of vitamin A by the infant is much higher than during pregnancy [1704]. The provitamin A carotenoid beta-carotene remains an important source of dietary vitamin A, and women are encouraged to obtain this by increasing their intake of darkly coloured vegetables and fruits. Postpartum supplementation with vitamin A has minimal effect on maternal or infant morbidity and is therefore not generally recommended [250]

## Vitamin B$_6$ requirements during breastfeeding

Weight gain and linear growth in early infancy have been shown to correlate with infant vitamin B$_6$ intake [362]. Infants with very low intake of vitamin B$_6$ may be at risk for the development of seizures [365]. Vitamin B$_6$ concentrations in human milk respond to changes in maternal intake [363], and it is therefore important to ensure that breastfeeding mothers consume adequate amounts of vitamin B$_6$ to supply to their infants. The IOM RDA for lactation is 2.0 mg/day.

Vitamin $B_6$ is widely distributed in foods, so supplementation is usually not required if the maternal diet is healthy and balanced. However, in women with low vitamin $B_6$ intake or status, supplementation with 2.5 mg/day pyridoxine-HCl provides adequate levels of vitamin $B_6$ in breast milk to support the growth of their breastfed infants [363].

## Vitamin $B_{12}$ requirements during breastfeeding

The vitamin $B_{12}$ content of breast milk is positively correlated with meat and fish consumption [1704]. Women who consume a strict vegetarian or vegan diet should be supplemented with vitamin $B_{12}$ during lactation to help insure adequate vitamin $B_{12}$ levels in their milk. If the mother is not sufficiently supplemented herself, breastfed infants of vegan mothers should receive vitamin $B_{12}$ supplementation, for the prevention of severe megaloblastic anaemia and neurological abnormalities associated with vitamin $B_{12}$ deficiency.

## Iron requirements during breastfeeding

The IOM recommendation for iron intake during lactation is lower than during pregnancy (see Table 36.1 in chapter 36). However, as many women enter pregnancy with insufficient iron stores, it is reasonable to consider the need to maintain similar iron intake to allow for recovery of iron stores after pregnancy. Despite the fact that breast milk contains little iron, full-term infants of well-nourished mothers generally have sufficient iron stores and receive enough iron from breast milk to satisfy their requirements through the first 4–6 months of life [1705]. Low-birthweight infants or those born to diabetic mothers may have reduced iron stores at birth [951]. At around 4–6 months, the infant's iron stores are depleted, and its need for iron simultaneously increases dramatically. At this point, the introduction of iron-rich complementary foods is strongly recommended (see 'Iron requirements during weaning').

## Folate requirements during breastfeeding

The folate content of human milk is conserved at the expense of maternal stores. Thus, most breastfed infants receive sufficient folate, except in cases of severe maternal folate deficiency. Lactating women planning or considering a subsequent pregnancy should continue to consume 400 µg folic acid/day as a supplement, although they should also ensure adequate vitamin $B_{12}$ intake to avoid the risk of masking deficiency for this vitamin, and possible associated neurological damage.

## Calcium requirements during breastfeeding

As in pregnancy, the maternal calcium status is tightly regulated by homeostatic mechanisms during lactation and is unrelated to dietary intake of calcium or vitamin D. Lactational bone loss from the mobilization of maternal skeletal calcium stores is transient and recovers after weaning unless calcium intake is very low. Adolescent mothers tend to have lower calcium intakes than adults and, if they are still growing themselves, they risk poor recovery of bone mineral density after lactation. Young mothers should therefore be advised to maintain or increase their dietary calcium intake to recommended levels (1,300 mg/day) during lactation to ensure their own long-term bone health [562].

### Zinc requirements during breastfeeding

Zinc is vital for infant development, and the demand for this trace mineral is high during lactation because zinc is preferentially concentrated in breast milk from maternal tissues. Maternal zinc status thus may be jeopardized by low intake, although dietary or supplementary zinc intake does not significantly influence the concentration of zinc in breast milk, which declines over the course of lactation irrespective of maternal consumption [1706]. Low-zinc diets are usually also poor in other nutrients, including iron and vitamin $B_{12}$, because they lack animal protein. Low-zinc status increases susceptibility to infections, so lactating mothers are advised to consume adequate levels of zinc in their diets or consume a multivitamin supplement containing zinc.

### Iodine requirements during breastfeeding

During lactation, iodine is concentrated in the mammary gland for excretion in breast milk, a process that is influenced by maternal iodine status. To protect against maternal deficiency, lactating women should consume an additional 50–70 µg/day of iodine above the recommendation of 200–220 µg/day during pregnancy by the WHO and the IOM [260, 867]. The iodine status of women varies widely by region, depending on the iodine levels in local soil, and the availability and use of iodized table salt. Most women in regions where salt iodization programmes are in effect have acceptable iodine status.

## Dieting during lactation

Postpartum weight retention is higher for women who were overweight or obese during pregnancy or whose gestational weight gain was high. For these women, breastfeeding has less of an effect on weight loss than it has in women who were normal weight in pregnancy [1686]. Overweight lactating women can safely exercise and restrict their energy intake by 500 kcal/day if they consume a well-balanced diet, decreasing the amount and proportion of fats, sweetened drinks, sweets, and snack foods that they consume. A small study of such an intervention (including exercise for 45 minutes/day, 4 days/week) showed increased maternal weight loss without obvious effects on infant well-being, although the dieting women had lower intakes of vitamin D and calcium, which consequently required supplementation [1707]. All women in the study, including those not restricting their energy intake, had low intakes of vitamins C and E. Overall, the study suggested that lactating women need to increase their consumption of fruits and vegetables as well as foods high in calcium and vitamin D; in addition, they may also need to take multivitamin supplements—particularly those women following a weight loss programme.

## Exposures during lactation

### Exposure to environmental contaminants during breastfeeding

Some environmental toxins accumulate in body fat, and there has been concern that they will enter the fat component of breast milk. It is advisable that breastfeeding women avoid high-level acute exposures to known toxic substances, as also advised during pregnancy (see chapter 30 for details). Although substances such as pesticides and herbicides have been detected in breast milk, their levels in most cases are lower that what is normally found in cow's milk. Thus, despite the possible contamination of breast milk from environmental chemicals, breastfeeding is still recommended, except in cases of acute high-level exposures [1690]. Some heavy metals have been detected in human milk, including lead, arsenic, mercury, and cadmium [1708]. Lead in particular remains a concern around the world, and women who are known to be exposed should consume extra iron and calcium either in their diets or via supplements in order to minimize the mobilization of lead from bone.

### Alcohol, drugs, and smoking during breastfeeding

Alcohol transfers readily into human milk, but also suppresses milk production. Heavy alcohol consumption should be discouraged during lactation. Mothers who ingest alcohol in moderate amounts should be advised to wait ~2 hours for each drink consumed before resuming breastfeeding [1709]. Marijuana use should also be discouraged, as some secretion into breast milk has been reported, and exposure of the infant may risk neurodevelopmental complications [1710, 1711].

Cigarette smoking is strongly discouraged during lactation, as it exposes infants to toxic xenobiotics in addition to nicotine, which can affect sleep patterns and feeding [1712]. Maternal smoking also alters the micronutrient composition of breast milk; for example, thiocyanate in cigarette smoke interferes with the transport of iodine into milk [1713]. Environmental cigarette smoke exposure is associated with wheeze and respiratory infection in infants and children [1714]. The use of drugs such as cocaine, methamphetamine, and heroin is clearly contraindicated during breastfeeding, as these substances can be transferred to the infant in breast milk and can cause serious adverse effects [318]. Passive exposure to the smoke of crack cocaine also poses a risk for the infant [1715].

## Use of prescribed drugs during breastfeeding

Women may be concerned about taking medications if they are breastfeeding. Thus, they may consider either not breastfeeding or stopping their medications in order to continue. However there are many common conditions that require drug treatment and which do not constitute a contraindication to breastfeeding, as exposure of the infant to the drugs via breast milk is minimal.

### Drugs for postpartum depression

Postpartum depression is a common condition affecting women after childbirth, and drug treatment is usually recommended. Breastfeeding should not be discouraged in women taking many of the common medications such as selective serotonin reuptake inhibitors, as transfer to breast milk and uptake by the infant has been shown to be low [1716, 1717]. Fluoxetine is the least preferred because of its longer half-life and therefore higher infant exposure, but women for whom this drug is the best choice to treat their condition are not advised to change to another drug. Women for whom benzodiazepines or other drugs for sedation/anxiety are warranted should be prescribed an agent with a short half-life and at the lowest effective dose and duration, in order to minimize infant exposure [1718].

### Pain medication during breastfeeding

Most nonsteroidal anti-inflammatory drugs, and acetaminophen, are suitable for use during lactation. However, the overuse of these agents should be discouraged. Opioids should be used with caution and only under the supervision of a physician [1718].

### Antihypertensives during breastfeeding

Some anti-hypertensive medications in the beta-adrenergic blocker class can cause hypotension, bradycardia, and lethargy in infants when used by breast-feeding mothers. However, angiotensin-converting enzyme inhibitors and calcium channel blockers have not raised concerns. Thus, despite some indication that diuretics reduce milk volume, these drugs are not contraindicated for lactating women [1718, 1719].

### Anti-infectives during breastfeeding

Many anti-infective agents are excreted into breast milk and have the potential to affect the breastfeeding infant. Most antibacterials, including penicillins, aminoglycosides, cephalosporins, and carbapenems, are suitable for use during lactation, though tetracyclines can cause tooth discolouration in infants [1720]. Of the antivirals, acyclovir has been most studied in lactating women and is considered to be compatible with breastfeeding [1721]. Because of a lack of safety data, most systemic antifungal agents, with the exception of fluconazole, are not recommended during breastfeeding [1722].

## Maternal stress during breastfeeding

Glucocorticoid levels rise in response to various forms of stress. Moreover, they are secreted in breast milk, via which they can affect infant behaviour and temperament, particularly among females [1565, 1566]. As in pregnancy, women who are breastfeeding should try to avoid stress and stressful situations as much as possible.

# Infant formulas

Women who wean their infants early or do not breast feed for medical or social reasons need advice from a health care professional on suitable formulas. Infant formula is devised as a breast milk substitute and can be used as such at least through the first year of life. Formula-fed infants require complementary foods at the same stage as breastfed infants (i.e. around 6 months; see 'Weaning and complementary foods').

Most infant formulas are based on cow's milk or soy and are designed to match as closely as possible the nutritional composition of breast milk. Protein hydrolysate formulas contain extensively hydrolysed proteins and are meant for babies with protein allergies or who do not tolerate regular cow's milk or soy-based formulas. Soy formula is suitable in some but not all cases of cow's milk protein allergy; otherwise, there are no particular benefits of soy formula, and there is some concern over the presence of phytoestrogens (isoflavones), which have been shown to cause changes in sexual development in animals [1723]. While this is still a matter of some debate and ambiguity, we suggest that soy formulas should be used only for specific medical indications, under the advice of a health care professional. Lactose-free formulas are usually not necessary, as true lactose intolerance is very rare in infants.

## Essential components and composition of infant formulas

An international expert group coordinated by the European Society of Paediatric Gastroenterology, Hepatology and Nutrition published recommendations for a global standard for the composition of infant formula, based on current scientific knowledge in 2005 [953]. Formula used in the first 6 months should meet the basic guidelines proposed, some of which are outlined below. The specific micronutrient recommendations are detailed in Table 38.1.

**Table 38.1** Recommended micronutrient composition of infant formula. Unless specifically stated, the amounts of vitamins, minerals, trace elements, and other components are appropriate for formulas based on either cow's milk protein or soy and are based on global standards developed by the European Society of Paediatric Gastroenterology, Hepatology and Nutrition [953]

| Micronutrient | Recommended amount in formula (per 100 kcal) | Comments |
|---|---|---|
| Vitamin A | 60–180 µg RE | Provided by retinol or retinyl esters. Carotenoid content should not be included in the calculation of vitamin A activity. |
| Vitamin $B_1$ (thiamine) | 60–300 µg | |
| Vitamin $B_2$ (riboflavin) | 300–400 µg | |
| Vitamin $B_3$ (niacin) | 300–1500 µg | As preformed niacin. |
| Vitamin $B_5$ (pantothenic acid) | 400–2000 µg | |
| Vitamin $B_6$ (pyridoxine) | 35–175 µg | |
| Vitamin $B_{12}$ (cobalamin) | 0.1–0.5 µg | |
| Vitamin C | 10–30 mg | High intakes may induce copper deficiency. |
| Vitamin D | 1–2.5 µg | As vitamin $D_3$; data on activity of vitamin $D_2$ in infants is lacking. |
| Vitamin E | 0.5–5 mg α-TE | Composition should not be less than 0.5 mg α-TE/g linoleic acid. |
| Vitamin K | 4–25 µg | |
| Folate | 10–50 µg | As folic acid. |
| Biotin | 1.5–7.5 µg | No agreed reference intake range. Human milk range = 0.75–1.3 µg/100 kcal. |
| Calcium[a] | 50–140 mg | Bioavailability is lower from cow's milk than human milk. |
| Chloride | 50–160 mg | |
| Choline | 7–50 mg | |
| Copper | 35–80 µg | |

**Table 38.1** (continued) Recommended micronutrient composition of infant formula. Unless specifically stated, the amounts of vitamins, minerals, trace elements, and other components are appropriate for formulas based on either cow's milk protein or soy and are based on global standards developed by the European Society of Paediatric Gastroenterology, Hepatology and Nutrition [953]

| Micronutrient | Recommended amount in formula (per 100 kcal) | Comments |
|---|---|---|
| Fluoride | ≤60 µg | Infants may be exposed from other sources (e.g. water). High exposure risks dental fluorosis. |
| Iodine | 10–50 µg | Recommended intakes range from 35 to130 µg/day. |
| Iron | 0.3–1.3 mg (cow's milk) 0.45–2 mg (soy) | Phytic acid in soy inhibits iron absorption. |
| L-Carnitine | ≥1.2 mg | |
| Magnesium | 5–15 mg | |
| Manganese | 1–50 µg | Higher manganese content may cause brain accumulation and adverse effects |
| Myoinositol | 4–40 mg | |
| Phosphorus[a] | 25–90 mg (cow's milk) 30–100 mg (soy) | Bioavailability is higher from cow's milk than from soy-based formula. |
| Potassium | 60–160 mg | |
| Selenium | 1–9 µg | Human milk content=0.8–3.3 µg/100 kcal. Very high intakes may cause adverse effects. |
| Sodium | 20–60 mg | |
| Zinc | 0.5–1.5 mg | |

RE = retinol equivalent; α-TE = alpha-tocopherol equivalent

[a] The calcium:phosphorus ratio (weight/weight) should be between 1:1 and 2:1

Source: Koletzko, B. et al., Global standard for the composition of infant formula: recommendations of an ESPGHAN coordinated international expert group, *Journal of Pediatric Gastroenterology and Nutrition*, Volume 41, Issue 5, pp.584–99, copyright © 2005 ESPGHAN Committee on Nutrition.

## Energy density of infant formulas

The energy density of infant formula should be in the range of 60–70kcal/100 mL to emulate the average energy density of human milk (65 kcal/100 mL) [953]. Formulas with substantially higher energy density will promote inappropriate weight gain, which can increase the risk of obesity later in life [1724]. Infants fed formulas with energy densities below the recommended range may exhibit low weight gain and may not be receiving some necessary dietary fats.

## Fatty acids in infant formulas

Previously, infant formula did not contain preformed arachidonic acid or DHA; rather, 18-carbon precursors to these long-chain polyunsaturated fatty acids (specifically, linoleic acid and alpha-linolenic acid) were present. However, it was noted that formula-fed infants, who need to either synthesize DHA from alpha-linolenic acid or utilize body stores, did not accumulate DHA to the same level as breastfed infants, who acquire DHA in their mothers' milk [165, 1725]. Human milk DHA levels correlate positively with visual development in breastfed infants [1726]. Trials of formula compositions containing doses of DHA between 0.3 per cent and 0.5 per cent of total fatty acids, and at least equal amounts of arachidonic acid, have consistently reported significant visual and cognitive benefits for term infants [1727]. The fatty acid composition of current formulas is now between 0.15 per cent and 0.32 per cent DHA, and between 0.4 per cent and 0.64 per cent arachidonic acid. Preterm infants may require additional long-chain polyunsaturated fatty acid supplementation.

## Protein content of infant formulas

Human milk has a high whey:casein ratio (70:30) as compared to cow's milk (18:82). This higher ratio promotes more rapid gastric emptying and makes human milk more digestible [1728]. Whey proteins also differ, so to match the whey:casein ratio of human milk, cow's milk formulas have a higher protein content than human milk and are supplemented with taurine, the second most abundant amino acid in human milk [1729]. The protein content of cow's milk infant formulas should be between 1.8 and 2.0 g/100 kcal and should not exceed 3.0 g/100 kcal. This includes formulas based on protein hydrolysates [953]. The protein content of soy-based formulas should be slightly higher than that of cow's milk formulas (minimum 2.25 g/100 kcal) to account for poorer digestibility but should also not exceed 3 g/100 kcal.

## Carbohydrates in infant formulas

Carbohydrates are an essential energy source for infants. The carbohydrate content of formulas should consist mainly of lactose, be between 9 and 14 g/100 kcal, and represent ~56 per cent of the energy content of the formulas [953]. Formulas should not contain glucose, sucrose, or fructose.

## Iron in infant formulas

Most infant formulas are fortified with iron, although the optimal amount remains a matter of debate, and fortification levels vary in different countries. The benefits of additional iron are dependent on the newborn's iron status. In infants who are iron replete, provision of iron-fortified formula may not be beneficial. Excess iron can interfere with zinc and copper absorption and may increase the risk of infection.

The suggestion of the international expert group coordinated by the European Society of Paediatric Gastroenterology, Hepatology and Nutrition was that infant formulas based on cow's milk be fortified with 0.3–1.3 mg iron/100 kcal. For infants with adequate iron stores, there is no additional benefit of iron above the minimum level. In areas with a high prevalence of iron deficiency, iron contents at the higher end of this range are appropriate [953].

## Other minerals and vitamins and additional components in infant formulas

The recommended composition of other minerals, vitamins, and additional components of infant formulas are outlined in Table 38.1.

## Follow-up formulas

Follow-up formulas are intended for older infants and young children. However, they are dispensable, as infant formula can be used for the first year, and cow's milk or other milks are appropriate after that time. Follow-up formulas should not be used prior to the introduction of complementary foods [1730].

# Weaning and complementary foods

## Timing of weaning

The timing of the introduction of complementary foods into the infant diet is determined by the nutritional adequacy of exclusive breastfeeding at different ages. Thus, the appropriate time for weaning will depend on the nutritional status of the mother and infant. The timing will also depend on the growth and development of the infant, and the readiness of the infant to accept a different feeding mode.

The concentrations of many nutrients in breast milk decline rapidly between 6 and 12 months of lactation. For example, breast milk may not provide sufficient iron and zinc for some infants between 4 and 6 months of age. This is a period of rapid growth for the infant, who begins to require additional dietary sources of these vital nutrients for continued healthy development. On a per body weight basis, the nutrient requirements at this stage are higher than any other time during the lifespan.

The 4–6 month window also appears to be critical for the introduction of complementary foods from the standpoint of allergen exposure, as delayed introduction of new foods can hinder the normal development of immune tolerance [1731, 1732]. Despite earlier belief that a delay in the introduction of solid foods would lessen the risk of atopic disorders, food sensitization was actually found to be more frequent in children whose first experience of solid foods was after 6 months of age [1733]. To reduce the risk of developing celiac disease, it is recommended that gluten-containing cereals be introduced by the age of 6 months, while maintaining breastfeeding to help reduce the risk of food allergy [1734]. On the other hand, very early introduction of solid foods (before 16 weeks) also increases the risk of developing allergic or autoimmune diseases.

From a growth perspective, the introduction of complementary foods earlier than 4 months may increase the rate of weight gain and the later risk of obesity, type 2 diabetes, and cardiovascular disease, while later introduction (after 6 months) can decrease growth velocity [1735]. Because formula-fed infants generally consume more energy than breastfed infants, their set point for energy demand is higher at weaning [1736]. Between 6 and 12 months of age, infants should consume between 800 and 1,000 kcal/day.

## Nutrient requirements during weaning

There are some nutrients, most notably iron, for which infant stores are a primary source and which are depleted over the course of extended breastfeeding. The specific nutrients must be acquired through complementary foods starting between 4 and 6 months of age. Infants also begin to require fibre in their diets, which is not present in breast milk. The specific nutrient requirements for infants beginning complementary feeding, and recommended foods and sequence, are discussed below. The British Dietetic Association recommends that infants from 6 months be given a supplement containing vitamins A, C, and D, unless they are consuming formula (500 mL/day).

### Fibre requirements during weaning

Prior to the introduction of complementary foods, breastfed infants consume no dietary fibre, as it is absent from human milk. Fibre becomes important in the diet as solid foods are introduced, to balance energy density and to provide protection against immunogenic agents by modifying the composition of colonic flora [1737]. Foods such as legumes, unprocessed grains, fruits, and vegetables are sources of fibre that can be introduced to infants during the weaning process, such that by 12 months of age, the infants are consuming 5 g fibre/day [1737]. However, there is a limit to the amount of fibre-rich foods that infants should consume, as a diet too high in fibre could diminish caloric intake and reduce the bioavailability of minerals and other nutrients.

The metabolic effects of fibre-containing foods are important for the infant's developing physiology and optimum metabolic function. Supplementing the infant's diet with vegetables prior to the introduction of animal-based foods may be preferable to establish an appropriate energy balance in the diet. A suggestion for the order of introduction of complementary foods is given in Table 38.2.

## Vitamin B$_6$ requirements during weaning

The vitamin B$_6$ status of breastfed infants of well-nourished mothers is generally adequate in the first 4 months, because gestationally accumulated stores supply some of the required nutrient to the infant. However, after 6 months the risk of low vitamin B$_6$ increases, even if the mother's status is adequate [361]. Many foods contain vitamin B$_6$, but infants who do not receive complementary foods after 6 months may require supplements of the vitamin.

## Vitamin B$_{12}$ requirements during weaning

The requirement for vitamin B$_{12}$ increases slightly (from 0.4 µg/day to 0.5 µg/day) during the second half of the infant's first year of life. If the infant has been breastfed by a vegetarian mother, its stores of the nutrient will likely be depleted by around 4 months of age. Thus, for these infants, supplementation with

**Table 38.2** Complementary foods and their approximate timing of introduction into the infant diet during continued breastfeeding

| Food | Infant age (months) |
| --- | --- |
| Rice, maize | 4 |
| Potato, carrot, lettuce | 4–5 |
| Apple pear, banana | 5–6 |
| Gluten-containing cereals | 5–6 |
| Meat, fish, chicken | 6 |
| Broccoli, cabbage | 7 |
| Legumes, breakfast cereals | 8 |
| Citrus fruits | 8–10 |
| Tomato, celery | 9–10 |
| Berries, nuts | 12 |

vitamin B$_{12}$ or the addition to the diet of animal-derived complementary foods will be required.

### Iron requirements during weaning

Once infants reach 6 months of age, their iron requirements increase substantially, to around 8–11 mg/day. At this stage, their iron stores from birth are also severely diminished or exhausted. Because of this, iron-rich foods such as meat and poultry should be introduced at around 6 months, or once the infant is eating pureed rice and vegetables.

### Zinc requirements during weaning

The zinc content of human milk declines rapidly during the first 6 months, and like iron, infant zinc stores are exhausted in most infants between 4 and 6 months of age. Zinc deficiency risk increases after 6 months of age and is associated with decreased growth velocity. Complementary foods are needed to provide adequate quantities of the mineral to support development and immune function. Weaning cereals containing zinc usually also contain phytates, which limit zinc absorption, so supplementation is sometimes necessary.

## Guidelines for the introduction of complementary foods during weaning

Guidelines on complementary feeding published by the WHO and the Pan American Health Organization recommend the daily or frequent consumption of meat, poultry, fish, or eggs—the main concern being the provision of adequate quantities of iron. However, the first complementary foods should be easily digestible foods such as pureed rice or maize. Continued breastfeeding throughout the period of introduction of solid foods is strongly recommended and should be encouraged in all women who are able to do so. New foods should be introduced in a gradual manner over a period of around 6 months, beginning with a small number of pureed semi-solid foods, followed by an increasingly greater range of tastes and textures as the infant begins to self-feed (see Table 38.2). From 1 year of age, a child should be capable of participating in family meals and eating at least some family foods.

### Food preferences and flavour learning during breastfeeding and weaning

Flavours of foods eaten by the mother during pregnancy are detectable in amniotic fluid and are sensed by the fetus. Similarly, the infant is exposed via breast milk to flavours in the mother's diet during lactation [12, 13]. Studies with formula-fed infants indicate a sensitive period spanning the first three postnatal months for acceptance of specific flavours. Flavour acceptance is very specific to the flavours experienced in the formulas, which can vary drastically depending on the content of free amino acids (e.g. protein hydrolysate formula vs standard cow's milk formula).

Flavours in formulas impact on taste preferences for food at weaning. For example, protein hydrolysate formulas, which have been shown to induce satiety at lower intakes than standard formulas, have a bitter taste that is perceived as unpleasant in older infants who did not experience this flavour in the first 3 months. Infants fed protein hydrolysate formulas have a greater preference for savoury vs sweet foods at weaning, as compared to infants fed with standard cow's milk formulas [13].

Unlike formula feeding, breastfeeding allows for a wide variety of flavour experiences as a function of food choices of the mother. Subsequently, these experiences can influence the infant's acceptance of new flavours when complementary foods are introduced. This highlights the importance of a varied diet for both pregnant and lactating women.

# References

1 Godfrey, K.M. and D.J. Barker, *Fetal nutrition and adult disease.* Am J Clin Nutr, 2000. **71**(5 Suppl):1344S–52S.

2 Barker, D.J., *The developmental origins of adult disease.* J Am Coll Nutr, 2004. **23**(6 Suppl):588S–595S.

3 Gluckman, P.D., and M. Hanson, eds., *Developmental Origins of Health and Disease.* 2006, Cambridge: Cambridge University Press.

4 Gluckman, P.D., M.A. Hanson, and A.S. Beedle, *Early life events and their consequences for later disease: a life history and evolutionary perspective.* Am J Hum Biol, 2007. **19**(1):1–19.

5 Gluckman, P.D. et al., *Effect of in utero and early-life conditions on adult health and disease.* N Engl J Med, 2008. **359**(1):61–73.

6 Wadhwa, P.D. et al., *Developmental origins of health and disease: brief history of the approach and current focus on epigenetic mechanisms.* Semin Reprod Med, 2009. **27**(5):358–68.

7 Newnham, J.P.R., Ross, M.G., eds, *Early Life Origins of Human Health and Disease.* 2009, Basel: Karger.

8 Lachapelle, M.Y. and G. Drouin, *Inactivation dates of the human and guinea pig vitamin C genes.* Genetica, 2011. **139**(2):199–207.

9 Cole, B.F. et al., *Folic acid for the prevention of colorectal adenomas: a randomized clinical trial.* JAMA, 2007. **297**(21):2351–9.

10 Sloan, N.L. et al., *The effect of prenatal dietary protein intake on birth weight.* Nutr Res, 2001. **21**(1):129–39.

11 Simpson, S.J. and D. Raubenheimer, *Obesity: the protein leverage hypothesis.* Obes Rev, 2005. **6**(2):133–42.

12 Mennella, J.A., C.P. Jagnow, and G.K. Beauchamp, *Prenatal and postnatal flavor learning by human infants.* Pediatrics, 2001. **107**(6):E88.

13 Beauchamp, G.K. and J.A. Mennella, *Flavor perception in human infants: development and functional significance.* Digestion, 2011. **83** (Suppl 1):1–6.

14 Kawai, M. and K. Kishi, *Adaptation of pancreatic islet B-cells during the last third of pregnancy: regulation of B-cell function and proliferation by lactogenic hormones in rats.* Eur J Endocrinol, 1999. **141**(4):419–25.

15 Parsons, J.A., T.C. Brelje, and R.L. Sorenson, *Adaptation of islets of Langerhans to pregnancy: increased islet cell proliferation and insulin secretion correlates with the onset of placental lactogen secretion.* Endocrinology, 1992. **130**(3):1459–66.

16 Herrera, E. and H. Ortega-Senovilla, *Disturbances in lipid metabolism in diabetic pregnancy—are these the cause of the problem?* Best Pract Res Clin Endocrinol Metab, 2010. **24**(4):515–25.

17 Ferrara, A. et al., *An increase in the incidence of gestational diabetes mellitus: Northern California, 1991–2000.* Obstet Gynecol, 2004. **103**(3):526–33.

18 Hunsberger, M., K.D. Rosenberg, and R.J. Donatelle, *Racial/ethnic disparities in gestational diabetes mellitus: findings from a population-based survey.* Womens Health Issues, 2010. **20**(5):323–8.

19 Rosenberg, T.J. et al., *Maternal obesity and diabetes as risk factors for adverse pregnancy outcomes: differences among 4 racial/ethnic groups.* Am J Public Health, 2005. **95**(9):1545–51.

20 Durnwald, C. and M. Landon, *Fetal links to chronic disease: the role of gestational diabetes mellitus.* Am J Perinatol, 2013. **30**(5):343–6.

21 Hadden, D.R., *Geographic, ethnic, and racial variations in the incidence of gestational diabetes mellitus.* Diabetes, 1985. **34** (Suppl 2):8–12.

22 Flores-le Roux, J.A. et al., *A prospective evaluation of neonatal hypoglycaemia in infants of women with gestational diabetes mellitus.* Diabetes Res Clin Pract, 2012. **97**(2): 217–22.

23 Metzger, B.E. et al., *Hyperglycemia and adverse pregnancy outcomes.* N Engl J Med, 2008. **358**(19):1991–2002.

24 Lapolla, A. et al., *New International Association of the Diabetes and Pregnancy Study Groups (IADPSG) recommendations for diagnosing gestational diabetes compared with former criteria: a retrospective study on pregnancy outcome.* Diabet Med, 2011. **28**(9):1074–7.

25 Metzger, B.E. et al., *International association of diabetes and pregnancy study groups recommendations on the diagnosis and classification of hyperglycemia in pregnancy.* Diabetes Care, 2010. **33**(3):676–82.

26 Lopaschuk, G.D., R.L. Collins-Nakai, and T. Itoi, *Developmental changes in energy substrate use by the heart.* Cardiovasc Res, 1992. **26**(12):1172–80.

27 Schieve, L.A., M.E. Cogswell, and K.S. Scanlon, *Trends in pregnancy weight gain within and outside ranges recommended by the Institute of Medicine in a WIC population.* Matern Child Health J, 1998. **2**(2):111–16.

28 Helms, E., C.C. Coulson, and S.L. Galvin, *Trends in weight gain during pregnancy: a population study across 16 years in North Carolina.* Am J Obstet Gynecol, 2006. **194**(5):e32–4.

29 Yajnik, C.S., *Nutrient-mediated teratogenesis and fuel-mediated teratogenesis: two pathways of intrauterine programming of diabetes.* Int J Gynaecol Obstet, 2009. **104** (Suppl 1):S27–31.

30 Bodnar, L.M. et al., *The impact of exposure misclassification on associations between prepregnancy BMI and adverse pregnancy outcomes.* Obesity (Silver Spring), 2010. **18**(11):2184–90.

31 Ensenauer, R. et al., *Effects of suboptimal or excessive gestational weight gain on childhood overweight and abdominal adiposity: results from a retrospective cohort study.* Int J Obes (Lond), 2013. **37**(4):505–512.

32 Ravelli, A.C. et al., *Glucose tolerance in adults after prenatal exposure to famine.* Lancet, 1998. **351**(9097):173–7.

33 Hult, M. et al., *Hypertension, diabetes and overweight: looming legacies of the Biafran famine.* PLoS ONE, 2010. **5**(10):e13582.

34  Wang, P.X. et al., *Impact of fetal and infant exposure to the Chinese Great Famine on the risk of hypertension in adulthood.* PLoS ONE, 2012. **7**(11):e49720.

35  Rayco-Solon, P., A.J. Fulford, and A.M. Prentice, *Maternal preconceptional weight and gestational length.* Am J Obstet Gynecol, 2005. **192**(4):1133–6.

36  Rayco-Solon, P., A.J. Fulford, and A.M. Prentice, *Differential effects of seasonality on preterm birth and intrauterine growth restriction in rural Africans.* Am J Clin Nutr, 2005. **81**(1):134–9.

37  Prentice, A.M. et al., *Critical windows for nutritional interventions against stunting.* Am J Clin Nutr, 2013. **97**(5):911–8.

38  Moore, S.E. et al., *Season of birth predicts mortality in rural Gambia.* Nature, 1997. **388**(6641):434.

39  Blair, S.N., M.J. LaMonte, and M.Z. Nichaman, *The evolution of physical activity recommendations: how much is enough?* Am J Clin Nutr, 2004. **79**(5):913S–20S.

40  Warburton, D.E., C.W. Nicol, and S.S. Bredin, *Health benefits of physical activity: the evidence.* CMAJ, 2006. **174**(6):801–9.

41  Saltin, B. and P.D. Gollnick, *Skeletal muscle adaptability: significance for metabolism and preformance.* Compr Physiol, 2011. **Suppl 27**:555–631.

42  Levine, J.A. and C.M. Kotz, *NEAT—non-exercise activity thermogenesis—egocentric & geocentric environmental factors vs. biological regulation.* Acta Physiol Scand, 2005. **184**(4):309–18.

43  Goldenberg, R.L., J.C. Hauth, and W.W. Andrews, *Intrauterine infection and preterm delivery.* N Engl J Med, 2000. **342**(20):1500–7.

44  Khlangwiset, P., G.S. Shephard, and F. Wu, *Aflatoxins and growth impairment: a review.* Crit Rev Toxicol, 2011. **41**(9):740–55.

45  Strategic Approach to International Chemicals Management, *Submission for a nominated new emerging policy issue for proposed actions on endocrine disrupting chemicals.* Third session of the International Conference on Chemicals Management (ICCM3), Nairobi 17–21 September 2012, SAICM/ICCM.3/INF/23. 2012, <http://www.saicm.org/images/saicm_documents/iccm/ICCM3/Meeting%20documents/INF%20Documents/ICCM3_INF23%20_Submission%20on%20EDC.doc>.

46  Grandjean, P. et al., *The faroes statement: human health effects of developmental exposure to chemicals in our environment.* Basic Clin Pharmacol Toxicol, 2008. **102**(2):73–5.

47  Barouki, R. et al., *Developmental origins of non-communicable disease: implications for research and public health.* Environ Health, 2012. **11**:42.

48  Schug, T.T. et al., *PPTOX III: environmental stressors in the developmental origins of disease—evidence and mechanisms.* Toxicol Sci, 2013. **131**(2):343–50.

49  Bloomfield, F.H., A.L. Jaquiery, and M.H. Oliver, *Nutritional regulation of fetal growth,* in J. Bhatia, Z.A. Bhutta, and S.C. Kalhan, eds., *Maternal and Child Nutrition: The First 1,000 Days. Nestle Nutr Inst Worshop Series, Vol. 74.* 2013, Basel: Nestec Ltd. Vevey/Karger AG, pp. 79–89.

50  Kalish, R.B. et al., *First trimester prediction of growth discordance in twin gestations.* Am J Obstet Gynecol, 2003. **189**(3):706–9.

51  Banks, C.L., S.M. Nelson, and P. Owen, *First and third trimester ultrasound in the prediction of birthweight discordance in dichorionic twins.* Eur J Obstet Gynecol Reprod Biol, 2008. **138**(1):34–8.

52  Gluckman, P.D. and M.A. Hanson, *Maternal constraint of fetal growth and its conse-quences.* Semin Fetal Neonatal Med, 2004. **9**(5):419–25.

53  Taveras, E.M. et al., *Weight status in the first 6 months of life and obesity at 3 years of age.* Pediatrics, 2009. **123**(4):1177–83.

54  Kuzawa, C.W., *Adipose tissue in human infancy and childhood: an evolutionary perspec-tive.* Am J Phys Anthropol, 1998. **107** (Suppl 27):177–209.

55  Kessler, J. et al., *Venous liver blood flow and regulation of human fetal growth: evidence from macrosomic fetuses.* Am J Obstet Gynecol, 2011. **204**(5):429.e1–7.

56  Gluckman, P.D. and M.A. Hanson, *Mismatch: Why Our World No Longer Fits Our Bod-ies.* 2006, Oxford: Oxford University Press.

57  Gluckman, P.D. and M.A. Hanson, *Living with the past: evolution, development, and patterns of disease.* Science, 2004. **305**(5691):1733–6.

58  Bateson, P. et al., *Developmental plasticity and human health.* Nature, 2004. **430**(6998):419–21.

59  Hanson, M. et al., *Developmental plasticity and developmental origins of non-communicable disease: theoretical considerations and epigenetic mechanisms.* Prog Biophys Mol Biol, 2011. **106**(1):272–80.

60  Gluckman, P.D. and M.A. Hanson, *Fat, Fate and Disease: Why Exercise and Diet Are Not Enough.* 2012, Oxford: Oxford University Press.

61  Vickers, M.H. and D.M. Sloboda, *Strategies for reversing the effects of metabolic disor-ders induced as a consequence of developmental programming.* Front Physiol, 2012. **3**:242.

62  Gluckman, P.D., M.A. Hanson, and F.M. Low, *The role of developmental plasticity and epigenetics in human health.* Birth Defects Res C Embryo Today, 2011. **93**(1):12–18.

63  Vickers, M.H. et al., *Neonatal leptin treatment reverses developmental programming.* Endocrinology, 2005. **146**(10):4211–16.

64  Gray, C. et al., *Pre-weaning growth hormone treatment reverses hypertension and endothelial dysfunction in adult male offspring of mothers undernourished during preg-nancy.* PLoS ONE, 2013. **8**(1):e53505.

65  Drake, A.J. and L. Liu, *Intergenerational transmission of programmed effects: public health consequences.* Trends Endocrinol Metab, 2010. **21**(4):206–13.

66  Ingelfinger, J.R., *Disparities in renal endowment: causes and consequences.* Adv Chronic Kidney Dis, 2008. **15**(2):107–14.

67  Langley-Evans, S.C. et al., *Intrauterine programming of hypertension: the role of the renin-angiotensin system.* Biochem Soc Trans, 1999. **27**(2):88–93.

68  Langley-Evans, S.C., S.J. Welham, and A.A. Jackson, *Fetal exposure to a maternal low protein diet impairs nephrogenesis and promotes hypertension in the rat.* Life Sci, 1999. **64**(11):965–74.

69  Institute of Medicine, *Dietary Reference Intakes: The Essential Guide to Nutrient Require-ments.* 2006, Washington, DC: The National Academies Press.

70  US Food and Drug Administration, *How to understand and use the nutrition facts label.* <http://www.fda.gov/food/ingredientspackaginglabeling/labelingnutrition/ucm274593. htm> accessed 28 Jan 2014.

71  UK Department of Health, Food Standards Agency, and British Retail Consortium, *Guide to creating a front of pack (FoP) nutrition label for pre-packed products sold through retail*

*outlets*. 2013, <https://www.gov.uk/government/uploads/system/uploads/attachment_data/file/300886/2902158_FoP_Nutrition_2014.pdf>.

72 Kind, K.L., V.M. Moore, and M.J. Davies, *Diet around conception and during pregnancy—effects on fetal and neonatal outcomes.* Reprod Biomed Online, 2006. **12**(5):532–41.

73 Zeisel, S.H., *Is maternal diet supplementation beneficial? Optimal development of infant depends on mother's diet.* Am J Clin Nutr, 2009. **89**(2):685S–7S.

74 Cleal, J.K. and R.M. Lewis, *The mechanisms and regulation of placental amino acid transport to the human foetus.* J Neuroendocrinol, 2008. **20**(4):419–26.

75 Larque, E., M. Ruiz-Palacios, and B. Koletzko, *Placental regulation of fetal nutrient supply.* Curr Opin Clin Nutr Metab Care, 2013. **16**(3):292–7.

76 Larque, E. et al., *Placental transfer of fatty acids and fetal implications.* Am J Clin Nutr, 2011. **94**(6 Suppl):1908S–13S.

77 Blumfield, M.L. et al., *Systematic review and meta-analysis of energy and macronutrient intakes during pregnancy in developed countries.* Nutr Rev, 2012. **70**(6):322–36.

78 Brion, M.J. et al., *Maternal macronutrient and energy intakes in pregnancy and offspring intake at 10 y: exploring parental comparisons and prenatal effects.* Am J Clin Nutr, 2010. **91**(3):748–56.

79 Blumfield, M.L. et al., *Dietary balance during pregnancy is associated with fetal adiposity and fat distribution.* Am J Clin Nutr, 2012. **96**(5):1032–41.

80 Almond, K. et al., *The influence of maternal protein nutrition on offspring development and metabolism: the role of glucocorticoids.* Proc Nutr Soc, 2012. **71**(1):198–203.

81 Petry, C.J. et al., *Diabetes in old male offspring of rat dams fed a reduced protein diet.* Int J Exp Diabetes Res, 2001. **2**(2):139–43.

82 Desai, M. et al., *Adult glucose and lipid metabolism may be programmed during fetal life.* Biochem Soc Trans, 1995. **23**(2):331–5.

83 Barker, D.J., *Adult consequences of fetal growth restriction.* Clin Obstet Gynecol, 2006. **49**(2):270–83.

84 Andreasyan, K. et al., *Higher maternal dietary protein intake in late pregnancy is associated with a lower infant ponderal index at birth.* Eur J Clin Nutr, 2007. **61**(4):498–508.

85 Zambrano, E. et al., *A low maternal protein diet during pregnancy and lactation has sex- and window of exposure-specific effects on offspring growth and food intake, glucose metabolism and serum leptin in the rat.* J Physiol, 2006. **571**(Pt 1):221–30.

86 Godfrey, K. et al., *Maternal nutrition in early and late pregnancy in relation to placental and fetal growth.* BMJ, 1996. **312**(7028):410–14.

87 Moore, V.M. et al., *Dietary composition of pregnant women is related to size of the baby at birth.* J Nutr, 2004. **134**(7):1820–6.

88 Shiell, A.W. et al., *High-meat, low-carbohydrate diet in pregnancy: relation to adult blood pressure in the offspring.* Hypertension, 2001. **38**(6):1282–8.

89 Imdad, A. and Z.A. Bhutta, *Effect of balanced protein energy supplementation during pregnancy on birth outcomes.* BMC Public Health, 2011. **11** (Suppl 3):S17.

90 Buckley, A.J. et al., *Altered body composition and metabolism in the male offspring of high fat-fed rats.* Metabolism, 2005. **54**(4):500–7.

91 Moses, R.G., J.L. Shand, and L.C. Tapsell, *The recurrence of gestational diabetes: could dietary differences in fat intake be an explanation?* Diabetes Care, 1997. **20**(11):1647–50.

92  Saldana, T.M., A.M. Siega-Riz, and L.S. Adair, *Effect of macronutrient intake on the development of glucose intolerance during pregnancy.* Am J Clin Nutr, 2004. **79**(3):479–86.

93  Ley, S.H. et al., *Effect of macronutrient intake during the second trimester on glucose metabolism later in pregnancy.* Am J Clin Nutr, 2011. **94**(5):1232–40.

94  Wang, Y. et al., *Dietary variables and glucose tolerance in pregnancy.* Diabetes Care, 2000. **23**(4):460–4.

95  Clapp, J.F., 3rd, *Maternal carbohydrate intake and pregnancy outcome.* Proc Nutr Soc, 2002. **61**(1):45–50.

96  Danielsen, I. et al., *Dietary glycemic index during pregnancy is associated with biomarkers of the metabolic syndrome in offspring at age 20 years.* PLoS ONE, 2013. **8**(5):e64887.

97  Rizkalla, S.W., *Health implications of fructose consumption: a review of recent data.* Nutr Metab (Lond), 2010. **7**:82.

98  Vuilleumier, S., *Worldwide production of high-fructose syrup and crystalline fructose.* Am J Clin Nutr, 1993. **58**(5):733S–6S.

99  Elliott, S.S. et al., *Fructose, weight gain, and the insulin resistance syndrome.* Am J Clin Nutr, 2002. **76**(5):911–22.

100  Bray, G.A., *How bad is fructose?* Am J Clin Nutr, 2007. **86**(4):895–6.

101  Vos, M.B. et al., *Dietary fructose consumption among US children and adults: the Third National Health and Nutrition Examination Survey.* Medscape J Med, 2008. **10**(7):160.

102  Bezerra, R.M. et al., *A high fructose diet affects the early steps of insulin action in muscle and liver of rats.* J Nutr, 2000. **130**(6):1531–5.

103  Luo, J. et al., *A fructose-rich diet decreases insulin-stimulated glucose incorporation into lipids but not glucose transport in adipocytes of normal and diabetic rats.* J Nutr, 1995. **125**(2):164–71.

104  Stanhope, K.L. et al., *Consuming fructose-sweetened, not glucose-sweetened, beverages increases visceral adiposity and lipids and decreases insulin sensitivity in overweight/ obese humans.* J Clin Invest, 2009. **119**(5):1322–34.

105  Thorburn, A.W. et al., *Fructose-induced in vivo insulin resistance and elevated plasma triglyceride levels in rats.* Am J Clin Nutr, 1989. **49**(6):1155–63.

106  Cambonie, G. et al., *Antenatal antioxidant prevents adult hypertension, vascular dysfunction, and microvascular rarefaction associated with in utero exposure to a low-protein diet.* Am J Physiol Regul Integr Comp Physiol, 2007. **292**(3):R1236–45.

107  Langley, S.C. and A.A. Jackson, *Increased systolic blood pressure in adult rats induced by fetal exposure to maternal low protein diets.* Clin Sci (Lond), 1994. **86**(2):217–22; discussion, 121.

108  Ludwig, D.S., K.E. Peterson, and S.L. Gortmaker, *Relation between consumption of sugar-sweetened drinks and childhood obesity: a prospective, observational analysis.* Lancet, 2001. **357**(9255):505–8.

109  Pollock, N.K. et al., *Greater fructose consumption is associated with cardiometabolic risk markers and visceral adiposity in adolescents.* J Nutr, 2012. **142**(2):251–7.

110  Teff, K.L. et al., *Dietary fructose reduces circulating insulin and leptin, attenuates postprandial suppression of ghrelin, and increases triglycerides in women.* J Clin Endocrinol Metab, 2004. **89**(6):2963–72.

111  Chen, L. et al., *Prospective study of pre-gravid sugar-sweetened beverage consumption and the risk of gestational diabetes mellitus.* Diabetes Care, 2009. **32**(12):2236–41.

112 Wong, A.C. and C.W. Ko, *Carbohydrate intake as a risk factor for biliary sludge and stones during pregnancy.* J Clin Gastroenterol, 2013. **47**(8):700–5.

113 Attili, A.F. et al., *Diet and gallstones in Italy: the cross-sectional MICOL results.* Hepatology, 1998. **27**(6):1492–8.

114 Misciagna, G. et al., *Diet, physical activity, and gallstones—a population-based, case-control study in southern Italy.* Am J Clin Nutr, 1999. **69**(1):120–6.

115 Scragg, R.K., A.J. McMichael, and P.A. Baghurst, *Diet, alcohol, and relative weight in gall stone disease: a case-control study.* Br Med J (Clin Res Ed), 1984. **288**(6424):1113–19.

116 Tandon, R.K. et al., *Dietary habits of gallstone patients in Northern India.* J Clin Gastroenterol, 1996. **22**(1):23–7.

117 Tsai, C.J. et al., *Glycemic load, glycemic index, and carbohydrate intake in relation to risk of cholecystectomy in women.* Gastroenterology, 2005. **129**(1):105–12.

118 Stokes, C.S., M. Krawczyk, and F. Lammert, *Gallstones: environment, lifestyle and genes.* Dig Dis, 2011. **29**(2):191–201.

119 Dekker, M.J. et al., *Fructose: a highly lipogenic nutrient implicated in insulin resistance, hepatic steatosis, and the metabolic syndrome.* Am J Physiol Endocrinol Metab, 2010. **299**(5):E685–94.

120 Havel, P.J., *Dietary fructose: implications for dysregulation of energy homeostasis and lipid/carbohydrate metabolism.* Nutr Rev, 2005. **63**(5):133–57.

121 Miller, A. and K. Adeli, *Dietary fructose and the metabolic syndrome.* Curr Opin Gastroenterol, 2008. **24**(2):204–9.

122 Tappy, L. et al., *Fructose and metabolic diseases: new findings, new questions.* Nutrition, 2010. **26**(11–2):1044–9.

123 Champ, M. and C. Hoebler, *Functional food for pregnant, lactating women and in perinatal nutrition: a role for dietary fibres?* Curr Opin Clin Nutr Metab Care, 2009. **12**(6):565–74.

124 Mozaffarian, D. et al., *Cereal, fruit, and vegetable fiber intake and the risk of cardiovascular disease in elderly individuals.* JAMA, 2003. **289**(13):1659–66.

125 Schulze, M.B. et al., *Glycemic index, glycemic load, and dietary fiber intake and incidence of type 2 diabetes in younger and middle-aged women.* Am J Clin Nutr, 2004. **80**(2):348–56.

126 Stampfer, M.J. et al., *Primary prevention of coronary heart disease in women through diet and lifestyle.* N Engl J Med, 2000. **343**(1):16–22.

127 Brown, L. et al., *Cholesterol-lowering effects of dietary fiber: a meta-analysis.* Am J Clin Nutr, 1999. **69**(1):30–42.

128 Lopez-Miranda, J., C. Williams, and D. Lairon, *Dietary, physiological, genetic and pathological influences on postprandial lipid metabolism.* Br J Nutr, 2007. **98**(3): 458–73.

129 McKeown, N.M., *Whole grain intake and insulin sensitivity: evidence from observational studies.* Nutr Rev, 2004. **62**(7 Pt 1):286–91.

130 Whelton, S.P. et al., *Effect of dietary fiber intake on blood pressure: a meta-analysis of randomized, controlled clinical trials.* J Hypertens, 2005. **23**(3):475–81.

131 Institute of Medicine, Food and Nutrition Board, *Dietary Reference Intakes for Energy, Carbohydrate, Fiber, Fat, Fatty Acids, Cholesterol, Protein, and Amino Acids.* 2005, Washington, DC: Institute of Medicine.

132 **Oken, E. et al.**, *Television, walking, and diet: associations with postpartum weight retention.* Am J Prev Med, 2007. **32**(4):305–11.

133 **Qiu, C. et al.**, *Dietary fiber intake in early pregnancy and risk of subsequent preeclampsia.* Am J Hypertens, 2008. **21**(8):903–9.

134 **Zhang, C. et al.**, *Dietary fiber intake, dietary glycemic load, and the risk for gestational diabetes mellitus.* Diabetes Care, 2006. **29**(10):2223–30.

135 **Tieu, J., C.A. Crowther, and P. Middleton,** *Dietary advice in pregnancy for preventing gestational diabetes mellitus.* Cochrane Database Syst Rev, 2008. **2**:CD006674.

136 **Frederick, I.O. et al.**, *Dietary fiber, potassium, magnesium and calcium in relation to the risk of preeclampsia.* J Reprod Med, 2005. **50**(5):332–44.

137 **Enquobahrie, D.A. et al.**, *Maternal plasma lipid concentrations in early pregnancy and risk of preeclampsia.* Am J Hypertens, 2004. **17**(7):574–81.

138 **Williams, M.A. and R. Mittendorf,** *Maternal morbidity,* in **M.B. Goldman and M. Hatch, eds.**, *Women and Health.* 2000, New York: Academic Press, pp. 172–81.

139 **Marlett, J. A. and J. L. Slavin,** *Position of the American Dietetic Association: health implications of dietary fiber.* J Am Diet Assoc, 1997. **97**(10):1157–9.

140 **Bhargava, A.**, *Fiber intakes and anthropometric measures are predictors of circulating hormone, triglyceride, and cholesterol concentrations in the women's health trial.* J Nutr, 2006. **136**(8):2249–54.

141 **Lindstrom, J. et al.**, *High-fibre, low-fat diet predicts long-term weight loss and decreased type 2 diabetes risk: the Finnish Diabetes Prevention Study.* Diabetologia, 2006. **49**(5):912–20.

142 **Drehmer, M. et al.**, *Fibre intake and evolution of BMI: from pre-pregnancy to postpartum.* Public Health Nutr, 2013. **16**(8):1403–13.

143 National Health and Medical Research Council, Department of Health and Ageing, *Nutrient Reference Values for Australia and New Zealand, Including Recommended Dietary Intakes.* 2006, Canberra: Australian Government.

144 **Huffman, S.L. et al.**, *Essential fats: how do they affect growth and development of infants and young children in developing countries? A literature review.* Matern Child Nutr, 2011. **7** (Suppl 3):44–65.

145 **Brenna, J.T.**, *Efficiency of conversion of alpha-linolenic acid to long chain n-3 fatty acids in man.* Curr Opin Clin Nutr Metab Care, 2002. **5**(2):127–32.

146 **Pawlosky, R.J. et al.**, *Physiological compartmental analysis of alpha-linolenic acid metabolism in adult humans.* J Lipid Res, 2001. **42**(8):1257–65.

147 **Vermunt, S.H. et al.**, *Effects of age and dietary n-3 fatty acids on the metabolism of [13C]-alpha-linolenic acid.* Lipids, 1999. **34** (Suppl):S127.

148 **Lattka, E. et al.**, *Do FADS genotypes enhance our knowledge about fatty acid related phenotypes?* Clin Nutr, 2010. **29**(3):277–87.

149 **Lattka, E. et al.**, *Genetic variants of the FADS1 FADS2 gene cluster as related to essential fatty acid metabolism.* Curr Opin Lipidol, 2010. **21**(1):64–9.

150 **Innis, S.M.**, *Fatty acids and early human development.* Early Hum Dev, 2007. **83**(12):761–6.

151 **Uauy, R. and A.D. Dangour,** *Fat and fatty acid requirements and recommendations for infants of 0–2 years and children of 2–18 years.* Ann Nutr Metab, 2009. **55**(1–3):76–96.

152 **Kris-Etherton, P.M. et al.**, *Polyunsaturated fatty acids in the food chain in the United States.* Am J Clin Nutr, 2000. **71**(1 Suppl):179S–88S.

153 Burdge, G.C. and P.C. Calder, *Dietary alpha-linolenic acid and health-related outcomes: a metabolic perspective.* Nutr Res Rev, 2006. **19**(1):26–52.

154 Gibson, R.A., B. Muhlhausler, and M. Makrides, *Conversion of linoleic acid and alpha-linolenic acid to long-chain polyunsaturated fatty acids (LCPUFAs), with a focus on pregnancy, lactation and the first 2 years of life.* Matern Child Nutr, 2011. **7** (Suppl 2):17–26.

155 Ehehalt, R. et al., *Uptake of long chain fatty acids is regulated by dynamic interaction of FAT/CD36 with cholesterol/sphingolipid enriched microdomains (lipid rafts).* BMC Cell Biol, 2008. **9**:45.

156 Larque, E. et al., *Docosahexaenoic acid supply in pregnancy affects placental expression of fatty acid transport proteins.* Am J Clin Nutr, 2006. **84**(4):853–61.

157 Zeijdner, E.E. et al., *Essential fatty acid status in plasma phospholipids of mother and neonate after multiple pregnancy.* Prostaglandins Leukot Essent Fatty Acids, 1997. **56**(5):395–401.

158 Otto, S.J. et al., *The postpartum docosahexaenoic acid status of lactating and nonlactating mothers.* Lipids, 1999. **34** (Suppl):S227.

159 Ailhaud, G. et al., *Temporal changes in dietary fats: role of n-6 polyunsaturated fatty acids in excessive adipose tissue development and relationship to obesity.* Prog Lipid Res, 2006. **45**(3):203–36.

160 Gibson, R.A. and G.M. Kneebone, *Fatty acid composition of human colostrum and mature breast milk.* Am J Clin Nutr, 1981. **34**(2):252–7.

161 Makrides, M. et al., *A randomized trial of different ratios of linoleic to alpha-linolenic acid in the diet of term infants: effects on visual function and growth.* Am J Clin Nutr, 2000. **71**(1):120–9.

162 Lauritzen, L. and S.E. Carlson, *Maternal fatty acid status during pregnancy and lactation and relation to newborn and infant status.* Matern Child Nutr, 2011. **7** (Suppl 2):41–58.

163 Farquharson, J. et al., *Infant cerebral cortex phospholipid fatty-acid composition and diet.* Lancet, 1992. **340**(8823):810–13.

164 Jamieson, E.C. et al., *Infant cerebellar gray and white matter fatty acids in relation to age and diet.* Lipids, 1999. **34**(10):1065–71.

165 Makrides, M. et al., *Fatty acid composition of brain, retina, and erythrocytes in breast- and formula-fed infants.* Am J Clin Nutr, 1994. **60**(2):189–94.

166 Ramakrishnan, U., *Fatty acid status and maternal mental health.* Matern Child Nutr, 2011. **7** (Suppl 2):99–111.

167 Carlson, S.E., *Docosahexaenoic acid supplementation in pregnancy and lactation.* Am J Clin Nutr, 2009. **89**(2):678S–84S.

168 Hibbeln, J.R., *Seafood consumption, the DHA content of mothers' milk and prevalence rates of postpartum depression: a cross-national, ecological analysis.* J Affect Disord, 2002. **69**(1–3):15–29.

169 Golding, J. et al., *High levels of depressive symptoms in pregnancy with low omega-3 fatty acid intake from fish.* Epidemiology, 2009. **20**(4):598–603.

170 Freeman, M.P. et al., *Omega-3 fatty acids and supportive psychotherapy for perinatal depression: a randomized placebo-controlled study.* J Affect Disord, 2008. **110**(1–2):142–8.

171 Su, K.P. et al., *Omega-3 fatty acids for major depressive disorder during pregnancy: results from a randomized, double-blind, placebo-controlled trial.* J Clin Psychiatry, 2008. **69**(4):644–51.

172 **Doornbos, B. et al.**, *Supplementation of a low dose of DHA or DHA + AA does not prevent peripartum depressive symptoms in a small population based sample.* Prog Neuropsychopharmacol Biol Psychiatry, 2009. **33**(1):49–52.

173 **Makrides, M. et al.**, *Effect of DHA supplementation during pregnancy on maternal depression and neurodevelopment of young children: a randomized controlled trial.* JAMA, 2010. **304**(15):1675–83.

174 **Badart-Smook, A. et al.**, *Fetal growth is associated positively with maternal intake of riboflavin and negatively with maternal intake of linoleic acid.* J Am Diet Assoc, 1997. **97**(8):867–70.

175 **Dirix, C.E., A.D. Kester, and G. Hornstra**, *Associations between neonatal birth dimensions and maternal essential and trans fatty acid contents during pregnancy and at delivery.* Br J Nutr, 2009. **101**(3):399–407.

176 **van Eijsden, M. et al.**, *Maternal n-3, n-6, and trans fatty acid profile early in pregnancy and term birth weight: a prospective cohort study.* Am J Clin Nutr, 2008. **87**(4):887–95.

177 **Carlson, S.E. et al.**, *Arachidonic acid status correlates with first year growth in preterm infants.* Proc Natl Acad Sci U S A, 1993. **90**(3):1073–7.

178 **Koletzko, B. and M. Braun**, *Arachidonic acid and early human growth: is there a relation?* Ann Nutr Metab, 1991. **35**(3):128–31.

179 **Donahue, S.M. et al.**, *Prenatal fatty acid status and child adiposity at age 3 y: results from a US pregnancy cohort.* Am J Clin Nutr, 2011. **93**(4):780–8.

180 **Much, D. et al.**, *Effect of dietary intervention to reduce the n-6/n-3 fatty acid ratio on maternal and fetal fatty acid profile and its relation to offspring growth and body composition at 1 year of age.* European J Clin Nutr, 2013. **67**(3):282–8.

181 **Ailhaud, G., P. Grimaldi, and R. Negrel**, *Cellular and molecular aspects of adipose tissue development.* Annu Rev Nutr, 1992. **12**(1):207–33.

182 **Massiera, F. et al.**, *A Western-like fat diet is sufficient to induce a gradual enhancement in fat mass over generations.* J Lipid Res, 2010. **51**(8):2352–61.

183 **Ailhaud, G. and P. Guesnet**, *Fatty acid composition of fats is an early determinant of childhood obesity: a short review and an opinion.* Obes Rev, 2004. **5**(1):21–6.

184 **Anderson, G.J. et al.**, *Can prenatal N-3 fatty acid deficiency be completely reversed after birth? Effects on retinal and brain biochemistry and visual function in rhesus monkeys.* Pediatr Res, 2005. **58**(5):865–72.

185 **Neuringer, M. et al.**, *Biochemical and functional effects of prenatal and postnatal omega 3 fatty acid deficiency on retina and brain in rhesus monkeys.* Proc Natl Acad Sci U S A, 1986. **83**(11):4021–5.

186 **Bakker, E.C. et al.**, *Relationship between long-chain polyunsaturated fatty acids at birth and motor function at 7 years of age.* Eur J Clin Nutr, 2009. **63**(4):499–504.

187 **Cheruku, S.R. et al.**, *Higher maternal plasma docosahexaenoic acid during pregnancy is associated with more mature neonatal sleep-state patterning.* Am J Clin Nutr, 2002. **76**(3):608–13.

188 **Colombo, J. et al.**, *Maternal DHA and the development of attention in infancy and toddlerhood.* Child Dev, 2004. **75**(4):1254–67.

189 **Hibbeln, J.R. et al.**, *Maternal seafood consumption in pregnancy and neurodevelopmental outcomes in childhood (ALSPAC study): an observational cohort study.* Lancet, 2007. **369**(9561):578–85.

190  Jacobson, J.L. et al., *Beneficial effects of a polyunsaturated fatty acid on infant development: evidence from the Inuit of Arctic Quebec.* J Pediatr, 2008. **152**(3):356–64.

191  Kannass, K.N., J. Colombo, and S.E. Carlson, *Maternal DHA levels and toddler free-play attention.* Dev Neuropsychol, 2009. **34**(2):159–74.

192  Mendez, M.A. et al., *Maternal fish and other seafood intakes during pregnancy and child neurodevelopment at age 4 years.* Public Health Nutr, 2009. **12**(10):1702–10.

193  Daniels, J.L. et al., *Fish intake during pregnancy and early cognitive development of offspring.* Epidemiology, 2004. **15**(4):394–402.

194  Gale, C.R. et al., *Oily fish intake during pregnancy—association with lower hyperactivity but not with higher full-scale IQ in offspring.* J Child Psychol Psychiatry, 2008. **49**(10):1061–8.

195  Oken, E. et al., *Maternal fish intake during pregnancy, blood mercury levels, and child cognition at age 3 years in a US cohort.* Am J Epidemiol, 2008. **167**(10):1171–81.

196  Williams, C. et al., *Stereoacuity at age 3.5 y in children born full-term is associated with prenatal and postnatal dietary factors: a report from a population-based cohort study.* Am J Clin Nutr, 2001. **73**(2):316–22.

197  Gould, J.F., L.G. Smithers, and M. Makrides, *The effect of maternal omega-3 (n23) LCPUFA supplementation during pregnancy on early childhood cognitive and visual development: a systematic review and meta-analysis of randomized controlled trials.* Am J Clin Nutr, 2013. **76**(4):189–203.

198  Black, P.N. and S. Sharpe, *Dietary fat and asthma: is there a connection?* Eur Respir J, 1997. **10**(1):6–12.

199  Hodge, L., J.K. Peat, and C. Salome, *Increased consumption of polyunsaturated oils may be a cause of increased prevalence of childhood asthma.* Aust N Z J Med, 1994. **24**(6):727.

200  Duchen, K. et al., *Human milk polyunsaturated long-chain fatty acids and secretory immunoglobulin A antibodies and early childhood allergy.* Pediatr Allergy Immunol, 2000. **11**(1):29–39.

201  Montes, R. et al., *Fatty-acid composition of maternal and umbilical cord plasma and early childhood atopic eczema in a Spanish cohort.* Eur J Clin Nutr, 2013. **67**(6), 658–63.

202  Pike, K.C. et al., *Maternal plasma phosphatidylcholine fatty acids and atopy and wheeze in the offspring at age of 6 years.* Clin Dev Immunol, 2012. **2012**:474613.

203  Kremmyda, L.S. et al., *Atopy risk in infants and children in relation to early exposure to fish, oily fish, or long-chain omega-3 fatty acids: a systematic review.* Clin Rev Allergy Immunol, 2011. **41**(1):36–66.

204  West, C.E., D.J. Videky, and S.L. Prescott, *Role of diet in the development of immune tolerance in the context of allergic disease.* Curr Opin Pediatr, 2010. **22**(5):635–41.

205  Palmer, D.J. et al., *Effect of n-3 long chain polyunsaturated fatty acid supplementation in pregnancy on infants' allergies in first year of life: randomised controlled trial.* BMJ, 2012. **344**:e184.

206  Calvani, M. et al, *Consumption of fish, butter and margarine during pregnancy and development of allergic sensitizations in the offspring: role of maternal atopy.* Pediatr Allergy Immunol, 2006. **17**(2):94–102.

207  Romieu, I. et al., *Maternal fish intake during pregnancy and atopy and asthma in infancy.* Clin Exp Allergy, 2007. **37**(4):518–25.

208 **Salam, M.T. et al.,** *Maternal fish consumption during pregnancy and risk of early childhood asthma.* J Asthma, 2005. **42**(6):513–8.

209 **Sausenthaler, S. et al.,** *Maternal diet during pregnancy in relation to eczema and allergic sensitization in the offspring at 2 y of age.* Am J Clin Nutr, 2007. **85**(2):530–7.

210 **Birch, E.E. et al.,** *The impact of early nutrition on incidence of allergic manifestations and common respiratory illnesses in children.* J Pediatr, 2010. **156**(6):902–6, 906.e1.

211 **Pastor, N. et al.,** *Infants fed docosahexaenoic acid- and arachidonic acid-supplemented formula have decreased incidence of bronchiolitis/bronchitis the first year of life.* Clin Pediatr (Phila), 2006. **45**(9):850–5.

212 **Minns, L.M. et al.,** *Toddler formula supplemented with docosahexaenoic acid (DHA) improves DHA status and respiratory health in a randomized, double-blind, controlled trial of US children less than 3 years of age.* Prostaglandins Leukot Essent Fatty Acids, 2010. **82**(4–6):287–93.

213 Food and Agriculture Organization of the United Nations, *Fats and fatty acids in human nutrition: report of an expert consultation. FAO Food and Nutrition Paper 91.* 2010, <http://www.fao.org/docrep/013/i1953e/i1953e00.pdf>.

214 EFSA Panel on Dietetic Products, Nutrition and Allergies, *Scientific Opinion on Dietary Reference Values for fats, including saturated fatty acids, polyunsaturated fatty acids, monounsaturated fatty acids, trans fatty acids, and cholesterol.* EFSA Journal, 2010. **8**(3):1461–568.

215 **Halldorsson, T.I. et al.,** *Linking exposure to polychlorinated biphenyls with fatty fish consumption and reduced fetal growth among Danish pregnant women: a cause for concern?* Am J Epidemiol, 2008. **168**(8):958–65.

216 **Association, A.P.,** *Mercury levels in fish.* <http://americanpregnancy.org/pregnancyhealth/fishmercury.htm> accessed 9 June 2013.

217 **Blomhoff, R. and H.K. Blomhoff,** *Overview of retinoid metabolism and function.* J Neurobiol, 2006. **66**(7):606–30.

218 **Kliewer, S.A. et al.,** *Retinoid X receptor interacts with nuclear receptors in retinoic acid, thyroid hormone and vitamin $D_3$ signalling.* Nature, 1992. **355**(6359):446–9.

219 **Blomhoff, R. et al.,** *Vitamin A metabolism: new perspectives on absorption, transport, and storage.* Physiol Rev, 1991. **71**(4):951–90.

220 **Blaner, W.S.,** *Retinol-binding protein: the serum transport protein for vitamin A.* Endocr Rev, 1989. **10**(3):308–16.

221 **Reijntjes, S. et al.,** *The control of morphogen signalling: regulation of the synthesis and catabolism of retinoic acid in the developing embryo.* Dev Biol, 2005. **285**(1):224–37.

222 World Health Organization, *Global prevalence of vitamin A deficiency in populations at risk 1995–2005.* 2009, <http://whqlibdoc.who.int/publications/2009/9789241598019_eng.pdf?ua=1>.

223 **Sommer, A.,** *Vitamin A Deficiency and its Consequences: A Field Guide to Detection and Control, Third Edition.* 1995, Geneva: World Health Organization.

224 **Rando, R.R.,** *The biochemistry of the visual cycle.* Chem Rev, 2001. **101**(7):1881–96.

225 **Clagett-Dame, M. and D. Knutson,** *Vitamin A in reproduction and development.* Nutrients, 2011. **3**(4):385–428.

226 **Lawson, N.D. and N. Berliner,** *Neutrophil maturation and the role of retinoic acid.* Exp Hematol, 1999. **27**(9):1355–67.

227  Stephensen, C.B., *Vitamin A, infection, and immune function.* Annu Rev Nutr, 2001. **21**:167–92.

228  Wiedermann, U. et al., *Increased translocation of Escherichia coli and development of arthritis in vitamin A-deficient rats.* Infect Immun, 1995. **63**(8):3062–8.

229  Rothman, K.J. et al., *Teratogenicity of high vitamin A intake.* N Engl J Med, 1995. **333**(21):1369–73.

230  Quadro, L. et al., *Pathways of vitamin A delivery to the embryo: insights from a new tunable model of embryonic vitamin A deficiency.* Endocrinology, 2005. **146**(10):4479–90.

231  World Health Organization and Food and Agriculture Organization of the United Nations, *Vitamin and Mineral Requirements in Human Nutrition, Second Edition.* 2004, Geneva: World Health Organization.

232  Wang, Y.Z. et al., *Concentrations of antioxidant vitamins in maternal and cord serum and their effect on birth outcomes.* J Nutr Sci Vitaminol (Tokyo), 2009. **55**(1):1–8.

233  Tielsch, J.M. et al., *Maternal night blindness during pregnancy is associated with low birthweight, morbidity, and poor growth in South India.* J Nutr, 2008. **138**(4):787–92.

234  Fawzi, W.W. et al., *Randomised trial of effects of vitamin supplements on pregnancy outcomes and T cell counts in HIV-1-infected women in Tanzania.* Lancet, 1998. **351**(9114):1477–82.

235  Christian, P. et al., *Effects of vitamin A and beta-carotene supplementation on birth size and length of gestation in rural Bangladesh: a cluster-randomized trial.* Am J Clin Nutr, 2013. **97**(1):188–94.

236  United Nations Standing Committee on Nutrition, *Progress in Nutrition: 6th Report on the World Nutrition Situation.* 2009, Geneva: World Health Organization.

237  van den Broek, N. et al., *Vitamin A supplementation during pregnancy for maternal and newborn outcomes.* Cochrane Database Syst Rev, 2010. **11**:CD008666.

238  Cox, S.E. et al., *Maternal vitamin A supplementation and immunity to malaria in pregnancy in Ghanaian primigravids.* Trop Med Int Health, 2005. **10**(12):1286–97.

239  Kumwenda, N. et al., *Antenatal vitamin A supplementation increases birth weight and decreases anemia among infants born to human immunodeficiency virus-infected women in Malawi.* Clin Infect Dis, 2002. **35**(5):618–24.

240  West, K.P., Jr. et al., *Effects of vitamin A or beta carotene supplementation on pregnancy-related mortality and infant mortality in rural Bangladesh: a cluster randomized trial.* JAMA, 2011. **305**(19):1986–95.

241  Kirkwood, B.R. et al., *Effect of vitamin A supplementation in women of reproductive age on maternal survival in Ghana (ObaapaVitA): a cluster-randomised, placebo-controlled trial.* Lancet, 2010. **375**(9726):1640–9.

242  Darlow, B.A. and P.J. Graham, *Vitamin A supplementation to prevent mortality and short- and long-term morbidity in very low birthweight infants.* Cochrane Database Syst Rev, 2011. **10**:CD000501.

243  Kolsteren, P. et al., *Treatment for iron deficiency anaemia with a combined supplementation of iron, vitamin A and zinc in women of Dinajpur, Bangladesh.* Eur J Clin Nutr, 1999. **53**(2):102–6.

244  Semba, R.D. et al., *Impact of vitamin A supplementation on anaemia and plasma erythropoietin concentrations in pregnant women: a controlled clinical trial.* Eur J Haematol, 2001. **66**(6):389–95.

245 van den Broek, N.R. et al., *Randomised trial of vitamin A supplementation in pregnant women in rural Malawi found to be anaemic on screening by HemoCue.* BJOG, 2006. **113**(5):569–76.

246 Stoltzfus, R.J. and B.A. Underwood, *Breast-milk vitamin A as an indicator of the vitamin A status of women and infants.* Bull World Health Organ, 1995. **73**(5):703–11.

247 Ross, A.C. and E.M. Gardner, *The function of vitamin A in cellular growth and differentiation, and its roles during pregnancy and lactation.* Adv Exp Med Biol, 1994. **352**:187–200.

248 Stoltzfus, R.J., *Vitamin A deficiency in the mother-infant dyad.* SCN News, 1994. **11**:25–7.

249 Stoltzfus, R.J. et al., *High dose vitamin A supplementation of breast-feeding Indonesian mothers: effects on the vitamin A status of mother and infant.* J Nutr, 1993. **123**(4):666–75.

250 Oliveira-Menegozzo, J.M. et al., *Vitamin A supplementation for postpartum women.* Cochrane Database Syst Rev, 2010. **10**:CD005944.

251 Inder, T.E. et al., *Plasma vitamin A levels in the very low birthweight infant—relationship to respiratory outcome.* Early Hum Dev, 1998. **52**(2):155–68.

252 Mayo-Wilson, E. et al., *Vitamin A supplements for preventing mortality, illness, and blindness in children aged under 5: systematic review and meta-analysis.* BMJ, 2011. **343**:d5094.

253 Li, E. and P. Tso, *Vitamin A uptake from foods.* Curr Opin Lipidol, 2003. **14**(3):241–7.

254 Leo, M.A. and C.S. Lieber, *Alcohol, vitamin A, and beta-carotene: adverse interactions, including hepatotoxicity and carcinogenicity.* Am J Clin Nutr, 1999. **69**(6):1071–85.

255 Deltour, L., H.L. Ang, and G. Duester, *Ethanol inhibition of retinoic acid synthesis as a potential mechanism for fetal alcohol syndrome.* FASEB J, 1996. **10**(9):1050–7.

256 Chan, A. et al., *Oral retinoids and pregnancy.* Med J Aust, 1996. **165**(3):164–7.

257 Miller, R.K. et al., *Periconceptional vitamin A use: how much is teratogenic?* Reprod Toxicol, 1998. **12**(1):75–88.

258 Voyles, L.M. et al., *High levels of retinol intake during the first trimester of pregnancy result from use of over-the-counter vitamin/mineral supplements.* J Am Diet Assoc, 2000. **100**(9):1068–70.

259 Adams, J. and E.J. Lammer, *Neurobehavioral teratology of isotretinoin.* Reprod Toxicol, 1993. **7**(2):175–7.

260 Institute of Medicine, Food and Nutrition Board, *Dietary Reference Intakes for Vitamin A, Vitamin K, Arsenic, Boron, Chromium, Copper, Iodine, Iron, Manganese, Molybdenum, Nickel, Silicon, Vanadium, and Zinc.* 2001, Washington, DC: The National Academies Press.

261 Gebhardt, S.E. and J.M. Holden, *Consequences of changes in the Dietary Reference Intakes for nutrient databases.* J Food Comp Anal, 2006. **19**(Suppl):S91–S95.

262 World Health Organization, *WHO Guideline: Vitamin A Supplementation in Pregnant Women.* 2011, Geneva: World Health Organization.

263 World Health Organization, *WHO Guideline: Vitamin A Supplementation in Postpartum Women.* 2011, Geneva: World Health Organization.

264 World Health Organization, *Report of the Consultation: Safe Vitamin A Dosage during Pregnancy and the First 6 Months Postpartum.* 1996, Geneva: World Health Organization.

265 SA Health, *Vitamin and mineral supplementation in pregnancy.* 2011, <http://www.sahealth.sa.gov.au/wps/wcm/connect/public+content/sa+health+internet/resources/policies/vitamin+and+mineral+supplementation+in+pregnancy+-+sa+perinatal+practice+guidelines>.

266 National Institute for Health and Clinical Excellence, *Antenatal Care: Routine Care for the Healthy Pregnant Woman. NICE Clinical Guidelines, No. 62.* 2008, London: RCOG Press.

267 Doets, E.L. et al., *Current micronutrient recommendations in Europe: towards understanding their differences and similarities.* Eur J Nutr, 2008. **47** (Suppl 1):17–40.

268 International Institute for Population Sciences and Macro International, *National family health survey-3 (NFHS-3), 2005–06, India: key findings.* 2007, Mumbai: International Institute for Population Sciences. <http://dhsprogram.com/pubs/pdf/SR128/SR128.pdf>.

269 Institute of Medicine, Food and Nutrition Board, *Dietary Reference Intakes: Thiamin, Riboflavin, Niacin, Vitamin B₆, Folate, Vitamin B₁₂, Pantothenic Acid, Biotin, and Choline.* 1998, Washington, DC: National Academy Press.

270 Rindi, G. and U. Laforenza, *Thiamine intestinal transport and related issues: recent aspects.* Proc Soc Exp Biol Med, 2000. **224**(4):246–55.

271 Ariaey-Nejad, M.R. et al., *Thiamin metabolism in man.* Am J Clin Nutr, 1970. **23**(6):764–78.

272 Bailey, A.L. et al., *Thiamin intake, erythrocyte transketolase (EC 2.2.1.1) activity and total erythrocyte thiamin in adolescents.* Br J Nutr, 1994. **72**(1):111–25.

273 Brin, M., *Erythrocyte as a biopsy tissue for functional evaluation of thiamine adequacy.* JAMA, 1964. **187**:762–6.

274 Talwar, D. et al., *Vitamin B(1) status assessed by direct measurement of thiamin pyrophosphate in erythrocytes or whole blood by HPLC: comparison with erythrocyte transketolase activation assay.* Clin Chem, 2000. **46**(5):704–10.

275 World Health Organization, United Nations High Commissioner for Refugees, *Thiamine Deficiency and its Prevention and Control in Major Emergencies.* 1999, Geneva: World Health Organization.

276 Tomasulo, P.A., R.M. Kater, and F.L. Iber, *Impairment of thiamine absorption in alcoholism.* Am J Clin Nutr, 1968. **21**(11):1341–4.

277 Isenberg-Grzeda, E., H.E. Kutner, and S.E. Nicolson, *Wernicke-Korsakoff-syndrome: under-recognized and under-treated.* Psychosomatics, 2012. **53**(6):507–16.

278 Butterworth, R.F. et al., *Thiamine deficiency and Wernicke's encephalopathy in AIDS.* Metab Brain Dis, 1991. **6**(4):207–12.

279 Cumming, R.G., P. Mitchell, and W. Smith, *Diet and cataract: the Blue Mountains Eye Study.* Ophthalmology, 2000. **107**(3):450–6.

280 Jacques, P.F. et al., *Long-term nutrient intake and 5-year change in nuclear lens opacities.* Arch Ophthalmol, 2005. **123**(4):517–26.

281 Tripathy, K., *Erythrocyte transketolase activity and thiamine transer across human placenta.* Am J Clin Nutr, 1968. **21**(7):739–42.

282 Heller, S., R.M. Salkeld, and W.F. Korner, *Vitamin B₁ status in pregnancy.* Am J Clin Nutr, 1974. **27**(11):1221–4.

283 van Stuijvenberg, M.E. et al., *The nutritional status and treatment of patients with hyperemesis gravidarum.* Am J Obstet Gynecol, 1995. **172**(5):1585–91.

284 Chitra, S. and K.V. Lath, *Wernicke's encephalopathy with visual loss in a patient with hyperemesis gravidarum.* J Assoc Physicians India, 2012. **60**:53–6.

285 Palacios-Marques, A. et al., *Wernicke's encephalopathy induced by hyperemesis gravidarum.* BMJ Case Rep, 2012. **99**(3):196–8.

286 Wyatt, D.T., D. Nelson, and R.E. Hillman, *Age-dependent changes in thiamin concentrations in whole blood and cerebrospinal fluid in infants and children.* Am J Clin Nutr, 1991. **53**(2):530–6.

287 Fattal-Valevski, A. et al., *Outbreak of life-threatening thiamine deficiency in infants in Israel caused by a defective soy-based formula.* Pediatrics, 2005. **115**(2):e233–8.

288 Fattal-Valevski, A. et al., *Epilepsy in children with infantile thiamine deficiency.* Neurology, 2009. **73**(11):828–33.

289 Attias, J. et al., *Auditory system dysfunction due to infantile thiamine deficiency: long-term auditory sequelae.* Audiol Neurootol, 2012. **17**(5):309–20.

290 Shamir, R., *Thiamine-deficient infant formula: what happened and what have we learned?* Ann Nutr Metab, 2012. **60**(3):185–7.

291 European Commission, *Commission Directive 2006/141/EC on infant formulae and follow on formulae and amending Directive 1999/21/EC. December 22, 2006.* 2006,<http://eur-lex.europa.eu/legal-content/EN/ALL/;jsessionid=RQQzTTypXDDx8wjntZx3VMF d2dP2bnhKlKhFdFy1SxVB34JLpx0p!1306593838?uri=CELEX:32006L0141>.

292 Burgess, R.C., *Deficiency diseases in prisoners of war at Changi, Singapore, February 1942 to August 1945.* Lancet, 1946. **2**(6421):411–8.

293 Lienhart, W.D., V. Gudipati, and P. Macheroux, *The human flavoproteome.* Arch Biochem Biophys, 2013. **535**(2), 150–62.

294 Ziegler, G.A. et al., *The structure of adrenodoxin reductase of mitochondrial P450 systems: electron transfer for steroid biosynthesis.* J Mol Biol, 1999. **289**(4):981–90.

295 McCormick, D.B., *Two interconnected B vitamins: riboflavin and pyridoxine.* Physiol Rev, 1989. **69**(4):1170–98.

296 Powers, H.J., *Riboflavin-iron interactions with particular emphasis on the gastrointestinal tract.* Proc Nutr Soc, 1995. **54**(2):509–17.

297 Powers, H.J. et al., *Correcting a marginal riboflavin deficiency improves hematologic status in young women in the United Kingdom (RIBOFEM).* Am J Clin Nutr, 2011. **93**(6):1274–84.

298 Powers, H.J., *Riboflavin (vitamin B-2) and health.* Am J Clin Nutr, 2003. **77**(6):1352–60.

299 Powers, H.J., *Current knowledge concerning optimum nutritional status of riboflavin, niacin and pyridoxine.* Proc Nutr Soc, 1999. **58**(2):435–40.

300 Wolf, G. and R.S. Rlin, *Inhibition of thyroid hormone induction of mitochondrial alpha-glycerophosphate dehydrogenase in riboflavin deficiency.* Endocrinology, 1970. **86**(6):1347–53.

301 Powers, H.J., B.M. Corfe, and E. Nakano, *Riboflavin in development and cell fate.* Subcell Biochem, 2012. **56**:229–45.

302 Olpin, S.E. and C.J. Bates, *Lipid metabolism in riboflavin-deficient rats. 1. Effect of dietary lipids on riboflavin status and fatty acid profiles.* Br J Nutr, 1982. **47**(3):577–96.

303 Kim, Y.S. and J.P. Lambooy, *Biochemical and physiological changes in the rat during riboflavin deprivation and supplementation.* J Nutr, 1969. **98**(4):467–76.

304 Natraj, U., S. George, and P. Kadam, *Isolation and partial characterisation of human riboflavin carrier protein and the estimation of its levels during human pregnancy.* J Reprod Immunol, 1988. **13**(1):1–16.

305 Prasad, P.D. et al., *Isolation and characterization of riboflavin carrier protein from human amniotic fluid.* Biochem Int, 1992. **27**(3):385–95.

306 Zempleni, J., G. Link, and I. Bitsch, *Intrauterine vitamin B$_2$ uptake of preterm and full-term infants.* Pediatr Res, 1995. **38**(4):585–91.

307 Bohn, H. and W. Winckler, *Isolation and characterization of a flavin-containing placental protein (PP3).* Arch Gynecol, 1987. **240**(4):201–6.

308 Bates, C.J. et al., *Riboflavin status in infants born in rural Gambia, and the effect of a weaning food supplement.* Trans R Soc Trop Med Hyg, 1982. **76**(2):253–8.

309 Heller, S., R.M. Salkeld, and W.F. Korner, *Riboflavin status in pregnancy.* Am J Clin Nutr, 1974. **27**(11):1225–30.

310 Vir, S.C., A.H. Love, and W. Thompson, *Riboflavin status during pregnancy.* Am J Clin Nutr, 1981. **34**(12):2699–705.

311 Bates, C.J. et al., *Riboflavin status in Gambian pregnant and lactating women and its implications for Recommended Dietary Allowances.* Am J Clin Nutr, 1981. **34**(5): 928–35.

312 Nail, P.A., M.R. Thomas, and R. Eakin, *The effect of thiamin and riboflavin supplementation on the level of those vitamins in human breast milk and urine.* Am J Clin Nutr, 1980. **33**(2):198–204.

313 Papathakis, P.C. and K.E. Pearson, *Food fortification improves the intake of all fortified nutrients, but fails to meet the estimated dietary requirements for vitamins A and B$_6$, riboflavin and zinc, in lactating South African women.* Public Health Nutr, 2012. **15**(10): 1810–7.

314 Ortega, R.M. et al., *Riboflavin levels in maternal milk: the influence of vitamin B$_2$ status during the third trimester of pregnancy.* J Am Coll Nutr, 1999. **18**(4):324–9.

315 Tan, K.L., M.T. Chow, and S.M. Karim, *Effect of phototherapy on neonatal riboflavin status.* J Pediatr, 1978. **93**(3):494–7.

316 Bates, C.J. et al., *Riboflavin status of adolescent vs elderly Gambian subjects before and during supplementation.* Am J Clin Nutr, 1989. **50**(4):825–9.

317 Kuizon, M.D. et al., *Riboflavin requirement of Filipino women.* Eur J Clin Nutr, 1992. **46**(4):257–64.

318 Kauffman, R.E. et al., *The transfer of drugs and other chemicals into human milk.* Pediatrics, 1994. **93**(1):137–50.

319 Berger, N.A., *Poly(ADP-ribose) in the cellular response to DNA damage.* Radiat Res, 1985. **101**(1):4–15.

320 Di Girolamo, M. et al., *Physiological relevance of the endogenous mono(ADP-ribosyl)ation of cellular proteins.* FEBS J, 2005. **272**(18):4565–75.

321 Bechgaard, H. and S. Jespersen, *GI absorption of niacin in humans.* J Pharm Sci, 1977. **66**(6):871–2.

322 Jacob, R.A. et al., *Biochemical markers for assessment of niacin status in young men: urinary and blood levels of niacin metabolites.* J Nutr, 1989. **119**(4):591–8.

323 Fu, C.S. et al., *Biochemical markers for assessment of niacin status in young men: levels of erythrocyte niacin coenzymes and plasma tryptophan.* J Nutr, 1989. **119**(12):1949–55.

324  Park, Y.K. et al., *Effectiveness of food fortification in the United States: the case of pellagra.* Am J Public Health, 2000. **90**(5):727–38.

325  Rose, D.P. and I.P. Braidman, *Excretion of tryptophan metabolites as affected by pregnancy, contraceptive steroids, and steroid hormones.* Am J Clin Nutr, 1971. **24**(6):673–83.

326  Wertz, A.W. et al., *Tryptophan-niacin relationships in pregnancy.* J Nutr, 1958. **64**(3):339–53.

327  Brown, R.R., M.J. Thornton, and J.M. Price, *The effect of vitamin supplementation on the urinary excretion of tryptophan metabolites by pregnant women.* J Clin Invest, 1961. **40**(4):617–23.

328  Wolf, H., *Hormonal alteration of efficiency of conversion of tryptophan to urinary metabolites of niacin in man.* Am J Clin Nutr, 1971. **24**(7):792–9.

329  Horwitt, M.K., A.E. Harper, and L.M. Henderson, *Niacin–tryptophan relationships for evaluating niacin equivalents.* Am J Clin Nutr, 1981. **34**(3):423–7.

330  Carter, E.G. and K.J. Carpenter, *The bioavailability for humans of bound niacin from wheat bran.* Am J Clin Nutr, 1982. **36**(5):855–61.

331  Gregory, J.F., 3rd, *Nutritional properties and significance of vitamin glycosides.* Annu Rev Nutr, 1998. **18**(1):277–96.

332  Dakshinamurti, S. and K. Dakshinamurti, *Vitamin $B_6$,* in J. Zempleni et al., eds., *Handbook of Vitamins, Fourth Edition.* 2007, Boca Raton: Taylor & Francis, pp. 315–359.

333  John, R.A., *Pyridoxal phosphate-dependent enzymes.* Biochim Biophys Acta, 1995. **1248**(2):81–96.

334  Schneider, G., H. Kack, and Y. Lindqvist, *The manifold of vitamin $B_6$ dependent enzymes.* Structure, 2000. **8**(1):R1–6.

335  Percudani, R. and A. Peracchi, *A genomic overview of pyridoxal-phosphate-dependent enzymes.* EMBO Rep, 2003. **4**(9):850–4.

336  Mason, J.B. and J.W. Miller, *The effects of vitamins $B_{12}$, $B_6$, and folate on blood homocysteine levels.* Ann N Y Acad Sci, 1992. **669**:197–203; discussion, 203–4.

337  Sturman, J.A. and L.T. Kremzner, *Polyamine biosynthesis and vitamin $B_6$ deficiency. Evidence for pyridoxal phosphate as coenzyme for S-adenosylmethionine decarboxylase.* Biochim Biophys Acta, 1974. **372**(1):162–70.

338  Bourquin, F., G. Capitani, and M.G. Grutter, *PLP-dependent enzymes as entry and exit gates of sphingolipid metabolism.* Protein Sci, 2011. **20**(9):1492–508.

339  Ink, S.L., H. Mehansho, and L.M. Henderson, *The binding of pyridoxal to hemoglobin.* J Biol Chem, 1982. **257**(9):4753–7.

340  Solomon, L.R., *Considerations in the use of $B_6$ vitamers in hematologic disorders: I. Red cell transport and metabolism of pyridoxal.* Blood, 1982. **59**(3):495–501.

341  Lumeng, L., A. Lui, and T.K. Li, *Plasma content of $B_6$ vitamens and its relationship to hepatic vitamin $B_6$ metabolism.* J Clin Invest, 1980. **66**(4):688–95.

342  Leklem, J.E., *Vitamin B-6: a status report.* J Nutr, 1990. **120** (Suppl 11):1503–7.

343  Centers for Disease Control and Prevention, Division of Laboratory Sciences, National Center for Environmental Health, *Second National Report on Biochemical Indicators of Diet and Nutrition in the US Population. Executive Summary.* 2012, Atlanta: Centers for Disease Control and Prevention.

344 **Roubenoff, R. et al.,** *Abnormal vitamin B₆ status in rheumatoid cachexia. Association with spontaneous tumor necrosis factor alpha production and markers of inflammation.* Arthritis Rheum, 1995. **38**(1):105–9.

345 **Saibeni, S. et al.,** *Low vitamin B(6) plasma levels, a risk factor for thrombosis, in inflammatory bowel disease: role of inflammation and correlation with acute phase reactants.* Am J Gastroenterol, 2003. **98**(1):112–7.

346 **Friso, S. et al.,** *Low plasma vitamin B-6 concentrations and modulation of coronary artery disease risk.* Am J Clin Nutr, 2004. **79**(6):992–8.

347 **Heller, S., R.M. Salkeld, and W.F. Korner,** *Vitamin B₆ status in pregnancy.* Am J Clin Nutr, 1973. **26**(12):1339–48.

348 **Hogeveen, M., H.J. Blom, and M. den Heijer,** *Maternal homocysteine and small-for-gestational-age offspring: systematic review and meta-analysis.* Am J Clin Nutr, 2012. **95**(1):130–6.

349 **Bergen, N.E. et al.,** *Homocysteine and folate concentrations in early pregnancy and the risk of adverse pregnancy outcomes: the Generation R Study.* BJOG, 2012. **119**(6):739–51.

350 **Furness, D. et al.,** *Folate, Vitamin B₁₂, Vitamin B₆ and homocysteine: impact on pregnancy outcome.* Matern Child Nutr, 2013. **9**(2):155–66.

351 **Ronnenberg, A.G. et al.,** *Preconception B-vitamin and homocysteine status, conception, and early pregnancy loss.* Am J Epidemiol, 2007. **166**(3):304–12.

352 **Vujkovic, M. et al.,** *The preconception Mediterranean dietary pattern in couples undergoing in vitro fertilization/intracytoplasmic sperm injection treatment increases the chance of pregnancy.* Fertil Steril, 2010. **94**(6):2096–101.

353 **Sahakian, V. et al.,** *Vitamin B₆ is effective therapy for nausea and vomiting of pregnancy: a randomized, double-blind placebo-controlled study.* Obstet Gynecol, 1991. **78**(1):33–6.

354 **Vutyavanich, T., S. Wongtra-ngan, and R. Ruangsri,** *Pyridoxine for nausea and vomiting of pregnancy: a randomized, double-blind, placebo-controlled trial.* Am J Obstet Gynecol, 1995. **173**(3 Pt 1):881–4.

355 **Matthews, A. et al.,** *Interventions for nausea and vomiting in early pregnancy.* Cochrane Database Syst Rev, 2010. **9**:CD007575.

356 American College of Obstetricians and Gynecologists, *ACOG Practice Bulletin #52: Nausea and vomiting in pregnancy.* Obstet Gynecol, 2004. **103**(4):803–14.

357 **Hisano, M. et al.,** *Vitamin B₆ deficiency and anemia in pregnancy.* Eur J Clin Nutr, 2010. **64**(2):221–3.

358 **Guilarte, T.R.,** *Vitamin B₆ and cognitive development: recent research findings from human and animal studies.* Nutr Rev, 1993. **51**(7):193–8.

359 **Musayev, F.N. et al.,** *Molecular basis of reduced pyridoxine 5'-phosphate oxidase catalytic activity in neonatal epileptic encephalopathy disorder.* J Biol Chem, 2009. **284**(45):30949–56.

360 **Borschel, M.W., A. Kirksey, and R.E. Hannemann,** *Effects of vitamin B₆ intake on nutriture and growth of young infants.* Am J Clin Nutr, 1986. **43**(1):7–15.

361 **Heiskanen, K. et al.,** *Risk of low vitamin B₆ status in infants breast-fed exclusively beyond six months.* J Pediatr Gastroenterol Nutr, 1996. **23**(1):38–44.

362 **Kang-Yoon, S.A. et al.,** *Vitamin B-6 status of breast-fed neonates: influence of pyridoxine supplementation on mothers and neonates.* Am J Clin Nutr, 1992. **56**(3):548–58.

363  Chang, S.J. and A. Kirksey, *Vitamin B$_6$ status of breast-fed infants in relation to pyridoxine HCl supplementation of mothers.* J Nutr Sci Vitaminol (Tokyo), 2002. **48**(1):10–7.

364  Nelson, E.M., *Association of vitamin B$_6$ deficiency with convulsions in infants.* Public Health Rep, 1956. **71**(5):445–8.

365  Bessey, O.A., D.J. Adam, and A.E. Hansen, *Intake of vitamin B$_6$ and infantile convulsions: a first approximation of requirements of pyridoxine in infants.* Pediatrics, 1957. **20**(1 Part 1):33–44.

366  McCullough, A.L. et al., *Vitamin B-6 status of Egyptian mothers: relation to infant behavior and maternal-infant interactions.* Am J Clin Nutr, 1990. **51**(6):1067–74.

367  Merrill, A.H., Jr. et al., *Metabolism of vitamin B-6 by human liver.* J Nutr, 1984. **114**(9):1664–74.

368  Morris, M.S. et al., *Plasma pyridoxal 5'-phosphate in the US population: the National Health and Nutrition Examination Survey, 2003–2004.* Am J Clin Nutr, 2008. **87**(5):1446–54.

369  Turner, R.E. et al., *Comparing nutrient intake from food to the estimated average requirements shows middle- to upper-income pregnant women lack iron and possibly magnesium.* J Am Diet Assoc, 2003. **103**(4):461–6.

370  European Communities, *Nutrient and Energy Intakes for the European Community. Report of the Scientific Committee for Food.* 1993, Brussels: European Commission.

371  Liu, Y.Y. et al., *Abnormal fatty acid composition of lymphocytes of biotin-deficient rats.* J Nutr Sci Vitaminol (Tokyo), 1994. **40**(3):283–8.

372  Bannister, D.W., *The biochemistry of fatty liver and kidney syndrome. Biotin-mediated restoration of hepatic gluconeogenesis in vitro and its relationship to pyruvate carboxylase activity.* Biochem J, 1976. **156**(1):167–73.

373  Hymes, J. and B. Wolf, *Biotinidase and its roles in biotin metabolism.* Clin Chim Acta, 1996. **255**(1):1–11.

374  Mock, N.I. et al., *Increased urinary excretion of 3-hydroxyisovaleric acid and decreased urinary excretion of biotin are sensitive early indicators of decreased biotin status in experimental biotin deficiency.* Am J Clin Nutr, 1997. **65**(4):951–8.

375  Mock, D.M. et al., *Biotin deficiency: an unusual complication of parenteral alimentation.* N Engl J Med, 1981. **304**(14):820–3.

376  Baez-Saldana, A. et al., *Biotin deficiency induces changes in subpopulations of spleen lymphocytes in mice.* Am J Clin Nutr, 1998. **67**(3):431–7.

377  Mock, D.M., *Marginal biotin deficiency is teratogenic in mice and perhaps humans: a review of biotin deficiency during human pregnancy and effects of biotin deficiency on gene expression and enzyme activities in mouse dam and fetus.* J Nutr Biochem, 2005. **16**(7):435–7.

378  Sealey, W.M. et al., *Smoking accelerates biotin catabolism in women.* Am J Clin Nutr, 2004. **80**(4):932–5.

379  Schenker, S. et al., *Human placental biotin transport: normal characteristics and effect of ethanol.* Alcohol Clin Exp Res, 1993. **17**(3):566–75.

380  Mock, D.M. et al., *Biotin status assessed longitudinally in pregnant women.* J Nutr, 1997. **127**(5):710–6.

381  Mock, D.M., *Marginal biotin deficiency is common in normal human pregnancy and is highly teratogenic in mice.* J Nutr, 2009. **139**(1):154–7.

382  Goldsmith, S.J. et al., *Biotin content of human milk during early lactational stages.* Nutr Res, 1982. **2**(5):579–83.

383 Mock, D.M., N.I. Mock, and J.A. Dankle, *Secretory patterns of biotin in human milk.* J Nutr, 1992. **122**(3):546–52.

384 Watanabe, T., *Morphological and biochemical effects of excessive amounts of biotin on embryonic development in mice.* Experientia, 1996. **52**(2):149–54.

385 Blom, H.J. and Y. Smulders, *Overview of homocysteine and folate metabolism. With special references to cardiovascular disease and neural tube defects.* J Inherit Metab Dis, 2011. **34**(1):75–81.

386 McCully, K.S., *Homocysteine, vitamins, and vascular disease prevention.* Am J Clin Nutr, 2007. **86**(5):1563S–8S.

387 Wang, X. et al., *Efficacy of folic acid supplementation in stroke prevention: a meta-analysis.* Lancet, 2007. **369**(9576):1876–82.

388 Wald, D.S., J.P. Bestwick, and N.J. Wald, *Homocysteine as a cause of ischemic heart disease: the door remains open.* Clin Chem, 2012. **58**(10):1488–90.

389 Crider, K.S. et al., *Folate and DNA methylation: a review of molecular mechanisms and the evidence for folate's role.* Adv Nutr, 2012. **3**(1):21–38.

390 Bird, A., *DNA methylation patterns and epigenetic memory.* Genes Dev, 2002. **16**(1):6–21.

391 Ehrlich, M. and M. Lacey, *DNA hypomethylation and hemimethylation in cancer.* Adv Exp Med Biol, 2013. **754**:31–56.

392 Metz, J., *Folates in megaloblastic anaemia.* Bull World Health Organ, 1963. **28**(4):517–29.

393 Green, R. and J.W. Miller, *Folate deficiency beyond megaloblastic anemia: hyperhomo-cysteinemia and other manifestations of dysfunctional folate status.* Semin Hematol, 1999. **36**(1):47–64.

394 Smithells, R.W. et al., *Apparent prevention of neural tube defects by periconceptional vitamin supplementation.* Arch Dis Child, 1981. **56**(12):911–8.

395 Smithells, R.W. et al., *Prevention of neural tube defect recurrences in Yorkshire: final report.* Lancet, 1989. **2**(8661):498–9.

396 Blom, H.J. et al., *Neural tube defects and folate: case far from closed.* Nat Rev Neurosci, 2006. **7**(9):724–31.

397 MRC Vitamin Study Research Group, *Prevention of neural tube defects: results of the Medical Research Council Vitamin Study.* Lancet, 1991. **338**(8760):131–7.

398 Czeizel, A.E. and I. Dudas, *Prevention of the first occurrence of neural-tube defects by periconceptional vitamin supplementation.* N Engl J Med, 1992. **327**(26):1832–5.

399 Czeizel, A.E., I. Dudas, and J. Metneki, *Pregnancy outcomes in a randomised controlled trial of periconceptional multivitamin supplementation. Final report.* Arch Gynecol Obstet, 1994. **255**(3):131–9.

400 Stabler, S.P., J. Lindenbaum, and R.H. Allen, *The use of homocysteine and other metabolites in the specific diagnosis of vitamin B-12 deficiency.* J Nutr, 1996. **126**(4 Suppl):1266S–72S.

401 Daly, L.E. et al., *Folate levels and neural tube defects. Implications for prevention.* JAMA, 1995. **274**(21):1698–702.

402 Yerby, M.S., *Management issues for women with epilepsy: neural tube defects and folic acid supplementation.* Neurology, 2003. **61**(6 Suppl 2):S23–6.

403 Rasmussen, S.A. et al., *Maternal obesity and risk of neural tube defects: a metaanalysis.* Am J Obstet Gynecol, 2008. **198**(6):611–9.

404  Stothard, K.J. et al., *Maternal overweight and obesity and the risk of congenital anomalies: a systematic review and meta-analysis.* JAMA, 2009. **301**(6):636–50.

405  Shaw, G.M., E.M. Velie, and D. Schaffer, *Risk of neural tube defect-affected pregnancies among obese women.* JAMA, 1996. **275**(14)p. 1093–6.

406  Ray, J.G. et al., *Greater maternal weight and the ongoing risk of neural tube defects after folic acid flour fortification.* Obstet Gynecol, 2005. **105**(2):261–5.

407  Werler, M.M. et al., *Prepregnant weight in relation to risk of neural tube defects.* JAMA, 1996. **275**(14):1089–92.

408  Tinker, S.C. et al., *Does obesity modify the association of supplemental folic acid with folate status among nonpregnant women of childbearing age in the United States?* Birth Defects Res A Clin Mol Teratol, 2012. **94**(10):749–55.

409  da Silva, V.R. et al., *Obesity affects short-term folate pharmacokinetics in women of childbearing age.* Int J Obes (Lond), 2013. **37**:1608–10.

410  Stern, S.J. et al., *Dosage requirements for periconceptional folic acid supplementation: accounting for BMI and lean body weight.* J Obstet Gynaecol Can, 2012. **34**(4):374–8.

411  Bar-Oz, B. et al., *Folate fortification and supplementation—are we there yet?* Reprod Toxicol, 2008. **25**(4):408–12.

412  Nguyen, P. et al., *Steady state folate concentrations achieved with 5 compared with 1.1 mg folic acid supplementation among women of childbearing age.* Am J Clin Nutr, 2009. **89**(3):844–52.

413  Ray, J.G. and C.A. Laskin, *Folic acid and homocyst(e)ine metabolic defects and the risk of placental abruption, pre-eclampsia and spontaneous pregnancy loss: A systematic review.* Placenta, 1999. **20**(7):519–29.

414  Nilsen, R.M. et al., *Folic acid and multivitamin supplement use and risk of placental abruption: a population-based registry study.* Am J Epidemiol, 2008. **167**(7):867–74.

415  Mignini, L.E. et al., *Mapping the theories of preeclampsia: the role of homocysteine.* Obstet Gynecol, 2005. **105**(2):411–25.

416  Makedos, G. et al., *Homocysteine, folic acid and $B_{12}$ serum levels in pregnancy complicated with preeclampsia.* Arch Gynecol Obstet, 2007. **275**(2):121–4.

417  Acilmis, Y.G. et al., *Homocysteine, folic acid and vitamin $B_{12}$ levels in maternal and umbilical cord plasma and homocysteine levels in placenta in pregnant women with preeclampsia.* J Obstet Gynaecol Res, 2011. **37**(1):45–50.

418  Hernandez-Diaz, S. et al., *Risk of gestational hypertension in relation to folic acid supplementation during pregnancy.* Am J Epidemiol, 2002. **156**(9):806–12.

419  Bukowski, R. et al., *Preconceptional folate supplementation and the risk of spontaneous preterm birth: a cohort study.* PLoS Med, 2009. **6**(5):e1000061.

420  Ek, J., *Plasma and red cell folate in mothers and infants in normal pregnancies. Relation to birth weight.* Acta Obstet Gynecol Scand, 1982. **61**(1):17–20.

421  Rao, S. et al., *Intake of micronutrient-rich foods in rural Indian mothers is associated with the size of their babies at birth: Pune Maternal Nutrition Study.* J Nutr, 2001. **131**(4):1217–24.

422  Bower, C. and F.J. Stanley, *Dietary folate as a risk factor for neural-tube defects: evidence from a case-control study in Western Australia.* Med J Aust, 1989. **150**(11):613–9.

423  Werler, M.M., S. Shapiro, and A.A. Mitchell, *Periconceptional folic acid exposure and risk of occurrent neural tube defects.* JAMA, 1993. **269**(10):1257–61.

424 Shaw, G.M. et al., *Periconceptional vitamin use, dietary folate, and the occurrence of neural tube defects*. Epidemiology, 1995. **6**(3):219–26.

425 Berry, R.J. et al., *Prevention of neural-tube defects with folic acid in China. China–U.S. Collaborative Project for Neural Tube Defect Prevention*. N Engl J Med, 1999. **341**(20):1485–90.

426 Laurence, K.M. et al., *Double-blind randomised controlled trial of folate treatment before conception to prevent recurrence of neural-tube defects*. Br Med J (Clin Res Ed), 1981. **282**(6275):1509–11.

427 De-Regil, L.M. et al., *Effects and safety of periconceptional folate supplementation for preventing birth defects*. Cochrane Database Syst Rev, 2010. **10**:CD007950.

428 Li, S. et al., *Folic acid use and nonsyndromic orofacial clefts in China: a prospective cohort study*. Epidemiology, 2012. **23**(3):423–32.

429 Czeizel, A.E., L. Timar, and A. Sarkozi, *Dose-dependent effect of folic acid on the prevention of orofacial clefts*. Pediatrics, 1999. **104**(6):e66.

430 Kelly, D., T. O'Dowd, and U. Reulbach, *Use of folic acid supplements and risk of cleft lip and palate in infants: a population-based cohort study*. Br J Gen Pract, 2012. **62**(600):e466–72.

431 Moretti, P. et al., *Brief report: autistic symptoms, developmental regression, mental retardation, epilepsy, and dyskinesias in CNS folate deficiency*. J Autism Dev Disord, 2008. **38**(6):1170–7.

432 Rodier, P.M. et al., *Embryological origin for autism: developmental anomalies of the cranial nerve motor nuclei*. J Comp Neurol, 1996. **370**(2):247–61.

433 Schmidt, R.J. et al., *Maternal periconceptional folic acid intake and risk of autism spectrum disorders and developmental delay in the CHARGE (CHildhood Autism Risks from Genetics and Environment) case-control study*. Am J Clin Nutr, 2012. **96**(1):80–9.

434 Roza, S.J. et al., *Maternal folic acid supplement use in early pregnancy and child behavioural problems: The Generation R Study*. Br J Nutr, 2010. **103**(3):445–52.

435 Steenweg-de Graaff, J. et al., *Maternal folate status in early pregnancy and child emotional and behavioral problems: the Generation R Study*. Am J Clin Nutr, 2012. **95**(6):1413–21.

436 EUROCAT Working Group, *Prevalence of neural tube defects in 20 regions of Europe and the impact of prenatal diagnosis, 1980–1986*. J Epidemiol Community Health, 1991. **45**(1):52–8.

437 Hall, J.G. et al., *Clinical, genetic, and epidemiological factors in neural tube defects*. Am J Hum Genet, 1988. **43**(6):827–37.

438 Li, Z. et al., *Extremely high prevalence of neural tube defects in a 4-county area in Shanxi Province, China*. Birth Defects Res A Clin Mol Teratol, 2006. **76**(4):237–40.

439 van der Put, N.M. et al., *Folate, homocysteine and neural tube defects: an overview*. Exp Biol Med (Maywood), 2001. **226**(4):243–70.

440 Kirke, P.N. et al., *Impact of the MTHFR C677T polymorphism on risk of neural tube defects: case-control study*. BMJ, 2004. **328**(7455):1535–6.

441 Wilcken, B. et al., *Geographical and ethnic variation of the 677C>T allele of 5,10 methylenetetrahydrofolate reductase (MTHFR): findings from over 7000 newborns from 16 areas world wide*. J Med Genet, 2003. **40**(8):619–25.

442 Moore, C.A. et al., *Elevated rates of severe neural tube defects in a high-prevalence area in northern China*. Am J Med Genet, 1997. **73**(2):113–8.

443 Shane, B., *Folate and vitamin B$_{12}$ metabolism: overview and interaction with riboflavin, vitamin B$_6$, and polymorphisms.* Food Nutr Bull, 2008. **29**(Suppl 1): S5–16; discussion, S17–9.

444 Shane, B. and E.L. Stokstad, *Vitamin B$_{12}$–folate interrelationships.* Annu Rev Nutr, 1985. **5**:115–41.

445 Yajnik, C.S. et al., *Vitamin B$_{12}$ and folate concentrations during pregnancy and insulin resistance in the offspring: the Pune Maternal Nutrition Study.* Diabetologia, 2008. **51**(1):29–38.

446 Kim, Y.I. et al., *Severe folate deficiency causes secondary depletion of choline and phosphocholine in rat liver.* J Nutr, 1994. **124**(11):2197–203.

447 Sauberlich, H.E. et al., *Folate requirement and metabolism in nonpregnant women.* Am J Clin Nutr, 1987. **46**(6):1016–28.

448 Yeung, L., Q. Yang, and R.J. Berry, *Contributions of total daily intake of folic acid to serum folate concentrations.* JAMA, 2008. **300**(21):2486–7.

449 Shuaibi, A.M., J.D. House, and G.P. Sevenhuysen, *Folate status of young Canadian women after folic acid fortification of grain products.* J Am Diet Assoc, 2008. **108**(12):2090–4.

450 Branum, A.M., R. Bailey, and B.J. Singer, *Dietary supplement use and folate status during pregnancy in the United States.* J Nutr, 2013. **143**(4), 486–92.

451 Botto, L.D. et al., *International retrospective cohort study of neural tube defects in relation to folic acid recommendations: are the recommendations working?* BMJ, 2005. **330**(7491):571.

452 Berry, R.J. et al., *Fortification of flour with folic acid.* Food Nutr Bull, 2010. **31**(Suppl 1):S22–35.

453 Stoll, C., Y. Alembik, and B. Dott, *Are the recommendations on the prevention of neural tube defects working?* Eur J Med Genet, 2006. **49**(6):461–5.

454 Tinker, S.C. et al., *Usual folic acid intakes: a modelling exercise assessing changes in the amount of folic acid in foods and supplements, National Health and Nutrition Examination Survey, 2003–2008.* Public Health Nutr, 2012. **15**(7):1216–27.

455 Daly, S. et al., *Minimum effective dose of folic acid for food fortification to prevent neural-tube defects.* Lancet, 1997. **350**(9092):1666–9.

456 Honein, M.A. et al., *Impact of folic acid fortification of the US food supply on the occurrence of neural tube defects.* JAMA, 2001. **285**(23):2981–6.

457 Persad, V.L. et al., *Incidence of open neural tube defects in Nova Scotia after folic acid fortification.* CMAJ, 2002. **167**(3):241–5.

458 Mills, J.L. and C. Signore, *Neural tube defect rates before and after food fortification with folic acid.* Birth Defects Res A Clin Mol Teratol, 2004. **70**(11):844–5.

459 Butterworth, C.E., Jr. and T. Tamura, *Folic acid safety and toxicity: a brief review.* Am J Clin Nutr, 1989. **50**(2):353–8.

460 Scientific Committee for Food, *Tolerable Upper Intake Levels for Vitamins and Minerals.* 2006, Brussels: European Food Safety Authority.

461 Tam, C., D. O'Connor, and G. Koren, *Circulating unmetabolized folic acid: relationship to folate status and effect of supplementation.* Obstet Gynecol Int, 2012. **2012**:485179.

462 Troen, A.M. et al., *Unmetabolized folic acid in plasma is associated with reduced natural killer cell cytotoxicity among postmenopausal women.* J Nutr, 2006. **136**(1):189–94.

463 Mason, J.B. et al., *A temporal association between folic acid fortification and an increase in colorectal cancer rates may be illuminating important biological principles: a hypothesis.* Cancer Epidemiol Biomarkers Prev, 2007. **16**(7):1325–9.

464 Vollset, S.E. et al., *Effects of folic acid supplementation on overall and site-specific cancer incidence during the randomised trials: meta-analyses of data on 50,000 individuals.* Lancet, 2013. **381**(9871):1029–36.

465 Hollingsworth, J.W. et al., *In utero supplementation with methyl donors enhances allergic airway disease in mice.* J Clin Invest, 2008. **118**(10):3462–9.

466 Haberg, S.E. et al., *Folic acid supplements in pregnancy and early childhood respiratory health.* Arch Dis Child, 2009. **94**(3):180–4.

467 Whitrow, M.J. et al., *Effect of supplemental folic acid in pregnancy on childhood asthma: a prospective birth cohort study.* Am J Epidemiol, 2009. **170**(12):1486–93.

468 Haberg, S.E. et al., *Maternal folate levels in pregnancy and asthma in children at age 3 years.* J Allergy Clin Immunol, 2011. **127**(1):262–4, 264.e1.

469 Magdelijns, F.J. et al., *Folic acid use in pregnancy and the development of atopy, asthma, and lung function in childhood.* Pediatrics, 2011. **128**(1):e135–44.

470 Matsui, E.C. and W. Matsui, *Higher serum folate levels are associated with a lower risk of atopy and wheeze.* J Allergy Clin Immunol, 2009. **123**(6):1253–9.e2.

471 Crider, K.S. et al., *Prenatal folic acid and risk of asthma in children: a systematic review and meta-analysis.* Am J Clin Nutr, 2013. **98**(5):1272–81.

472 Huot, P.S. et al., *High folic acid intake during pregnancy lowers body weight and reduces femoral area and strength in female rat offspring.* J Osteoporosis, 2013. **2013**:154109.

473 Lumley, J. et al., *Periconceptional supplementation with folate and/or multivitamins for preventing neural tube defects.* Cochrane Database Syst Rev, 2001. **3**:CD001056.

474 Stevenson, R.E. et al., *Decline in prevalence of neural tube defects in a high-risk region of the United States.* Pediatrics, 2000. **106**(4):677–83.

475 Ray, J.G. et al., *Association of neural tube defects and folic acid food fortification in Canada.* Lancet, 2002. **360**(9350):2047–8.

476 Sayed, A.R. et al., *Decline in the prevalence of neural tube defects following folic acid fortification and its cost-benefit in South Africa.* Birth Defects Res A Clin Mol Teratol, 2008. **82**(4):211–6.

477 Chen, B.H. et al., *NTD prevalences in central California before and after folic acid fortification.* Birth Defects Res A Clin Mol Teratol, 2008. **82**(8):547–52.

478 Centers for Disease Control and Prevention, *Spina bifida and anencephaly before and after folic acid mandate—United States, 1995–1996 and 1999–2000.* MMWR Morb Mortal Wkly Rep., 2004. **53**(17):362–5.

479 Centers for Disease Control and Prevention, *Recommendations for the Use of Folic Acid to Reduce the Number of Cases of Spina Bifida and Other Neural Tube Defects.* MMWR Recomm Rep, 1992. **41**(RR–14).

480 Centers for Disease Control and Prevention, Division of Birth Defects, National Center on Birth Defects and Developmental Disabilities, *Folic acid, recommendations.* <http://www.cdc.gov/ncbddd/folicacid/recommendations.html> accessed 8 March 2013.

481 US Preventive Services Task Force, *Folic acid for the prevention of neural tube defects: U.S. Preventive Services Task Force recommendation statement.* Ann Intern Med, 2009. **150**(9):626–31.

482 Wilson, R.D. et al., *Pre-conceptional vitamin/folic acid supplementation 2007: the use of folic acid in combination with a multivitamin supplement for the prevention of neural tube defects and other congenital anomalies.* J Obstet Gynaecol Can, 2007. **29**(12):1003–26.

483 Modder, J. and K.J. Fitzsimons, *CMACE/RCOG Joint Guideline on the management of women with obesity in pregnancy.* 2010, <http://www.rcog.org.uk/files/rcog-corp/CMACERCOGJointGuidelineManagementWomenObesityPregnancya.pdf>.

484 Scientific Advisory Committee on Nutrition, *Paper for discussion: CMACE/RCOG Joint Guideline on the management of women with obesity in pregnancy: recommendation on high dose folic acid supplements.* SACN/SMCN/10/09. 2010, <http://www.sacn.gov.uk/pdfs/SMCN1009%20-%20RCOGCMACE%20folic%20acid%20suppl%20in%20obese%20pregnancy%20f%E2%80%A6.pdf>.

485 Flegal, K.M. et al., *Overweight and obesity in the United States: prevalence and trends, 1960–1994.* Int J Obes Relat Metab Disord, 1998. **22**(1):39–47.

486 Mokdad, A.H. et al., *The spread of the obesity epidemic in the United States, 1991–1998.* JAMA, 1999. **282**(16):1519–22.

487 Roth, J.R., J.G. Lawrence, and T.A. Bobik, *Cobalamin (coenzyme $B_{12}$): synthesis and biological significance.* Annu Rev Microbiol, 1996. **50**:137–81.

488 Pfohl-Leszkowicz, A., G. Keith, and G. Dirheimer, *Effect of cobalamin derivatives on in vitro enzymatic DNA methylation: methylcobalamin can act as a methyl donor.* Biochemistry, 1991. **30**(32):8045–51.

489 Quadros, E.V., *Advances in the understanding of cobalamin assimilation and metabolism.* Br J Haematol, 2010. **148**(2):195–204.

490 Carmel, R. et al., *Update on cobalamin, folate, and homocysteine.* Hematology Am Soc Hematol Educ Program, 2003. **2003**(1):62–81.

491 Thorpe, S.J. et al., *A Proposed International Standard for Vitamin $B_{12}$ and Serum Folate. Report of the International Collaborative Study to Evaluate a Batch of Lyophilised Serum for $B_{12}$ and Folate Content.* 2005, Geneva: World Health Organization.

492 de Benoist, B., *Conclusions of a WHO Technical Consultation on folate and vitamin $B_{12}$ deficiencies.* Food Nutr Bull, 2008. **29**(2 Suppl):S238–44.

493 Savage, D.G. et al., *Sensitivity of serum methylmalonic acid and total homocysteine determinations for diagnosing cobalamin and folate deficiencies.* Am J Med, 1994. **96**(3):239–46.

494 Nexo, E. and E. Hoffmann-Lucke, *Holotranscobalamin, a marker of vitamin B-12 status: analytical aspects and clinical utility.* Am J Clin Nutr, 2011. **94**(1):359S–65S.

495 Dali-Youcef, N. and E. Andres, *An update on cobalamin deficiency in adults.* QJM, 2009. **102**(1):17–28.

496 Yetley, E.A. et al., *Biomarkers of vitamin B-12 status in NHANES: a roundtable summary.* Am J Clin Nutr, 2011. **94**(1):313S–21S.

497 Herrmann, W. and R. Obeid, *Utility and limitations of biochemical markers of vitamin $B_{12}$ deficiency.* Eur J Clin Invest, 2013. **43**(3):231–7.

498 Snow, C.F., *Laboratory diagnosis of vitamin $B_{12}$ and folate deficiency: a guide for the primary care physician.* Arch Intern Med, 1999. **159**(12):1289–98.

499 Carmel, R. et al., *Food cobalamin malabsorption occurs frequently in patients with unexplained low serum cobalamin levels.* Arch Intern Med, 1988. **148**(8):1715–9.

500 Hvas, A.M. and E. Nexo, *Diagnosis and treatment of vitamin $B_{12}$ deficiency—an update.* Haematologica, 2006. **91**(11):1506–12.

501 Lindenbaum, J. and C.S. Lieber, *Alcohol-induced malabsorption of vitamin $B_{12}$ in man.* Nature, 1969. **224**(5221):806.

502 Linnell, J.C. et al., *Effects of smoking on metabolism and excretion of vitamin $B_{12}$.* Br Med J, 1968. **2**(5599):215–6.

503 Hoffbrand, A.V. and B.F. Jackson, *Correction of the DNA synthesis defect in vitamin $B_{12}$ deficiency by tetrahydrofolate: evidence in favour of the methyl-folate trap hypothesis as the cause of megaloblastic anaemia in vitamin $B_{12}$ deficiency.* Br J Haematol, 1993. **83**(4):643–7.

504 Healton, E.B. et al., *Neurologic aspects of cobalamin deficiency.* Medicine (Baltimore), 1991. **70**(4):229–45.

505 Bottiglieri, T., *Folate, vitamin $B_{12}$, and neuropsychiatric disorders.* Nutr Rev, 1996. **54**(12):382–90.

506 Dwarkanath, P. et al., *High folate and low vitamin B-12 intakes during pregnancy are associated with small-for-gestational age infants in South Indian women: a prospective observational cohort study.* Am J Clin Nutr, 2013. **98**(6):1450–8.

507 Robertson, J.A. and N.D. Gallagher, *Increased intestinal uptake of cobalamin in pregnancy does not require synthesis of new receptors.* Biochim Biophys Acta, 1983. **757**(2):145–50.

508 Hellegers, A. et al., *Vitamin $B_{12}$ absorption in pregnancy and in the newborn.* Am J Clin Nutr, 1957. **5**(3):327–31.

509 Fernandes-Costa, F. and J. Metz, *Levels of transcobalamins I, II, and III during pregnancy and in cord blood.* Am J Clin Nutr, 1982. **35**(1):87–94.

510 Pardo, J. et al., *Evaluation of low serum vitamin B(12) in the non-anaemic pregnant patient.* Hum Reprod, 2000. **15**(1):224–6.

511 Frery, N. et al., *Vitamin $B_{12}$ among parturients and their newborns and its relationship with birthweight.* Eur J Obstet Gynecol Reprod Biol, 1992. **45**(3):155–63.

512 Baker, S.J. et al., *Vitamin-$B_{12}$ deficiency in pregnancy and the puerperium.* Br Med J, 1962. **1**(5293):1658–61.

513 Vaz Pinto, A. et al., *Folic acid and vitamin $B_{12}$ determination in fetal liver.* Am J Clin Nutr, 1975. **28**(10):1085–6.

514 Pardo, J., L. Gindes, and R. Orvieto, *Cobalamin (vitamin $B_{12}$) metabolism during pregnancy.* Int J Gynaecol Obstet, 2004. **84**(1):77–8.

515 Schorah, C.J., R.W. Smithells, and J. Scott, *Vitamin $B_{12}$ and anencephaly.* Lancet, 1980. **315**(8173):880.

516 Kirke, P.N. et al., *Maternal plasma folate and vitamin $B_{12}$ are independent risk factors for neural tube defects.* Q J Med, 1993. **86**(11):703–8.

517 Gardiki-Kouidou, P. and M.J. Seller, *Amniotic fluid folate, vitamin $B_{12}$ and transcobalamins in neural tube defects.* Clin Genet, 1988. **33**(6):441–8.

518 Groenen, P.M. et al., *Marginal maternal vitamin $B_{12}$ status increases the risk of offspring with spina bifida.* Am J Obstet Gynecol, 2004. **191**(1):11–17.

519 Ray, J.G. et al., *Vitamin $B_{12}$ and the risk of neural tube defects in a folic-acid-fortified population.* Epidemiology, 2007. **18**(3):362–6.

520 Molloy, A.M. et al., *Maternal vitamin $B_{12}$ status and risk of neural tube defects in a population with high neural tube defect prevalence and no folic Acid fortification.* Pediatrics, 2009. **123**(3):917–23.

521 Specker, B.L. et al., *Increased urinary methylmalonic acid excretion in breast-fed infants of vegetarian mothers and identification of an acceptable dietary source of vitamin B-12.* Am J Clin Nutr, 1988. **47**(1):89–92.

522 Graham, S.M., O.M. Arvela, and G.A. Wise, *Long-term neurologic consequences of nutritional vitamin $B_{12}$ deficiency in infants.* J Pediatr, 1992. **121**(5 Pt 1):710–14.

523 Rosenblatt, D.S. and V.M. Whitehead, *Cobalamin and folate deficiency: acquired and hereditary disorders in children.* Semin Hematol, 1999. **36**(1):19–34.

524 Dagnelie, P.C., W.A. van Staveren, and H. van den Berg, *Vitamin B-12 from algae appears not to be bioavailable.* Am J Clin Nutr, 1991. **53**(3):695–7.

525 Zeisel, S.H. and J.K. Blusztajn, *Choline and human nutrition.* Annu Rev Nutr, 1994. **14**:269–96.

526 Jacob, R.A. et al., *Folate nutriture alters choline status of women and men fed low choline diets.* J Nutr, 1999. **129**(3):712–17.

527 Zeisel, S.H. et al., *Choline, an essential nutrient for humans.* FASEB J, 1991. **5**(7):2093–8.

528 Zeisel, S.H. et al., *Concentrations of choline-containing compounds and betaine in common foods.* J Nutr, 2003. **133**(5):1302–7.

529 Fischer, L.M. et al., *Ad libitum choline intake in healthy individuals meets or exceeds the proposed adequate intake level.* J Nutr, 2005. **135**(4):826–9.

530 Fischer, L.M. et al., *Sex and menopausal status influence human dietary requirements for the nutrient choline.* Am J Clin Nutr, 2007. **85**(5):1275–85.

531 Ozarda Ilcol, Y., G. Uncu, and I.H. Ulus, *Free and phospholipid-bound choline concentrations in serum during pregnancy, after delivery and in newborns.* Arch Physiol Biochem, 2002. **110**(5):393–9.

532 Jiang, X. et al., *A higher maternal choline intake among third-trimester pregnant women lowers placental and circulating concentrations of the antiangiogenic factor fms-like tyrosine kinase-1 (sFLT1).* FASEB J, 2013. **27**(3):1245–53.

533 Jiang, X. et al., *Maternal choline intake alters the epigenetic state of fetal cortisol-regulating genes in humans.* FASEB J, 2012. **26**(8):3563–74.

534 Yan, J. et al., *Pregnancy alters choline dynamics: results of a randomized trial using stable isotope methodology in pregnant and nonpregnant women.* Am J Clin Nutr, 2013. **98**(6):1459–67.

535 Molloy, A.M. et al., *Choline and homocysteine interrelations in umbilical cord and maternal plasma at delivery.* Am J Clin Nutr, 2005. **82**(4):836–42.

536 Vollset, S.E. et al., *Plasma total homocysteine, pregnancy complications, and adverse pregnancy outcomes: the Hordaland Homocysteine study.* Am J Clin Nutr, 2000. **71**(4):962–8.

537 Murphy, M.M. and J.D. Fernandez-Ballart, *Homocysteine in pregnancy.* Adv Clin Chem, 2011. **53**:105–37.

538 Shaw, G.M. et al., *Periconceptional dietary intake of choline and betaine and neural tube defects in offspring.* Am J Epidemiol, 2004. **160**(2):102–9.

539 Shaw, G.M. et al., *Choline and risk of neural tube defects in a folate-fortified population.* Epidemiology, 2009. **20**(5):714–19.

540 Craciunescu, C.N., A.R. Johnson, and S.H. Zeisel, *Dietary choline reverses some, but not all, effects of folate deficiency on neurogenesis and apoptosis in fetal mouse brain.* J Nutr, 2010. **140**(6):1162–6.

541 Cermak, J.M. et al., *Prenatal availability of choline modifies development of the hippocampal cholinergic system.* FASEB J, 1998. **12**(3):349–57.

542 Zeisel, S.H., *The fetal origins of memory: the role of dietary choline in optimal brain development.* J Pediatr, 2006. **149**(5 Suppl):S131–6.

543 Guo-Ross, S.X. et al., *Prenatal choline supplementation protects against postnatal neurotoxicity.* J Neurosci, 2002. **22**(1):RC195.

544 Cheatham, C.L. et al., *Phosphatidylcholine supplementation in pregnant women consuming moderate-choline diets does not enhance infant cognitive function: a randomized, double-blind, placebo-controlled trial.* Am J Clin Nutr, 2012. **96**(6):1465–72.

545 Yang, E.K. et al., *Rat and human mammary tissue can synthesize choline moiety via the methylation of phosphatidylethanolamine.* Biochem J, 1988. **256**(3):821–8.

546 Holmes-McNary, M.Q. et al., *Choline and choline esters in human and rat milk and in infant formulas.* Am J Clin Nutr, 1996. **64**(4):572–6.

547 Fischer, L.M. et al., *Choline intake and genetic polymorphisms influence choline metabolite concentrations in human breast milk and plasma.* Am J Clin Nutr, 2010. **92**(2):336–46.

548 Mellott, T.J. et al., *Prenatal choline availability modulates hippocampal and cerebral cortical gene expression.* FASEB J, 2007. **21**(7):1311–23.

549 Zeisel, S.H., *Epigenetic mechanisms for nutrition determinants of later health outcomes.* Am J Clin Nutr, 2009. **89**(5):1488S–93S.

550 Rosen, C.J. et al., *The nonskeletal effects of vitamin D: an Endocrine Society scientific statement.* Endocr Rev, 2012. **33**(3):456–92.

551 Feldman, D., J.W. Pike, and J.S. Adams, *Vitamin D. Third Edition.* Vol. 1. 2011, London: Elsevier/Academic Press.

552 Zehnder, D. et al., *The ontogeny of 25-hydroxyvitamin D(3) 1alpha-hydroxylase expression in human placenta and decidua.* Am J Pathol, 2002. **161**(1):105–14.

553 Heaney, R.P., *Vitamin D in health and disease.* Clin J Am Soc Nephrol, 2008. **3**(5):1535–41.

554 Procopio, M. and G. Borretta, *Derangement of glucose metabolism in hyperparathyroidism.* J Endocrinol Invest, 2003. **26**(11):1136–42.

555 Bikle, D.D., *Vitamin D regulation of immune function.* Vitam Horm, 2011. **86**:1–21.

556 Chiu, K.C. et al., *Hypovitaminosis D is associated with insulin resistance and beta cell dysfunction.* Am J Clin Nutr, 2004. **79**(5):820–5.

557 Hypponen, E. et al., *Intake of vitamin D and risk of type 1 diabetes: a birth-cohort study.* Lancet, 2001. **358**(9292):1500–3.

558 Erkkola, M. et al., *Maternal vitamin D intake during pregnancy is inversely associated with asthma and allergic rhinitis in 5-year-old children.* Clin Exp Allergy, 2009. **39**(6):875–82.

559 Camargo, C.A., Jr. et al., *Maternal intake of vitamin D during pregnancy and risk of recurrent wheeze in children at 3 y of age.* Am J Clin Nutr, 2007. **85**(3):788–95.

560 Weiss, S.T. and A.A. Litonjua, *The in utero effects of maternal vitamin D deficiency: how it results in asthma and other chronic diseases.* Am J Respir Crit Care Med, 2011. **183**(10):1286–7.

561 Hypponen, E. et al., *Does vitamin D supplementation in infancy reduce the risk of pre-eclampsia?* Eur J Clin Nutr, 2007. **61**(9):1136–9.

562 Institute of Medicine, *Dietary Reference Intakes for Calcium and Vitamin D*. 2011, Washington, DC: The National Academies Press.

563 **Priemel, M. et al.**, *Bone mineralization defects and vitamin D deficiency: histomorphometric analysis of iliac crest bone biopsies and circulating 25-hydroxyvitamin D in 675 patients.* J Bone Miner Res, 2010. **25**(2):305–12.

564 **Burgi, A.A. et al.**, *High serum 25-hydroxyvitamin D is associated with a low incidence of stress fractures.* J Bone Miner Res, 2011. **26**(10):2371–7.

565 **Heaney, R.P. et al.**, *Calcium absorption varies within the reference range for serum 25-hydroxyvitamin D.* J Am Coll Nutr, 2003. **22**(2):142–6.

566 **Heaney, R.P. et al.**, *Human serum 25-hydroxycholecalciferol response to extended oral dosing with cholecalciferol.* Am J Clin Nutr, 2003. **77**(1):204–10.

567 **Bischoff-Ferrari, H.A. et al.**, *Prevention of nonvertebral fractures with oral vitamin D and dose dependency: a meta-analysis of randomized controlled trials.* Arch Intern Med, 2009. **169**(6):551–61.

568 **Garland, C.F. et al.**, *Vitamin D for cancer prevention: global perspective.* Ann Epidemiol, 2009. **19**(7):468–83.

569 **Ritchie, L.D. et al.**, *A longitudinal study of calcium homeostasis during human pregnancy and lactation and after resumption of menses.* Am J Clin Nutr, 1998. **67**(4):693–701.

570 **Abrams, S.A.**, *In utero physiology: role in nutrient delivery and fetal development for calcium, phosphorus, and vitamin D.* Am J Clin Nutr, 2007. **85**(2):604S–7S.

571 Institute of Medicine, Food and Nutrition Board, *Dietary Reference Intakes for Calcium, Phosphorus, Magnesium, Vitamin D, and Fluoride.* 1997, Washington, DC: The National Academies Press.

572 **Viljakainen, H.T. et al.**, *Maternal vitamin D status determines bone variables in the newborn.* J Clin Endocrinol Metab, 2010. **95**(4):1749–57.

573 **Weiler, H. et al.**, *Vitamin D deficiency and whole-body and femur bone mass relative to weight in healthy newborns.* CMAJ, 2005. **172**(6):757–61.

574 **Lawlor, D.A. et al.**, *Association of maternal vitamin D status during pregnancy with bone-mineral content in offspring: a prospective cohort study.* Lancet, 2013. **381**(9884):2176–83.

575 **Lucas, R.M. et al.**, *Future health implications of prenatal and early-life vitamin D status.* Nutr Rev, 2008. **66**(12):710–20.

576 **Mulligan, M.L. et al.**, *Implications of vitamin D deficiency in pregnancy and lactation.* Am J Obstet Gynecol, 2010. **202**(5):429.e1–9.

577 **Aloia, J.F. et al.**, *Vitamin D intake to attain a desired serum 25-hydroxyvitamin D concentration.* Am J Clin Nutr, 2008. **87**(6):1952–8.

578 **Holick, M.F.**, *Vitamin D deficiency.* N Engl J Med, 2007. **357**(3):266–81.

579 **Tzotzas, T. et al.**, *Rising serum 25-hydroxy-vitamin D levels after weight loss in obese women correlate with improvement in insulin resistance.* J Clin Endocrinol Metab, 2010. **95**(9):4251–7.

580 **Reinehr, T. et al.**, *Vitamin D status and parathyroid hormone in obese children before and after weight loss.* Eur J Endocrinol, 2007. **157**(2):225–32.

581 **Wortsman, J. et al.**, *Decreased bioavailability of vitamin D in obesity.* Am J Clin Nutr, 2000. **72**(3):690–3.

582 Holick, M.F. et al., *Evaluation, treatment, and prevention of vitamin D deficiency: an Endocrine Society clinical practice guideline.* J Clin Endocrinol Metab, 2011. **96**(7):1911–30.

583 Josefson, J.L. et al., *Maternal obesity and vitamin D sufficiency are associated with cord blood vitamin D insufficiency.* J Clin Endocrinol Metab, 2013. **98**(1):114–19.

584 Hamilton, S.A. et al., *Profound vitamin D deficiency in a diverse group of women during pregnancy living in a sun-rich environment at latitude 32 degrees N.* Int J Endocrinol, 2010. **2010**:917428.

585 Hollis, B.W. et al., *Vitamin D supplementation during pregnancy: double-blind, randomized clinical trial of safety and effectiveness.* J Bone Miner Res, 2011. **26**(10): 2341–57.

586 Johnson, D.D. et al., *Vitamin D deficiency and insufficiency is common during pregnancy.* Am J Perinatol, 2011. **28**(1):7–12.

587 Ginde, A.A. et al., *Vitamin D insufficiency in pregnant and nonpregnant women of childbearing age in the United States.* Am J Obstet Gynecol, 2010. **202**(5):436.e1–8.

588 Bodnar, L.M. et al., *Maternal vitamin D deficiency increases the risk of preeclampsia.* J Clin Endocrinol Metab, 2007. **92**(9):3517–22.

589 Baker, A.M. et al., *A nested case-control study of midgestation vitamin D deficiency and risk of severe preeclampsia.* J Clin Endocrinol Metab, 2010. **95**(11):5105–9.

590 Robinson, C.J. et al., *Plasma 25-hydroxyvitamin D levels in early-onset severe preeclampsia.* Am J Obstet Gynecol, 2010. **203**(4):366.e1–6.

591 Powe, C.E. et al., *First trimester vitamin D, vitamin D binding protein, and subsequent preeclampsia.* Hypertension, 2010. **56**(4):758–63.

592 Seely, E.W. et al., *Lower serum ionized calcium and abnormal calciotropic hormone levels in preeclampsia.* J Clin Endocrinol Metab, 1992. **74**(6):1436–40.

593 Shand, A.W. et al., *Maternal vitamin D status in pregnancy and adverse pregnancy outcomes in a group at high risk for pre-eclampsia.* BJOG, 2010. **117**(13):1593–8.

594 Wei, S.Q. et al., *Longitudinal vitamin D status in pregnancy and the risk of preeclampsia.* BJOG, 2012. **119**(7):832–9.

595 Haugen, M. et al., *Vitamin D supplementation and reduced risk of preeclampsia in nulliparous women.* Epidemiology, 2009. **20**(5):720–6.

596 Rothers, J. et al., *Cord blood 25-hydroxyvitamin D levels are associated with aeroallergen sensitization in children from Tucson, Arizona.* J Allergy Clin Immunol, 2011. **128**(5):1093–9.e1–5.

597 Gale, C.R. et al., *Maternal vitamin D status during pregnancy and child outcomes.* Eur J Clin Nutr, 2008. **62**(1):68–77.

598 Matheu, V. et al., *Dual effects of vitamin D-induced alteration of TH1/TH2 cytokine expression: enhancing IgE production and decreasing airway eosinophilia in murine allergic airway disease.* J Allergy Clin Immunol, 2003. **112**(3):585–92.

599 Jones, A.P. et al., *Vitamin D and allergic disease: sunlight at the end of the tunnel?* Nutrients, 2012. **4**(1):13–28.

600 Devereux, G. et al., *Maternal vitamin D intake during pregnancy and early childhood wheezing.* Am J Clin Nutr, 2007. **85**(3):853–9.

601 Camargo, C.A., Jr. et al., *Cord-blood 25-hydroxyvitamin D levels and risk of respiratory infection, wheezing, and asthma.* Pediatrics, 2011. **127**(1):e180–7.

602 **Dunlop, A.L. et al.**, *Maternal vitamin D, folate, and polyunsaturated fatty acid status and bacterial vaginosis during pregnancy.* Infect Dis Obstet Gynecol, 2011. **2011**:216217.

603 **French, A.L. et al.**, *The association of HIV status with bacterial vaginosis and vitamin D in the United States.* J Womens Health (Larchmt), 2011. **20**(10):1497–503.

604 **Boucher, B.J.**, *Is vitamin D status relevant to metabolic syndrome?* Dermatoendocrinol, 2012. **4**(2):212–24.

605 **Clifton-Bligh, R.J., P. McElduff, and A. McElduff**, *Maternal vitamin D deficiency, ethnicity and gestational diabetes.* Diabet Med, 2008. **25**(6):678–84.

606 **Parlea, L. et al.**, *Association between serum 25-hydroxyvitamin D in early pregnancy and risk of gestational diabetes mellitus.* Diabet Med, 2012. **29**(7):e25–32.

607 **Zhang, C. et al.**, *Maternal plasma 25-hydroxyvitamin D concentrations and the risk for gestational diabetes mellitus.* PLoS ONE, 2008. **3**(11):e3753.

608 **Asemi, Z. et al.**, *Effects of vitamin D supplementation on glucose metabolism, lipid concentrations, inflammation, and oxidative stress in gestational diabetes: a double-blind randomized controlled clinical trial.* Am J Clin Nutr, 2013. **98**(6):1425–32.

609 **Gernand, A.D. et al.**, *Maternal serum 25-hydroxyvitamin D and measures of newborn and placental weight in a U.S. multicenter cohort study.* J Clin Endocrinol Metab, 2013. **98**(1):398–404.

610 **Leffelaar, E.R., T.G. Vrijkotte, and M. van Eijsden**, *Maternal early pregnancy vitamin D status in relation to fetal and neonatal growth: results of the multi-ethnic Amsterdam Born Children and their Development cohort.* Br J Nutr, 2010. **104**(1):108–17.

611 **Crozier, S.R. et al.**, *Maternal vitamin D status in pregnancy is associated with adiposity in the offspring: findings from the Southampton Women's Survey.* Am J Clin Nutr, 2012. **96**(1):57–63.

612 **Agic, A. et al.**, *Relative expression of 1,25-dihydroxyvitamin $D_3$ receptor, vitamin D 1 alpha-hydroxylase, vitamin D 24-hydroxylase, and vitamin D 25-hydroxylase in endometriosis and gynecologic cancers.* Reprod Sci, 2007. **14**(5):486–97.

613 **Nangia, A.K. et al.**, *Testicular maturation arrest to testis cancer: spectrum of expression of the vitamin D receptor and vitamin D treatment in vitro.* J Urol, 2007. **178**(3 Pt 1): 1092–6.

614 **Lerchbaum, E. and B. Obermayer-Pietsch**, *Vitamin D and fertility: a systematic review.* Eur J Endocrinol, 2012. **166**(5):765–78.

615 **Webb, A.R. and O. Engelsen**, *Calculated ultraviolet exposure levels for a healthy vitamin D status.* Photochem Photobiol, 2006. **82**(6):1697–703.

616 **Terushkin, V. et al.**, *Estimated equivalency of vitamin D production from natural sun exposure versus oral vitamin D supplementation across seasons at two US latitudes.* J Am Acad Dermatol, 2010. **62**(6):929.e1–9.

617 **Gilchrest, B.A.**, *Sun protection and Vitamin D: three dimensions of obfuscation.* J Steroid Biochem Mol Biol, 2007. **103**(3–5):655–63.

618 **Murphy, S.P. and D.H. Calloway**, *Nutrient intakes of women in NHANES II, emphasizing trace minerals, fiber, and phytate.* J Am Diet Assoc, 1986. **86**(10):1366–72.

619 **Biancuzzo, R.M. et al.**, *Fortification of orange juice with vitamin D(2) or vitamin D(3) is as effective as an oral supplement in maintaining vitamin D status in adults.* Am J Clin Nutr, 2010. **91**(6):1621–6.

620 **Armas, L.A., B.W. Hollis, and R.P. Heaney**, *Vitamin $D_2$ is much less effective than vitamin $D_3$ in humans.* J Clin Endocrinol Metab, 2004. **89**(11):5387–91.

621 Tripkovic, L. et al., *Comparison of vitamin D₂ and vitamin D₃ supplementation in rais-ing serum 25-hydroxyvitamin D status: a systematic review and meta-analysis.* Am J Clin Nutr, 2012. **95**(6):1357–64.

622 Mulligan, G.B. and A. Licata, *Taking vitamin D with the largest meal improves absorp-tion and results in higher serum levels of 25-hydroxyvitamin D.* J Bone Miner Res, 2010. **25**(4):928–30.

623 Reddy, K.K. and B.A. Gilchrest, *What is all this commotion about vitamin D?* J Invest Dermatol, 2010. **130**(2):321–6.

624 De-Regil, L.M. et al., *Vitamin D supplementation for women during pregnancy.* Cochrane Database Syst Rev, 2012. **2**:CD008873.

625 Brooke, O.G. et al., *Vitamin D supplements in pregnant Asian women: effects on calcium status and fetal growth.* Br Med J, 1980. **280**(6216):751–4.

626 Delvin, E.E. et al., *Vitamin D supplementation during pregnancy: effect on neonatal cal-cium homeostasis.* J Pediatr, 1986. **109**(2):328–34.

627 Mallet, E. et al., *Vitamin D supplementation in pregnancy: a controlled trial of two meth-ods.* Obstet Gynecol, 1986. **68**(3):300–4.

628 Marya, R.K. et al., *Effect of vitamin D supplementation during pregnancy on foetal growth.* Indian J Med Res, 1988. **88**:488–92.

629 Yu, C.K. et al., *Vitamin D deficiency and supplementation during pregnancy.* Clin Endo-crinol (Oxf), 2009. **70**(5):685–90.

630 Marya, R.K., S. Rathee, and M. Manrow, *Effect of calcium and vitamin D supplementa-tion on toxaemia of pregnancy.* Gynecol Obstet Invest, 1987. **24**(1):38–42.

631 Hollis, B.W., *Circulating 25-hydroxyvitamin D levels indicative of vitamin D sufficiency: implications for establishing a new effective dietary intake recommendation for vitamin D.* J Nutr, 2005. **135**(2):317–22.

632 Holick, M.F., *Resurrection of vitamin D deficiency and rickets.* J Clin Invest, 2006. **116**(8):2062–72.

633 Haggerty, L.L., *Maternal supplementation for prevention and treatment of vitamin D deficiency in exclusively breastfed infants.* Breastfeed Med, 2011. **6**(3):137–44.

634 Hollis, B.W. and C.L. Wagner, *Vitamin D requirements during lactation: high-dose maternal supplementation as therapy to prevent hypovitaminosis D for both the mother and the nursing infant.* Am J Clin Nutr, 2004. **80**(6 Suppl):1752S–8S.

635 Majid Molla, A. et al., *Risk factors for nutritional rickets among children in Kuwait.* Pediatr Int, 2000. **42**(3):280–4.

636 Specker, B.L. et al., *Prospective study of vitamin D supplementation and rickets in China.* J Pediatr, 1992. **120**(5):733–9.

637 Wagner, C.L. and F.R. Greer, *Prevention of rickets and vitamin D deficiency in infants, children, and adolescents.* Pediatrics, 2008. **122**(5):1142–52.

638 Cancela, L., N. Le Boulch, and L. Miravet, *Relationship between the vitamin D content of maternal milk and the vitamin D status of nursing women and breast-fed infants.* J Endocrinol, 1986. **110**(1):43–50.

639 Wagner, C.L. et al., *High-dose vitamin D₃ supplementation in a cohort of breastfeeding mothers and their infants: a 6-month follow-up pilot study.* Breastfeed Med, 2006. **1**(2):59–70.

640 Rothberg, A.D. et al., *Maternal-infant vitamin D relationships during breast-feeding.* J Pediatr, 1982. **101**(4):500–3.

641 Pittard, W.B., 3rd et al., *How much vitamin D for neonates?* Am J Dis Child, 1991. **145**(10):1147–9.

642 Cooke, R. et al., *Vitamin D and mineral metabolism in the very low birth weight infant receiving 400 IU of vitamin D.* J Pediatr, 1990. **116**(3):423–8.

643 Greer, F.R. and S. Marshall, *Bone mineral content, serum vitamin D metabolite concentrations, and ultraviolet B light exposure in infants fed human milk with and without vitamin D₂ supplements.* J Pediatr, 1989. **114**(2):204–12.

644 Zeghoud, F. et al., *Subclinical vitamin D deficiency in neonates: definition and response to vitamin D supplements.* Am J Clin Nutr, 1997. **65**(3):771–8.

645 Abrams, S.A. et al., *Effects of ethnicity and vitamin D supplementation on vitamin D status and changes in bone mineral content in infants.* BMC Pediatr, 2012. **12**:6.

646 Koo, W.W. et al., *Effect of three levels of vitamin D intake in preterm infants receiving high mineral-containing milk.* J Pediatr Gastroenterol Nutr, 1995. **21**(2):182–9.

647 Vieth, R., *Vitamin D supplementation, 25-hydroxyvitamin D concentrations, and safety.* Am J Clin Nutr, 1999. **69**(5):842–56.

648 Luxwolda, M.F. et al., *Traditionally living populations in East Africa have a mean serum 25-hydroxyvitamin D concentration of 115 nmol/l.* Br J Nutr, 2012. **108**(9):1557–61.

649 Vieth, R., *Vitamin D and cancer mini-symposium: the risk of additional vitamin D.* Ann Epidemiol, 2009. **19**(7):441–5.

650 ACOG Committee on Obstetric Practice, *ACOG Committee Opinion No. 495: Vitamin D: screening and supplementation during pregnancy.* Obstet Gynecol, 2011. **118**(1):197–8.

651 National Collaborating Centre for Women's and Children's Health, *Antenatal Care: Routine Care for the Healthy Pregnant Woman.* 2008, London: RCOG Press.

652 World Health Organization, *WHO Guideline: Vitamin D Supplementation in Pregnant Women.* 2012, Geneva: World Health Organization.

653 American Academy of Pediatrics. Committee on Environmental Health, *Ultraviolet light: a hazard to children.* Pediatrics, 1999. **104**(2 Pt 1):328–33.

654 European Society of Paediatric Gastroenterology and Nutrition, *ESPGAN Committee on nutrition of the preterm infant: nutrition and feeding of preterm infants.* Acta Paediatr Scand Suppl, 1987. **336**:1–14.

655 Southern Health, *Vitamin D in pregnancy and the term newborn guideline.* 2009, <http://www.southernhealth.org.au/ icms_docs/3569_Vitamin_D_in_pregnancy _ and_breastfeeding_guideline.pdf>.

656 Munns, C. et al., *Prevention and treatment of infant and childhood vitamin D deficiency in Australia and New Zealand: a consensus statement.* Med J Aust, 2006. **185**(5):268–72.

657 Stenflo, J. and J.W. Suttie, *Vitamin K-dependent formation of gamma-carboxyglutamic acid.* Annu Rev Biochem, 1977. **46**:157–72.

658 Suttie, J.W., *Synthesis of vitamin K-dependent proteins.* FASEB J, 1993. **7**(5):445–52.

659 Stafford, D.W., *The vitamin K cycle.* J Thromb Haemost, 2005. **3**(8):1873–8.

660 Vermeer, C., K.S. Jie, and M.H. Knapen, *Role of vitamin K in bone metabolism.* Annu Rev Nutr, 1995. **15**:1–22.

661 Sokoll, L.J. and J.A. Sadowski, *Comparison of biochemical indexes for assessing vitamin K nutritional status in a healthy adult population.* Am J Clin Nutr, 1996. **63**(4):566–73.

662 Widdershoven, J. et al., *Four methods compared for measuring des-carboxy-prothrombin (PIVKA-II).* Clin Chem, 1987. **33**(11):2074–8.

663  Ramotar, K. et al., *Production of menaquinones by intestinal anaerobes.* J Infect Dis, 1984. **150**(2):213–18.

664  Shevchuk, Y.M. and J.M. Conly, *Antibiotic-associated hypoprothrombinemia: a review of prospective studies, 1966–1988.* Rev Infect Dis, 1990. **12**(6):1109–26.

665  Shearer, M.J., *Vitamin K metabolism and nutriture.* Blood Rev, 1992. **6**(2):92–104.

666  Chuansumrit, A. et al., *Prevalence of subclinical vitamin K deficiency in Thai newborns: relationship to maternal phylloquinone intakes and delivery risk.* Arch Dis Child Fetal Neonatal Ed, 2010. **95**(2):F104–8.

667  Cornelissen, M. et al., *Increased incidence of neonatal vitamin K deficiency resulting from maternal anticonvulsant therapy.* Am J Obstet Gynecol, 1993. **168**(3 Pt 1):923–8.

668  Cornelissen, M. et al., *Supplementation of vitamin K in pregnant women receiving anticonvulsant therapy prevents neonatal vitamin K deficiency.* Am J Obstet Gynecol, 1993. **168**(3 Pt 1):884–8.

669  Hall, J.G., R.M. Pauli, and K.M. Wilson, *Maternal and fetal sequelae of anticoagulation during pregnancy.* Am J Med, 1980. **68**(1):122–40.

670  Schaefer, C. et al., *Vitamin K antagonists and pregnancy outcome. A multi-centre prospective study.* Thromb Haemost, 2006. **95**(6):949–57.

671  Booth, S.L. and J.W. Suttie, *Dietary intake and adequacy of vitamin K.* J Nutr, 1998. **128**(5):785–8.

672  Shearer, M.J., X. Fu, and S.L. Booth, *Vitamin K nutrition, metabolism, and requirements: current concepts and future research.* Adv Nutr, 2012. **3**(2):182–95.

673  Olson, R.E., *The function and metabolism of vitamin K.* Annu Rev Nutr, 1984. **4**:281–337.

674  Gijsbers, B.L., K.S. Jie, and C. Vermeer, *Effect of food composition on vitamin K absorption in human volunteers.* Br J Nutr, 1996. **76**(2):223–9.

675  Groenen-van Dooren, M.M. et al., *Bioavailability of phylloquinone and menaquinones after oral and colorectal administration in vitamin K-deficient rats.* Biochem Pharmacol, 1995. **50**(6):797–801.

676  Yan, L. et al., *Effect of apolipoprotein E genotype on vitamin K status in healthy older adults from China and the UK.* Br J Nutr, 2005. **94**(6):956–61.

677  Newborn, A.A.o.P.C.o.F.a., *Controversies concerning vitamin K and the newborn. American Academy of Pediatrics Committee on Fetus and Newborn.* Pediatrics, 2003. **112**(1 Pt 1):191–2.

678  Hansen, K.N. and F. Ebbesen, *Neonatal vitamin K prophylaxis in Denmark: three years' experience with oral administration during the first three months of life compared with one oral administration at birth.* Acta Paediatr, 1996. **85**(10):1137–9.

679  Gracy, R.W. et al., *Reactive oxygen species: the unavoidable environmental insult?* Mutat Res, 1999. **428**(1–2):17–22.

680  Johnston, C.S., C.G. Meyer, and J.C. Srilakshmi, *Vitamin C elevates red blood cell glutathione in healthy adults.* Am J Clin Nutr, 1993. **58**(1):103–5.

681  Prasad, A.S. et al., *Antioxidant effect of zinc in humans.* Free Radic Biol Med, 2004. **37**(8):1182–90.

682  Weeks, B.S., M.S. Hanna, and D. Cooperstein, *Dietary selenium and selenoprotein function.* Med Sci Monit, 2012. **18**(8):RA127–32.

683  Coassin, M., F. Ursini, and A. Bindoli, *Antioxidant effect of manganese.* Arch Biochem Biophys, 1992. **299**(2):330–3.

684 Shoji, H. and B. Koletzko, *Oxidative stress and antioxidant protection in the perinatal period.* Curr Opin Clin Nutr Metab Care, 2007. **10**(3):324–8.

685 Myatt, L. and X. Cui, *Oxidative stress in the placenta.* Histochem Cell Biol, 2004. **122**(4):369–82.

686 Mueller, A. et al., *Placental defence is considered sufficient to control lipid peroxidation in pregnancy.* Med Hypotheses, 2005. **64**(3):553–7.

687 Davidge, S.T. et al., *Sera antioxidant activity in uncomplicated and preeclamptic pregnancies.* Obstet Gynecol, 1992. **79**(6):897–901.

688 Sagol, S., E. Ozkinay, and S. Ozsener, *Impaired antioxidant activity in women with preeclampsia.* Int J Gynaecol Obstet, 1999. **64**(2):121–7.

689 Wisdom, S.J. et al., *Antioxidant systems in normal pregnancy and in pregnancy-induced hypertension.* Am J Obstet Gynecol, 1991. **165**(6 Pt 1):1701–4.

690 Mikhail, M.S. et al., *Preeclampsia and antioxidant nutrients: decreased plasma levels of reduced ascorbic acid, alpha-tocopherol, and beta-carotene in women with preeclampsia.* Am J Obstet Gynecol, 1994. **171**(1):150–7.

691 Zhang, C. et al., *Plasma concentrations of carotenoids, retinol, and tocopherols in preeclamptic and normotensive pregnant women.* Am J Epidemiol, 2001. **153**(6):572–80.

692 Eriksson, U.J. and L.A. Borg, *Diabetes and embryonic malformations. Role of substrate-induced free-oxygen radical production for dysmorphogenesis in cultured rat embryos.* Diabetes, 1993. **42**(3):411–19.

693 Baynes, J.W. and S.R. Thorpe, *Role of oxidative stress in diabetic complications: a new perspective on an old paradigm.* Diabetes, 1999. **48**(1):1–9.

694 Yan, S.D. et al., *Enhanced cellular oxidant stress by the interaction of advanced glycation end products with their receptors/binding proteins.* J Biol Chem, 1994. **269**(13):9889–97.

695 Yang, X. et al., *Maternal antioxidant treatments prevent diabetes-induced alterations of mitochondrial morphology in rat embryos.* Anat Rec, 1998. **251**(3):303–15.

696 McCance, D.R. et al., *Vitamins C and E for prevention of pre-eclampsia in women with type 1 diabetes (DAPIT): a randomised placebo-controlled trial.* Lancet, 2010. **376**(9737):259–66.

697 Scholl, T.O. and T.P. Stein, *Oxidant damage to DNA and pregnancy outcome.* J Matern Fetal Med, 2001. **10**(3):182–5.

698 Potdar, N. et al., *First-trimester increase in oxidative stress and risk of small-for-gestational-age fetus.* BJOG, 2009. **116**(5):637–42.

699 Georas, S.N. et al., *T-helper cell type-2 regulation in allergic disease.* Eur Respir J, 2005. **26**(6):1119–37.

700 Miyake, Y. et al., *Consumption of vegetables, fruit, and antioxidants during pregnancy and wheeze and eczema in infants.* Allergy, 2010. **65**(6):758–65.

701 Nwaru, B.I. et al., *Intake of antioxidants during pregnancy and the risk of allergies and asthma in the offspring.* Eur J Clin Nutr, 2011. **65**(8):937–43.

702 Haenen, G.R. et al., *Peroxynitrite scavenging by flavonoids.* Biochem Biophys Res Commun, 1997. **236**(3):591–3.

703 Chen, J.W. et al., *Structure-activity relationship of natural flavonoids in hydroxyl radical-scavenging effects.* Acta Pharmacol Sin, 2002. **23**(7):667–72.

704 Williams, R.J., J.P. Spencer, and C. Rice-Evans, *Flavonoids: antioxidants or signalling molecules?* Free Radic Biol Med, 2004. **36**(7):838–49.

705 Lotito, S.B. et al., *Metabolic conversion of dietary flavonoids alters their anti-inflammatory and antioxidant properties.* Free Radic Biol Med, 2011. **51**(2):454–63.

706 Halliwell, B., *Are polyphenols antioxidants or pro-oxidants? What do we learn from cell culture and in vivo studies?* Arch Biochem Biophys, 2008. **476**(2):107–12.

707 Skopinski, P. et al., *Chocolate feeding of pregnant mice influences length of limbs of their progeny.* Pol J Vet Sci, 2003. **6**(3 Suppl):57–9.

708 Zielinsky, P. et al., *Maternal consumption of polyphenol-rich foods in late pregnancy and fetal ductus arteriosus flow dynamics.* J Perinatol, 2010. **30**(1):17–21.

709 Zielinsky, P. et al., *Fetal ductal constriction caused by maternal ingestion of green tea in late pregnancy: an experimental study.* Prenat Diagn, 2012. **32**(10):921–6.

710 Zielinsky, P. et al., *Reversal of fetal ductal constriction after maternal restriction of polyphenol-rich foods: an open clinical trial.* J Perinatol, 2012. **32**(8):574–9.

711 Olson, J.A. and N.I. Krinsky, *Introduction: the colorful, fascinating world of the carotenoids: important physiologic modulators.* FASEB J, 1995. **9**(15):1547–50.

712 Burton, G.W., *Antioxidant action of carotenoids.* J Nutr, 1989. **119**(1):109–11.

713 Lowe, G.M., K. Vlismas, and A.J. Young, *Carotenoids as prooxidants?* Mol Aspects Med, 2003. **24**(6):363–9.

714 Lowe, G.M. et al., *Lycopene and beta-carotene protect against oxidative damage in HT29 cells at low concentrations but rapidly lose this capacity at higher doses.* Free Radic Res, 1999. **30**(2):141–51.

715 Zhang, P. and S.T. Omaye, *DNA strand breakage and oxygen tension: effects of beta-carotene, alpha-tocopherol and ascorbic acid.* Food Chem Toxicol, 2001. **39**(3):239–46.

716 Yeh, S.L. and M.L. Hu, *Induction of oxidative DNA damage in human foreskin fibroblast Hs68 cells by oxidized beta-carotene and lycopene.* Free Radic Res, 2001. **35**(2):203–13.

717 Williams, M.A. et al., *Plasma carotenoids, retinol, tocopherols, and lipoproteins in preeclamptic and normotensive pregnant Zimbabwean women.* Am J Hypertens, 2003. **16**(8):665–72.

718 Institute of Medicine, Food and Nutrition Board., *Dietary Reference Intakes for VItamin C, Vitamin E, Selenium and Carotenoids.* 2000, Washington, DC: The National Academies Press.

719 Tveden-Nyborg, P. et al., *Maternal vitamin C deficiency during pregnancy persistently impairs hippocampal neurogenesis in offspring of guinea pigs.* PLoS ONE, 2012. **7**(10):e48488.

720 Dror, D.K. and L.H. Allen, *Interventions with vitamins $B_6$, $B_{12}$ and C in pregnancy.* Paediatr Perinat Epidemiol, 2012. **26** (Suppl 1):55–74.

721 Byerley, L.O. and A. Kirksey, *Effects of different levels of vitamin C intake on the vitamin C concentration in human milk and the vitamin C intakes of breast-fed infants.* Am J Clin Nutr, 1985. **41**(4):665–71.

722 Blanchard, J., T.N. Tozer, and M. Rowland, *Pharmacokinetic perspectives on megadoses of ascorbic acid.* Am J Clin Nutr, 1997. **66**(5):1165–71.

723 Nienhuis, A.W., *Vitamin C and iron.* N Engl J Med, 1981. **304**(3):170–1.

724 Schectman, G., J.C. Byrd, and H.W. Gruchow, *The influence of smoking on vitamin C status in adults.* Am J Public Health, 1989. **79**(2):158–62.

725 Australian National Health and Medical Research Council and the New Zealand Ministry of Health, *Nutrient reference values for Australia and New Zealand: vitamin C.* <http://www.nrv.gov.au/nutrients/vitamin-c> accessed 8 May 2013.

726 Packer, J.E., T.F. Slater, and R.L. Willson, *Direct observation of a free radical interaction between vitamin E and vitamin C.* Nature, 1979. **278**(5706):737–8.

727 Zingg, J.M. and A. Azzi, *Non-antioxidant activities of vitamin E.* Curr Med Chem, 2004. **11**(9):1113–33.

728 Vardi, M., N.S. Levy, and A.P. Levy, *Vitamin E in the prevention of cardiovascular disease- the importance of proper patient selection.* J Lipid Res, 2013. **54**(9), 2307–14.

729 Traber, M.G., B. Frei, and J.S. Beckman, *Vitamin E revisited: do new data validate benefits for chronic disease prevention?* Curr Opin Lipidol, 2008. **19**(1):30–8.

730 Sokol, R.J., *Vitamin E and neurologic deficits.* Adv Pediatr, 1990. **37**:119–48.

731 Ford, E.S. and A. Sowell, *Serum alpha-tocopherol status in the United States population: findings from the Third National Health and Nutrition Examination Survey.* Am J Epidemiol, 1999. **150**(3):290–300.

732 Fulgoni, V.L., 3rd et al., *Foods, fortificants, and supplements: where do Americans get their nutrients?* J Nutr, 2011. **141**(10):1847–54.

733 Traber, M.G. and I. Jialal, *Measurement of lipid-soluble vitamins—further adjustment needed?* Lancet, 2000. **355**(9220):2013–4.

734 Horwitt, M.K. et al., *Relationship between tocopherol and serum lipid levels for determination of nutritional adequacy.* Ann N Y Acad Sci, 1972. **203**:223–36.

735 Dreyfuss, M.L. et al., *Determinants of low birth weight among HIV-infected pregnant women in Tanzania.* Am J Clin Nutr, 2001. **74**(6):814–26.

736 Jagadeesan, V. and K. Prema, *Plasma tocopherol and lipid levels in mother and umbilical cord; influence on birth weight.* Br J Obstet Gynaecol, 1980. **87**(10):908–10.

737 Scholl, T.O. et al., *Vitamin E: maternal concentrations are associated with fetal growth.* Am J Clin Nutr, 2006. **84**(6):1442–8.

738 Department of Health, *Dietary reference values for food energy and nutrients for the United Kingdom. Report of the Panel on Dietary Reference Values of the Committee on Medical Aspects of Food Policy.* Rep Health Soc Subj (Lond), 1991. **41**:1–210.

739 Takahashi, O., H. Ichikawa, and M. Sasaki, *Hemorrhagic toxicity of d-alpha-tocopherol in the rat.* Toxicology, 1990. **63**(2):157–65.

740 Miller, E.R., 3rd et al., *Meta-analysis: high-dosage vitamin E supplementation may increase all-cause mortality.* Ann Intern Med, 2005. **142**(1):37–46.

741 Smedts, H.P. et al., *High maternal vitamin E intake by diet or supplements is associated with congenital heart defects in the offspring.* BJOG, 2009. **116**(3):416–23.

742 Boskovic, R. et al., *Pregnancy outcome following high doses of Vitamin E supplementation.* Reprod Toxicol, 2005. **20**(1):85–8.

743 Duckworth, S., H.D. Mistry, and L.C. Chappell, *Vitamin supplementation in pregnancy.* The Obstetrician & Gynaecologist, 2012. **14**(3):175–8.

744 Australian National Health and Medical Research Council and the New Zealand Ministry of Health, *Nutrient reference values for Australia and New Zealand: vitamin E.* <http://www.nrv.gov.au/nutrients/vitamin-e.htm> accessed 10 May 2013.

745 Chan, A.C., *Partners in defense, vitamin E and vitamin C.* Can J Physiol Pharmacol, 1993. **71**(9):725–31.

746 Chappell, L.C. et al., *Effect of antioxidants on the occurrence of pre-eclampsia in women at increased risk: a randomised trial.* Lancet, 1999. **354**(9181):810–6.

747  Villar, J. et al., *World Health Organisation multicentre randomised trial of supplementation with vitamins C and E among pregnant women at high risk for pre-eclampsia in populations of low nutritional status from developing countries.* BJOG, 2009. **116**(6):780–8.

748  Poston, L. et al., *Vitamin C and vitamin E in pregnant women at risk for pre-eclampsia (VIP trial): randomised placebo-controlled trial.* Lancet, 2006. **367**(9517):1145–54.

749  Xu, H. et al., *An international trial of antioxidants in the prevention of preeclampsia (INTAPP).* Am J Obstet Gynecol, 2010. **202**(3):239.e1–239.e10.

750  Roberts, J.M. et al., *Vitamins C and E to prevent complications of pregnancy-associated hypertension.* N Engl J Med, 2010. **362**(14):1282–91.

751  Klemmensen, A. et al., *Intake of vitamin C and E in pregnancy and risk of pre-eclampsia: prospective study among 57 346 women.* BJOG, 2009. **116**(7):964–74.

752  Woods, J.R., Jr., M.A. Plessinger, and R.K. Miller, *Vitamins C and E: missing links in preventing preterm premature rupture of membranes?* Am J Obstet Gynecol, 2001. **185**(1):5–10.

753  Casanueva, E. et al., *Vitamin C supplementation to prevent premature rupture of the chorioamniotic membranes: a randomized trial.* Am J Clin Nutr, 2005. **81**(4):859–63.

754  Mercer, B.M. et al., *The impact of vitamin C supplementation in pregnancy and in vitro upon fetal membrane strength and remodeling.* Reprod Sci, 2010. **17**(7):685–95.

755  Swaney, P., J. Thorp, and I. Allen, *Vitamin C supplementation in pregnancy—does it decrease rates of preterm birth? A systematic review.* Am J Perinatol, 2013. **31**(2):91–8.

756  Bartfai, L. et al., *Rate of preterm birth in pregnant women with vitamin E treatment: a population-based study.* J Matern Fetal Neonatal Med, 2012. **25**(6):575–80.

757  Greenough, A. et al., *Respiratory outcomes in early childhood following antenatal vitamin C and E supplementation.* Thorax, 2010. **65**(11):998–1003.

758  West, C.E. et al., *Associations between maternal antioxidant intakes in pregnancy and infant allergic outcomes.* Nutrients, 2012. **4**(11):1747–58.

759  Moyer, M.W., *The myth of antioxidants.* Sci Am, 2013. **308**(2):62–7.

760  Scientific Advisory Committee of the RCOG, *Opinion Paper 16: Vitamin Supplementation in Pregnancy.* 2009, London: Royal College of Obstetricians and Gynaecologists.

761  National Institute for Health and Clinical Excellence, *Hypertension in Pregnancy: The Management of Hypertensive Disorders during Pregnancy.* 2010, London: NICE.

762  Nordin, B.E.C. *Calcium in health and disease.* Food, Nutrition and Agriculture, 1997. **1997**:13–26.

763  Johnston, C.C., Jr. et al., *Calcium supplementation and increases in bone mineral density in children.* N Engl J Med, 1992. **327**(2):82–7.

764  Nieves, J.W. et al., *Calcium potentiates the effect of estrogen and calcitonin on bone mass: review and analysis.* Am J Clin Nutr, 1998. **67**(1):18–24.

765  Abrams, S.A. et al., *Differences in calcium absorption and kinetics between black and white girls aged 5–16 years.* J Bone Miner Res, 1995. **10**(5):829–33.

766  Brown, E.M., *Chapter 24—Vitamin D and the calcium-sensing receptor*, in D.P. Feldman and J.W. Adams, eds., *Vitamin D, Third Edition.* 2011, San Diego: Academic Press, pp. 425–56.

767  Jorde, R. et al., *Relation between low calcium intake, parathyroid hormone, and blood pressure.* Hypertension, 2000. **35**(5):1154–9.

768 Lab Tests Online, *Calcium: the test.* <http://www.labtestsonline.org/understanding/analytes/calcium/tab/test> accessed 1 July 2014.

769 Olausson, H. et al., *Calcium economy in human pregnancy and lactation.* Nutr Res Rev, 2012. **25**(1):40–67.

770 Ulrich, U. et al., *Bone remodeling and bone mineral density during pregnancy.* Arch Gynecol Obstet, 2003. **268**(4):309–16.

771 Kovacs, C.S., *Calcium and bone metabolism during pregnancy and lactation.* J Mammary Gland Biol Neoplasia, 2005. **10**(2):105–18.

772 Oliveri, B. et al., *Mineral and bone mass changes during pregnancy and lactation.* Nutrition, 2004. **20**(2):235–40.

773 Vargas Zapata, C.L. et al., *Calcium homeostasis during pregnancy and lactation in Brazilian women with low calcium intakes: a longitudinal study.* Am J Clin Nutr, 2004. **80**(2):417–22.

774 Koo, W.W. et al., *Maternal calcium supplementation and fetal bone mineralization.* Obstet Gynecol, 1999. **94**(4):577–82.

775 Laboissiere, F.P.B., F.F.; Rodrigues, R.B; King, J.C.; Donangelo, C.M., *Calium homeostasis in primiparae and multiparae pregnant woment with marginal calcium intakes and response to a 7-day calcium supplementation trial.* Nutr Res, 2000. **20**(9):1229–39.

776 Janakiraman, V. et al., *Calcium supplements and bone resorption in pregnancy: a randomized crossover trial.* Am J Prev Med, 2003. **24**(3):260–4.

777 Liu, Z. et al., *Effect of milk and calcium supplementation on bone density and bone turnover in pregnant Chinese women: a randomized controlled trail.* Arch Gynecol Obstet, 2011. **283**(2):205–11.

778 Jarjou, L.M. et al., *Effect of calcium supplementation in pregnancy on maternal bone outcomes in women with a low calcium intake.* Am J Clin Nutr, 2010. **92**(2):450–7.

779 Raman, L. et al., *Effect of calcium supplementation to undernourished mothers during pregnancy on the bone density of the bone density of the neonates.* Am J Clin Nutr, 1978. **31**(3):466–9.

780 Abalos, E. et al., *Effects of calcium supplementation on fetal growth in mothers with deficient calcium intake: a randomised controlled trial.* Paediatr Perinat Epidemiol, 2010. **24**(1):53–62.

781 Jarjou, L.M. et al., *Randomized, placebo-controlled, calcium supplementation study in pregnant Gambian women: effects on breast-milk calcium concentrations and infant birth weight, growth, and bone mineral accretion in the first year of life.* Am J Clin Nutr, 2006. **83**(3):657–66.

782 Belizan, J.M. and J. Villar, *The relationship between calcium intake and edema-, proteinuria-, and hypertension-getosis: an hypothesis.* Am J Clin Nutr, 1980. **33**(10):2202–10.

783 Hofmeyr, G.J. et al., *Calcium supplementation during pregnancy for preventing hypertensive disorders and related problems.* Cochrane Database Syst Rev, 2010. **8**:CD001059.

784 Imdad, A., A. Jabeen, and Z.A. Bhutta, *Role of calcium supplementation during pregnancy in reducing risk of developing gestational hypertensive disorders: a meta-analysis of studies from developing countries.* BMC Public Health, 2011. **11** (Suppl 3):S18.

785 Villar, J. et al., *World Health Organization randomized trial of calcium supplementation among low calcium intake pregnant women.* Am J Obstet Gynecol, 2006. **194**(3):639–49.

786 **Trumbo, P.R. and K.C. Ellwood,** *Supplemental calcium and risk reduction of hypertension, pregnancy-induced hypertension, and preeclampsia: an evidence-based review by the US Food and Drug Administration.* Nutr Rev, 2007. **65**(2):78–87.

787 **Villar, J. and J.T. Repke,** *Calcium supplementation during pregnancy may reduce preterm delivery in high-risk populations.* Am J Obstet Gynecol, 1990. **163**(4 Pt 1):1124–31.

788 **Bergel, E. and A.J. Barros,** *Effect of maternal calcium intake during pregnancy on children's blood pressure: a systematic review of the literature.* BMC Pediatr, 2007. **7**:15.

789 **Prentice, A. et al.,** *Calcium requirements of lactating Gambian mothers: effects of a calcium supplement on breast-milk calcium concentration, maternal bone mineral content, and urinary calcium excretion.* Am J Clin Nutr, 1995. **62**(1):58–67.

790 **Abrams, S.A., J. Wen, and J.E. Stuff,** *Absorption of calcium, zinc, and iron from breast milk by five- to seven-month-old infants.* Pediatr Res, 1997. **41**(3):384–90.

791 **Hicks, P.D. et al.,** *Total calcium absorption is similar from infant formulas with and without prebiotics and exceeds that in human milk-fed infants.* BMC Pediatr, 2012. **12**:118.

792 **Specker, B.L. et al.,** *Randomized trial of varying mineral intake on total body bone mineral accretion during the first year of life.* Pediatrics, 1997. **99**(6):E12.

793 **Sowers, M. et al.,** *Biochemical markers of bone turnover in lactating and nonlactating postpartum women.* J Clin Endocrinol Metab, 1995. **80**(7):2210–6.

794 **Laskey, M.A. et al.,** *Bone changes after 3 mo of lactation: influence of calcium intake, breast-milk output, and vitamin D-receptor genotype.* Am J Clin Nutr, 1998. **67**(4):685–92.

795 **Lopez, J.M. et al.,** *Bone turnover and density in healthy women during breastfeeding and after weaning.* Osteoporos Int, 1996. **6**(2):153–9.

796 **Aggarwal, V. et al.,** *Role of calcium deficiency in development of nutritional rickets in Indian children: a case control study.* J Clin Endocrinol Metab, 2012. **97**(10):3461–6.

797 **DeLucia, M.C., M.E. Mitnick, and T.O. Carpenter,** *Nutritional rickets with normal circulating 25-hydroxyvitamin D: a call for reexamining the role of dietary calcium intake in North American infants.* J Clin Endocrinol Metab, 2003. **88**(8):3539–45.

798 **Thacher, T.D. and S.A. Abrams,** *Relationship of calcium absorption with 25(OH)D and calcium intake in children with rickets.* Nutr Rev, 2010. **68**(11):682–8.

799 **Meyer, H.E. et al.,** *Dietary factors and the incidence of hip fracture in middle-aged Norwegians. A prospective study.* Am J Epidemiol, 1997. **145**(2):117–23.

800 **Clements, M.R., L. Johnson, and D.R. Fraser,** *A new mechanism for induced vitamin D deficiency in calcium deprivation.* Nature, 1987. **325**(6099):62–5.

801 **Canada, H.,** *Vitamin D and calcium: updated dietary reference intakes.* <http://www.hc-sc.gc.ca/fn-an/nutrition/vitamin/vita-d-eng.php> accessed 20 Dec 2012.

802 **Mouratidou, T. et al.,** *Dietary assessment of a population of pregnant women in Sheffield, UK.* Br J Nutr, 2006. **96**(5):929–35.

803 National Institute of Nutrition, Indian Council of Medical Research, *Nutrient Requirements and Recommended Dietary Allowances for Indians: A Report of the Expert Group of the Indian Council of Medical Research 2009.* 2010, Hyderabad: National Institute of Nutrition, Indian Council of Medical Research.

804 **Nordin, B.E. et al.,** *The nature and significance of the relationship between urinary sodium and urinary calcium in women.* J Nutr, 1993. **123**(9):1615–22.

805 Dawson-Hughes, B., *Interaction of dietary calcium and protein in bone health in humans.* J Nutr, 2003. **133**(3):852S–4S.

806 Greger, J.L., *Nondigestible carbohydrates and mineral bioavailability.* J Nutr, 1999. **129**(7):1434S–5S.

807 DeSantiago, S. et al., *Negative calcium balance during lactation in rural Mexican women.* Am J Clin Nutr, 2002. **76**(4):845–51.

808 Armas, L.A. et al., *Chronic dietary fiber supplementation with wheat dextrin does not inhibit calcium and magnesium absorption in premenopausal and postmenopausal women.* J Int Med Res, 2011. **39**(5):1824–33.

809 Hallberg, L. et al., *Calcium and iron absorption: mechanism of action and nutritional importance.* Eur J Clin Nutr, 1992. **46**(5):317–27.

810 Bolland, M.J. et al., *Calcium supplements with or without vitamin D and risk of cardiovascular events: reanalysis of the Women's Health Initiative limited access dataset and meta-analysis.* BMJ, 2011. **342**:d2040.

811 Bolland, M.J. et al., *Calcium and vitamin D supplements and health outcomes: a reanalysis of the Women's Health Initiative (WHI) limited-access data set.* Am J Clin Nutr, 2011. **94**(4):1144–9.

812 Abrahamsen, B. and O. Sahota, *Do calcium plus vitamin D supplements increase cardiovascular risk?* BMJ, 2011. **342**:d2080.

813 Prince, R.L., K. Zhu, and J.R. Lewis, *Evidence of harm is unconvincing.* BMJ, 2011. **342**:d3541.

814 Metcalfe, A.V. and B.E. Nordin, *A reanalysis too far?* BMJ, 2011. **342**:d3538.

815 American Pregnancy Association, *Pregnancy nutrition.* <http://americanpregnancy.org/pregnancyhealth/pregnancynutrition.html> accessed 1 July 2014.

816 World Health Organization, *Prevention and Management of Osteoporosis: Report of a WHO Scientific Group. WHO Technical Report Series.* 2003, Geneva: World Health Organization.

817 Hetzel, B.S., *Iodine and neuropsychological development.* J Nutr, 2000. **130**(2S Suppl):493S–5S.

818 Pemberton, H.N., J.A. Franklyn, and M.D. Kilby, *Thyroid hormones and fetal brain development.* Minerva Ginecol, 2005. **57**(4):367–78.

819 Glinoer, D., *The importance of iodine nutrition during pregnancy.* Public Health Nutr, 2007. **10**(12A):1542–6.

820 Liberman, C.S. et al., *Circulating iodide concentrations during and after pregnancy.* J Clin Endocrinol Metab, 1998. **83**(10):3545–9.

821 Vejbjerg, P. et al., *Estimation of iodine intake from various urinary iodine measurements in population studies.* Thyroid, 2009. **19**(11):1281–6.

822 Davidson, J., *An epidemic of nonexistent iodine deficiency due to inappropriate urine iodide testing and reference ranges.* N Z Med J, 2009. **122**(1291):109–10.

823 Lazarus, J.H., *Thyroid function in pregnancy.* Br Med Bull, 2011. **97**:137–48.

824 Glinoer, D., *The regulation of thyroid function during normal pregnancy: importance of the iodine nutrition status.* Best Pract Res Clin Endocrinol Metab, 2004. **18**(2):133–52.

825 Zimmermann, M.B., *Iodine deficiency in pregnancy and the effects of maternal iodine supplementation on the offspring: a review.* Am J Clin Nutr, 2009. **89**(2):668S–72S.

826  Casey, B.M. et al., *Subclinical hypothyroidism and pregnancy outcomes*. Obstet Gynecol, 2005. **105**(2):239–45.

827  Benhadi, N. et al., *Higher maternal TSH levels in pregnancy are associated with increased risk for miscarriage, fetal or neonatal death*. Eur J Endocrinol, 2009. **160**(6):985–91.

828  Dillon, J.C. and J. Milliez, *Reproductive failure in women living in iodine deficient areas of West Africa*. BJOG, 2000. **107**(5):631–6.

829  Chaouki, M.L. and M. Benmiloud, *Prevention of iodine deficiency disorders by oral administration of lipiodol during pregnancy*. Eur J Endocrinol, 1994. **130**(6):547–51.

830  DeLong, G.R. et al., *Effect on infant mortality of iodination of irrigation water in a severely iodine-deficient area of China*. Lancet, 1997. **350**(9080):771–3.

831  Cao, X.Y. et al., *Timing of vulnerability of the brain to iodine deficiency in endemic cretinism*. N Engl J Med, 1994. **331**(26):1739–44.

832  Mason, J.B. et al., *Iodine fortification is related to increased weight-for-age and birthweight in children in Asia*. Food Nutr Bull, 2002. **23**(3):292–308.

833  Delange, F., *Screening for congenital hypothyroidism used as an indicator of the degree of iodine deficiency and of its control*. Thyroid, 1998. **8**(12):1185–92.

834  Melse-Boonstra, A. and N. Jaiswal, *Iodine deficiency in pregnancy, infancy and childhood and its consequences for brain development*. Best Pract Res Clin Endocrinol Metab, 2010. **24**(1):29–38.

835  Bleichrodt, N. and M.P. Born, *A metaanalysis of research on iodine and its relationship to cognitive development*, in J.B. Stanbury, ed., *The Damaged Brain of Iodine Deficiency*. 1994, New York: Cognizant Communication Corporation, pp. 195–200.

836  Qian, M. et al., *The effects of iodine on intelligence in children: a meta-analysis of studies conducted in China*. Asia Pac J Clin Nutr, 2005. **14**(1):32–42.

837  Haddow, J.E. et al., *Maternal thyroid deficiency during pregnancy and subsequent neuropsychological development of the child*. N Engl J Med, 1999. **341**(8):549–55.

838  Berbel, P. et al., *Delayed neurobehavioral development in children born to pregnant women with mild hypothyroxinemia during the first month of gestation: the importance of early iodine supplementation*. Thyroid, 2009. **19**(5):511–9.

839  Velasco, I. et al., *Effect of iodine prophylaxis during pregnancy on neurocognitive development of children during the first two years of life*. J Clin Endocrinol Metab, 2009. **94**(9):3234–41.

840  van den Hove, M.F. et al., *Hormone synthesis and storage in the thyroid of human preterm and term newborns: effect of thyroxine treatment*. Biochimie, 1999. **81**(5):563–70.

841  Azizi, F. and P. Smyth, *Breastfeeding and maternal and infant iodine nutrition*. Clin Endocrinol (Oxf), 2009. **70**(5):803–9.

842  Spitzweg, C. et al., *Analysis of human sodium iodide symporter gene expression in extrathyroidal tissues and cloning of its complementary deoxyribonucleic acids from salivary gland, mammary gland, and gastric mucosa*. J Clin Endocrinol Metab, 1998. **83**(5):1746–51.

843  Leung, A.M. et al., *Breastmilk iodine concentrations following acute dietary iodine intake*. Thyroid, 2012. **22**(11):1176–80.

844  Zimmermann, M.B., *The effects of iodine deficiency in pregnancy and infancy*. Paediatr Perinat Epidemiol, 2012. **26** (Suppl 1):108–17.

845 Pharoah, P.O., I.H. Buttfield, and B.S. Hetzel, *Neurological damage to the fetus resulting from severe iodine deficiency during pregnancy.* Lancet, 1971. **297**(7694):308–10.

846 Thilly, C.H. et al., *Fetal hypothyroidism and maternal thyroid status in severe endemic goiter.* J Clin Endocrinol Metab, 1978. **47**(2):354–60.

847 Pharoah, P.O., *Iodine-supplementation trials.* Am J Clin Nutr, 1993. **57**(2):276S–9S.

848 Romano, R. et al., *The effects of iodoprophylaxis on thyroid size during pregnancy.* Am J Obstet Gynecol, 1991. **164**(2):482–5.

849 Pedersen, K.M. et al., *Amelioration of some pregnancy-associated variations in thyroid function by iodine supplementation.* J Clin Endocrinol Metab, 1993. **77**(4):1078–83.

850 Glinoer, D. et al., *A randomized trial for the treatment of mild iodine deficiency during pregnancy: maternal and neonatal effects.* J Clin Endocrinol Metab, 1995. **80**(1):258–69.

851 Liesenkotter, K.P. et al., *Earliest prevention of endemic goiter by iodine supplementation during pregnancy.* Eur J Endocrinol, 1996. **134**(4):443–8.

852 Zhou, S.J. et al., *Effect of iodine supplementation in pregnancy on child development and other clinical outcomes: a systematic review of randomized controlled trials.* Am J Clin Nutr, 2013. **98**(5):1241–54.

853 Nohr, S.B. et al., *Postpartum thyroid dysfunction in pregnant thyroid peroxidase antibody-positive women living in an area with mild to moderate iodine deficiency: is iodine supplementation safe?* J Clin Endocrinol Metab, 2000. **85**(9):3191–8.

854 Flachowsky, G., *Iodine in animal nutrition and iodine transfer from feed into food of animal origin.* Lohmann Information, 2007. **42**(2):47–59.

855 M. Andersson et al., eds., *Iodine Deficiency in Europe: A Continuing Public Health Problem.* 2007, Geneva: World Health Organization, UNICEF.

856 Azizi, F. et al., *Urinary iodine excretion in pregnant women residing in areas with adequate iodine intake.* Public Health Nutr, 2003. **6**(1):95–8.

857 Yan, Y.Q. et al., *Attention to the hiding iodine deficiency in pregnant and lactating women after universal salt iodization: a multi-community study in China.* J Endocrinol Invest, 2005. **28**(6):547–53.

858 Marchioni, E. et al., *Iodine deficiency in pregnant women residing in an area with adequate iodine intake.* Nutrition, 2008. **24**(5):458–61.

859 Oguz Kutlu, A. and C. Kara, *Iodine deficiency in pregnant women in the apparently iodine-sufficient capital city of Turkey.* Clin Endocrinol (Oxf), 2012. **77**(4):615–20.

860 Andersson, M., V. Karumbunathan, and M.B. Zimmermann, *Global iodine status in 2011 and trends over the past decade.* J Nutr, 2012. **142**(4):744–50.

861 Expert Group on Vitamins and Minerals, *Safe Upper Levels for Vitamins and Minerals.* 2003, London: Food Standards Agency.

862 Sang, Z. et al., *Thyroid dysfunction during late gestation is associated with excessive iodine intake in pregnant women.* J Clin Endocrinol Metab, 2012. **97**(8):E1363–9.

863 Nishiyama, S. et al., *Transient hypothyroidism or persistent hyperthyrotropinemia in neonates born to mothers with excessive iodine intake.* Thyroid, 2004. **14**(12):1077–83.

864 Connelly, K.J. et al., *Congenital hypothyroidism caused by excess prenatal maternal iodine ingestion.* J Pediatr, 2012. **161**(4):760–2.

865 Emder, P.J. and M.M. Jack, *Iodine-induced neonatal hypothyroidism secondary to maternal seaweed consumption: a common practice in some Asian cultures to promote breast milk supply.* J Paediatr Child Health, 2011. **47**(10):750–2.

866 National Health and Medical Research Council, *NHMRC Public Statement: Iodine Supplementation for Pregnant and Breastfeeding Women.* 2010, Canberra: Australian Government.

867 **Andersson, M. et al.**, *Prevention and control of iodine deficiency in pregnant and lactating women and in children less than 2-years-old: conclusions and recommendations of the Technical Consultation.* Public Health Nutr, 2007. **10**(12A):1606–11.

868 **De Groot, L. et al.**, *Management of thyroid dysfunction during pregnancy and postpartum: an Endocrine Society clinical practice guideline.* J Clin Endocrinol Metab, 2012. **97**(8):2543–65.

869 **Stagnaro-Green, A. et al.**, *Guidelines of the American Thyroid Association for the diagnosis and management of thyroid disease during pregnancy and postpartum.* Thyroid, 2011. **21**(10):1081–125.

870 **Becker, D.V. et al.**, *Iodine supplementation for pregnancy and lactation-United States and Canada: recommendations of the American Thyroid Association.* Thyroid, 2006. **16**(10):949–51.

871 **Leung, A.M., E.N. Pearce, and L.E. Braverman,** *Iodine content of prenatal multivitamins in the United States.* N Engl J Med, 2009. **360**(9):939–40.

872 **Kohgo, Y. et al.**, *Body iron metabolism and pathophysiology of iron overload.* Int J Hematol, 2008. **88**(1):7–15.

873 **Finberg, K.E.**, *Unraveling mechanisms regulating systemic iron homeostasis.* Hematology Am Soc Hematol Educ Program, 2011. **2011**:532–7.

874 **Andrews, N.C. and P.J. Schmidt,** *Iron homeostasis.* Annu Rev Physiol, 2007. **69**:69–85.

875 **Ganz, T.,** *Hepcidin—a regulator of intestinal iron absorption and iron recycling by macrophages.* Best Pract Res Clin Haematol, 2005. **18**(2):171–82.

876 **Koulaouzidis, A. et al.**, *Soluble transferrin receptors and iron deficiency, a step beyond ferritin. A systematic review.* J Gastrointestin Liver Dis, 2009. **18**(3):345–52.

877 **Szoke, D. and M. Panteghini,** *Diagnostic value of transferrin.* Clin Chim Acta, 2012. **413**(15–6):1184–9.

878 **Firkin, F. and B. Rush,** *Interpretation of biochemical tests for iron deficiency: diagnostic difficulties related to limitations of individual tests.* Aust Prescr, 1997. **20**:74–6.

879 **Pasricha, S.R. et al.**, *Serum hepcidin as a diagnostic test of iron deficiency in premenopausal female blood donors.* Haematologica, 2011. **96**(8):1099–105.

880 **McLean, E. et al.**, *Worldwide prevalence of anaemia, WHO Vitamin and Mineral Nutrition Information System, 1993–2005.* Public Health Nutr, 2009. **12**(4):444–54.

881 **Lynch, S.,** *Improving the assessment of iron status.* Am J Clin Nutr, 2011. **93**(6):1188–9.

882 Vitamin and Mineral Nutrition Information System, *Haemoglobin Concentrations for the Diagnosis of Anaemia and Assessment of Severity.* 2011, Geneva: World Health Organization.

883 **Bothwell, T.H.**, *Iron requirements in pregnancy and strategies to meet them.* Am J Clin Nutr, 2000. **72**(1 Suppl):257S–64S.

884 Joint FAO/WHO Expert Consultation on Human Vitamin and Mineral Requirements, *Human Vitamin and Mineral Requirements. Report of a Joint FAO/WHO Expert Consulation, Bangkok, Thailand.* 2001, Rome: FAO.

885 **Milman, N.**, *Oral iron prophylaxis in pregnancy: not too little and not too much!* J Pregnancy, 2012. **2012**:514345.

886  Shao, J. et al., *Maternal serum ferritin concentration is positively associated with new-born iron stores in women with low ferritin status in late pregnancy.* J Nutr, 2012. **142**(11):2004–9.

887  World Health Organization, WHO Guideline: Intermittent Iron and Folic Acid Supplementation to Non-anaemic Pregnant Women. 2012, Geneva: World Health Oganization.

888  Brooker, S., P.J. Hotez, and D.A. Bundy, *Hookworm-related anaemia among pregnant women: a systematic review.* PLoS Negl Trop Dis, 2008. **2**(9):e291.

889  Oregon Evidence-based Practice Center, *Screening for Iron Deficiency Anemia in Childhood and Pregnancy: Update of the 1996 U.S. Preventive Task Force Review. Evidence Syntheses, No. 40.* 2006, Rockville: Agency for Healthcare Research and Quality.

890  Scholl, T.O., *Maternal iron status: relation to fetal growth, length of gestation, and iron endowment of the neonate.* Nutr Rev, 2011. **69** (Suppl 1):S23–9.

891  Georgieff, M.K. et al., *Abnormal iron distribution in infants of diabetic mothers: spectrum and maternal antecedents.* J Pediatr, 1990. **117**(3):455–61.

892  Allen, L.H., *Biological mechanisms that might underlie iron's effects on fetal growth and preterm birth.* J Nutr, 2001. **131**(2S-2):581S–9S.

893  Lieberman, E. et al., *Association of maternal hematocrit with premature labor.* Am J Obstet Gynecol, 1988. **159**(1):107–14.

894  Scholl, T.O. et al., *Anemia vs iron deficiency: increased risk of preterm delivery in a prospective study.* Am J Clin Nutr, 1992. **55**(5):985–8.

895  Hindmarsh, P.C. et al., *Effect of early maternal iron stores on placental weight and structure.* Lancet, 2000. **356**(9231):719–23.

896  Barker, D.J. et al., *Fetal and placental size and risk of hypertension in adult life.* BMJ, 1990. **301**(6746):259–62.

897  Alwan, N.A. et al., *Dietary iron intake during early pregnancy and birth outcomes in a cohort of British women.* Hum Reprod, 2011. **26**(4):911–9.

898  Lozoff, B., *Early iron deficiency has brain and behavior effects consistent with dopaminergic dysfunction.* J Nutr, 2011. **141**(4):740S–746S.

899  Lozoff, B. et al., *Long-lasting neural and behavioral effects of iron deficiency in infancy.* Nutr Rev, 2006. **64**(5 Pt 2):S34–43; discussion, S72–91.

900  Rao, R. et al., *Fetal and neonatal iron deficiency causes volume loss and alters the neuro-chemical profile of the adult rat hippocampus.* Nutr Neurosci, 2011. **14**(2):59–65.

901  Wu, L.L. et al., *Effect of perinatal iron deficiency on myelination and associated behaviors in rat pups.* Behav Brain Res, 2008. **188**(2):263–70.

902  Carter, R.C. et al., *Iron deficiency anemia and cognitive function in infancy.* Pediatrics, 2010. **126**(2):e427–34.

903  Lozoff, B. et al., *Dose-response relationships between iron deficiency with or without anemia and infant social-emotional behavior.* J Pediatr, 2008. **152**(5):696–702, 702.31–3.

904  Algarin, C. et al., *Iron deficiency anemia in infancy: long-lasting effects on auditory and visual system functioning.* Pediatr Res, 2003. **53**(2):217–23.

905  Peirano, P.D. et al., *Sleep and neurofunctions throughout child development: lasting effects of early iron deficiency.* J Pediatr Gastroenterol Nutr, 2009. **48** (Suppl 1): S8–15.

906 **Zimmermann, M.B. and J. Kohrle,** *The impact of iron and selenium deficiencies on iodine and thyroid metabolism: biochemistry and relevance to public health.* Thyroid, 2002. **12**(10):867–78.

907 **Soares, N.N. et al.,** *Iron deficiency anemia and iron stores in adult and adolescent women in pregnancy.* Acta Obstet Gynecol Scand, 2010. **89**(3):343–9.

908 **Blickstein, I., R. Goldschmit, and S. Lurie,** *Hemoglobin levels during twin vs. singleton pregnancies. Parity makes the difference.* J Reprod Med, 1995. **40**(1):47–50.

909 **Luke, B.,** *Nutrition and multiple gestation.* Semin Perinatol, 2005. **29**(5):349–54.

910 **Pinhas-Hamiel, O. et al.,** *Greater prevalence of iron deficiency in overweight and obese children and adolescents.* Int J Obes Relat Metab Disord, 2003. **27**(3):416–18.

911 **Brotanek, J.M. et al.,** *Iron deficiency in early childhood in the United States: risk factors and racial/ethnic disparities.* Pediatrics, 2007. **120**(3):568–75.

912 **Sultan, A.N. and R.W. Zuberi,** *Late weaning: the most significant risk factor in the development of iron deficiency anaemia at 1–2 years of age.* J Ayub Med Coll Abbottabad, 2003. **15**(2):3–7.

913 **Fernandez-Gaxiola, A.C. and L.M. De-Regil,** *Intermittent iron supplementation for reducing anaemia and its associated impairments in menstruating women.* Cochrane Database Syst Rev, 2011. **12**:CD009218.

914 **Olsen, A. et al.,** *Failure of twice-weekly iron supplementation to increase blood haemoglobin and serum ferritin concentrations: results of a randomized controlled trial.* Ann Trop Med Parasitol, 2006. **100**(3):251–63.

915 **Pena-Rosas, J.P. and F.E. Viteri,** *Effects and safety of preventive oral iron or iron + folic acid supplementation for women during pregnancy.* Cochrane Database Syst Rev, 2009. **4**:CD004736.

916 **Yakoob, M.Y. and Z.A. Bhutta,** *Effect of routine iron supplementation with or without folic acid on anemia during pregnancy.* BMC Public Health, 2011. **11** (Suppl 3):S21.

917 **Cockell, K.A., D.C. Miller, and H. Lowell,** *Application of the Dietary Reference Intakes in developing a recommendation for pregnancy iron supplements in Canada.* Am J Clin Nutr, 2009. **90**(4):1023–8.

918 **Health Canada,** *Prenatal nutrition guidelines for health professionals—iron contributes to a healthy pregnancy.* 2009, <http://www.hc-sc.gc.ca/fn-an/alt_formats/hpfb-dgpsa/pdf/pubs/iron-fer-eng.pdf>.

919 **Thomsen, J.K. et al.,** *Low dose iron supplementation does not cover the need for iron during pregnancy.* Acta Obstet Gynecol Scand, 1993. **72**(2):93–8.

920 United Nations Children's Fund, World Health Organization, and United Nations University, *Composition of a Multi-micronutrient Supplement to be Used in Pilot Programmes Among Pregnant Women in Developing Countries: Report of a United Nations Children's Fund (UNICEF), World Health Organization (WHO), United Nations University (UNU) Workshop.* 1999, New York: UNICEF/WHO/UNU.

921 **Shah, P.S. et al.,** *Effects of prenatal multimicronutrient supplementation on pregnancy outcomes: a meta-analysis.* CMAJ, 2009. **180**(12):E99–108.

922 **Christian, P. et al.,** *Antenatal and postnatal iron supplementation and childhood mortality in rural Nepal: a prospective follow-up in a randomized, controlled community trial.* Am J Epidemiol, 2009. **170**(9):1127–36.

923  Mills, R.J. and M.W. Davies, *Enteral iron supplementation in preterm and low birth weight infants.* Cochrane Database Syst Rev, 2012. 3:CD005095.

924  Berglund, S.K. et al., *Effects of iron supplementation of LBW infants on cognition and behavior at 3 years.* Pediatrics, 2013. **131**(1):47–55.

925  Hulten, L. et al., *Iron absorption from the whole diet. Relation to meal composition, iron requirements and iron stores.* Eur J Clin Nutr, 1995. **49**(11):794–808.

926  Swensen, A.R., L.J. Harnack, and J.A. Ross, *Nutritional assessment of pregnant women enrolled in the Special Supplemental Program for Women, Infants, and Children (WIC).* J Am Diet Assoc, 2001. **101**(8):903–8.

927  Hunt, J.R. and Z.K. Roughead, *Nonheme-iron absorption, fecal ferritin excretion, and blood indexes of iron status in women consuming controlled lactoovovegetarian diets for 8 wk.* Am J Clin Nutr, 1999. **69**(5):944–52.

928  Melamed, N. et al., *Iron supplementation in pregnancy—does the preparation matter?* Arch Gynecol Obstet, 2007. **276**(6):601–4.

929  Coplin, M. et al., *Tolerability of iron: a comparison of bis-glycino iron II and ferrous sulfate.* Clin Ther, 1991. **13**(5):606–12.

930  Frykman, E. et al., *Side effects of iron supplements in blood donors: superior tolerance of heme iron.* J Lab Clin Med, 1994. **123**(4):561–4.

931  Gill, S.K., C. Maltepe, and G. Koren, *The effectiveness of discontinuing iron-containing prenatal multivitamins on reducing the severity of nausea and vomiting of pregnancy.* J Obstet Gynaecol, 2009. **29**(1):13–16.

932  Gill, S.K., P. Nguyen, and G. Koren, *Adherence and tolerability of iron-containing prenatal multivitamins in pregnant women with pre-existing gastrointestinal conditions.* J Obstet Gynaecol, 2009. **29**(7):594–8.

933  Nchito, M. et al., *Iron supplementation increases small intestine permeability in primary schoolchildren in Lusaka, Zambia.* Trans R Soc Trop Med Hyg, 2006. **100**(8):791–4.

934  Dandona, P. et al., *Insulin resistance and iron overload.* Ann Clin Biochem, 1983. **20** (Pt 2):77–9.

935  Qiu, C. et al., *Gestational diabetes mellitus in relation to maternal dietary heme iron and nonheme iron intake.* Diabetes Care, 2011. **34**(7):1564–9.

936  Chan, K.K. et al., *Iron supplement in pregnancy and development of gestational diabetes—a randomised placebo-controlled trial.* BJOG, 2009. **116**(6):789–97; discussion, 797–8.

937  Rajpathak, S. et al., *Iron intake and the risk of type 2 diabetes in women: a prospective cohort study.* Diabetes Care, 2006. **29**(6):1370–6.

938  Ziaei, S. et al., *A randomised placebo-controlled trial to determine the effect of iron supplementation on pregnancy outcome in pregnant women with haemoglobin > or = 13.2 g/dl.* BJOG, 2007. **114**(6):684–8.

939  Steen, D.L. et al., *Prognostic evaluation of catalytic iron in patients with acute coronary syndromes.* Clin Cardiol, 2013. **36**(3):139–45.

940  Stevens, R.G. et al., *Moderate elevation of body iron level and increased risk of cancer occurrence and death.* Int J Cancer, 1994. **56**(3):364–9.

941  Knuppel, R.A. et al., *Oxidative stress and antioxidants: preterm birth and preterm infants,* in J. Morrison, ed., *Preterm Birth—Mother and Child.* 2012, Rijeka: InTech, pp. 125–50.

942 Lozoff, B. et al., *Iron-fortified vs low-iron infant formula: developmental outcome at 10 years*. Arch Pediatr Adolesc Med, 2012. **166**(3):208–15.

943 Becroft, D.M., M.R. Dix, and K. Farmer, *Intramuscular iron-dextran and susceptibility of neonates to bacterial infections. In vitro studies*. Arch Dis Child, 1977. **52**(10):778–81.

944 Litovitz, T. and A. Manoguerra, *Comparison of pediatric poisoning hazards: an analysis of 3.8 million exposure incidents. A report from the American Association of Poison Control Centers*. Pediatrics, 1992. **89**(6 Pt 1):999–1006.

945 Food and Drug Administration, Health and Human Services, *Iron-containing supplements and drugs; label warning statements and unit-dose packaging requirements; removal of regulations for unit-dose packaging requirements for dietary supplements and drugs. Final rule; removal of regulatory provisions in response to court order*. Fed Regist, 2003. **68**(201):59714–15.

946 de Benoist, B. et al., eds., *Worldwide Prevalence of Anaemia 1993–2005. WHO Global Database on Anaemia*. 2008, Geneva: World Health Organization.

947 Centers for Disease Control and Prevention, *Recommendations to prevent and control iron deficiency in the United States*. MMWR Recomm Rep, 1998. **47**(RR-3):1–29.

948 American Congress and Obstetric and Gynecologists, *ACOG Practice Bulletin No. 95: anemia in pregnancy*. Obstet Gynecol, 2008. **112**(1):201–7.

949 US Department of Agriculture, and US Department of Health and Human Services, *Dietary Guidelines for Americans 2010*. 2010, Washington, DC: US Government Printing Office.

950 Pavord, S. et al., *UK guidelines on the management of iron deficiency in pregnancy*. Br J Haematol, 2012. **156**(5):588–600.

951 Baker, R.D., F.R. Greer, and Committee on Nutrition American Academy of Pediatrics, *Diagnosis and prevention of iron deficiency and iron-deficiency anemia in infants and young children (0–3 years of age)*. Pediatrics, 2010. **126**(5):1040–50.

952 Domellof, M., *Iron requirements in infancy*. Ann Nutr Metab, 2011. **59**(1):59–63.

953 Koletzko, B. et al., *Global standard for the composition of infant formula: recommendations of an ESPGHAN coordinated international expert group*. J Pediatr Gastroenterol Nutr, 2005. **41**(5):584–99.

954 Wester, P.O., *Magnesium*. Am J Clin Nutr, 1987. **45**(5 Suppl):1305–12.

955 Rude, R.K., *Magnesium deficiency: a cause of heterogeneous disease in humans*. J Bone Miner Res, 1998. **13**(4):749–58.

956 Fatemi, S. et al., *Effect of experimental human magnesium depletion on parathyroid hormone secretion and 1,25-dihydroxyvitamin D metabolism*. J Clin Endocrinol Metab, 1991. **73**(5):1067–72.

957 Arnaud, M.J., *Update on the assessment of magnesium status*. Br J Nutr, 2008. **99** (Suppl 3):S24–36.

958 Guerrero-Romero, F. and M. Rodriguez-Moran, *Low serum magnesium levels and metabolic syndrome*. Acta Diabetol, 2002. **39**(4):209–13.

959 Chacko, S.A. et al., *Magnesium supplementation, metabolic and inflammatory markers, and global genomic and proteomic profiling: a randomized, double-blind, controlled, crossover trial in overweight individuals*. Am J Clin Nutr, 2011. **93**(2):463–73.

960 Rodriguez-Hernandez, H. et al., *Oral magnesium supplementation decreases alanine aminotransferase levels in obese women*. Magnes Res, 2010. **23**(2):90–6.

961  Lopez-Ridaura, R. et al., *Magnesium intake and risk of type 2 diabetes in men and women.* Diabetes Care, 2004. **27**(1):134–40.

962  Song, Y. et al., *Dietary magnesium intake in relation to plasma insulin levels and risk of type 2 diabetes in women.* Diabetes Care, 2004. **27**(1):59–65.

963  Kao, W.H. et al., *Serum and dietary magnesium and the risk for type 2 diabetes mellitus: the Atherosclerosis Risk in Communities Study.* Arch Intern Med, 1999. **159**(18):2151–9.

964  Rodriguez-Moran, M. and F. Guerrero-Romero, *Oral magnesium supplementation improves insulin sensitivity and metabolic control in type 2 diabetic subjects: a randomized double-blind controlled trial.* Diabetes Care, 2003. **26**(4):1147–52.

965  Liao, F., A.R. Folsom, and F.L. Brancati, *Is low magnesium concentration a risk factor for coronary heart disease? The Atherosclerosis Risk in Communities (ARIC) Study.* Am Heart J, 1998. **136**(3):480–90.

966  Ascherio, A. et al., *A prospective study of nutritional factors and hypertension among US men.* Circulation, 1992. **86**(5):1475–84.

967  Witteman, J.C. et al., *A prospective study of nutritional factors and hypertension among US women.* Circulation, 1989. **80**(5):1320–7.

968  Witteman, J.C. et al., *Reduction of blood pressure with oral magnesium supplementation in women with mild to moderate hypertension.* Am J Clin Nutr, 1994. **60**(1):129–35.

969  Shechter, M. et al., *Effects of oral magnesium therapy on exercise tolerance, exercise-induced chest pain, and quality of life in patients with coronary artery disease.* Am J Cardiol, 2003. **91**(5):517–21.

970  Pokan, R. et al., *Oral magnesium therapy, exercise heart rate, exercise tolerance, and myocardial function in coronary artery disease patients.* Br J Sports Med, 2006. **40**(9):773–8.

971  Appel, L.J. et al., *A clinical trial of the effects of dietary patterns on blood pressure. DASH Collaborative Research Group.* N Engl J Med, 1997. **336**(16):1117–24.

972  Rude, R.K., F.R. Singer, and H.E. Gruber, *Skeletal and hormonal effects of magnesium deficiency.* J Am Coll Nutr, 2009. **28**(2):131–41.

973  Tranquilli, A.L. et al., *Calcium, phosphorus and magnesium intakes correlate with bone mineral content in postmenopausal women.* Gynecol Endocrinol, 1994. **8**(1):55–8.

974  Odabasi, E. et al., *Magnesium, zinc, copper, manganese, and selenium levels in postmenopausal women with osteoporosis. Can magnesium play a key role in osteoporosis?* Ann Acad Med Singapore, 2008. **37**(7):564–7.

975  Sojka, J.E. and C.M. Weaver, *Magnesium supplementation and osteoporosis.* Nutr Rev, 1995. **53**(3):71–4.

976  Tsang, R.C., *Neonatal magnesium disturbances.* Am J Dis Child, 1972. **124**(2):282–93.

977  Kamal, S. et al., *Serum magnesium level in preterm labour.* Indian J Pathol Microbiol, 2003. **46**(2):271–3.

978  Newman, V., J.T. Fullerton, and P.O. Anderson, *Clinical advances in the management of severe nausea and vomiting during pregnancy.* J Obstet Gynecol Neonatal Nurs, 1993. **22**(6):483–90.

979  Bardicef, M. et al., *Extracellular and intracellular magnesium depletion in pregnancy and gestational diabetes.* Am J Obstet Gynecol, 1995. **172**(3):1009–13.

980  Wibell, L., M. Gebre-Medhin, and G. Lindmark, *Magnesium and zinc in diabetic pregnancy.* Acta Paediatr Scand Suppl, 1985. **74** (s320):100–6.

981 Peacock, J.M. et al., *Relationship of serum and dietary magnesium to incident hypertension: the Atherosclerosis Risk in Communities (ARIC) Study.* Ann Epidemiol, 1999. **9**(3):159–65.

982 Indumati, V.K., M.V.; Sheela, M.K., *The role of serum electrolytes in pregnancy induced hypertension.* Journal of Clinical and Diagnostic Research, 2011. **5**(1):66–9.

983 Li, S. and H. Tian, *[Oral low-dose magnesium gluconate preventing pregnancy induced hypertension].* Zhonghua Fu Chan Ke Za Zhi, 1997. **32**(10):613–15.

984 Sibai, B.M., M.A. Villar, and E. Bray, *Magnesium supplementation during pregnancy: a double-blind randomized controlled clinical trial.* Am J Obstet Gynecol, 1989. **161**(1):115–19.

985 Makrides, M. and C.A. Crowther, *Magnesium supplementation in pregnancy.* Cochrane Database Syst Rev, 2001. **4**:CD000937.

986 Altman, D. et al., *Do women with pre-eclampsia, and their babies, benefit from magnesium sulphate? The Magpie Trial: a randomised placebo-controlled trial.* Lancet, 2002. **359**(9321):1877–90.

987 Bhat, S. et al., *Hypomagnesemia as a marker for preterm labour and its association with socio economic status.* J Invest Biochem Year, 2012. **1**(1):24–30.

988 Spatling, L. and G. Spatling, *Magnesium supplementation in pregnancy. A double-blind study.* Br J Obstet Gynaecol, 1988. **95**(2):120–5.

989 Han, S., C.A. Crowther, and V. Moore, *Magnesium maintenance therapy for preventing preterm birth after threatened preterm labour.* Cochrane Database Syst Rev, 2010. 7:CD000940.

990 Yang, C.Y. et al., *Magnesium in drinking water and the risk of delivering a child of very low birth weight.* Magnes Res, 2002. **15**(3–4):207–13.

991 Himpens, E. et al., *Prevalence, type, distribution, and severity of cerebral palsy in relation to gestational age: a meta-analytic review.* Dev Med Child Neurol, 2008. **50**(5):334–40.

992 Doyle, L.W. et al., *Magnesium sulphate for women at risk of preterm birth for neuroprotection of the fetus.* Cochrane Database Syst Rev, 2009. **1**:CD004661.

993 Harrison, V., S. Fawcus, and E. Jordaan, *Magnesium supplementation and perinatal hypoxia: outcome of a parallel group randomised trial in pregnancy.* BJOG, 2007. **114**(8):994–1002.

994 Tobias, J.H. et al., *Bone mass in childhood is related to maternal diet in pregnancy.* Osteoporos Int, 2005. **16**(12):1731–41.

995 Jones, G., M.D. Riley, and T. Dwyer, *Maternal diet during pregnancy is associated with bone mineral density in children: a longitudinal study.* Eur J Clin Nutr, 2000. **54**(10):749–56.

996 Yin, J. et al., *The association between maternal diet during pregnancy and bone mass of the children at age 16.* Eur J Clin Nutr, 2010. **64**(2):131–7.

997 Dahle, L.O. et al., *The effect of oral magnesium substitution on pregnancy-induced leg cramps.* Am J Obstet Gynecol, 1995. **173**(1):175–80.

998 Nygaard, I.H. et al., *Does oral magnesium substitution relieve pregnancy-induced leg cramps?* Eur J Obstet Gynecol Reprod Biol, 2008. **141**(1):23–6.

999 Supakatisant, C. and V. Phupong, *Oral magnesium for relief in pregnancy-induced leg cramps: a randomised controlled trial.* Matern Child Nutr, 2012. doi: 10.1111/j.1740-8709.2012.00440.x.

1000 **Koebnick, C. et al.**, *Long-term effect of a plant-based diet on magnesium status during pregnancy*. Eur J Clin Nutr, 2005. **59**(2):219–25.

1001 **Skajaa, K., I. Dorup, and B.M. Sandstrom,** *Magnesium intake and status and pregnancy outcome in a Danish population*. Br J Obstet Gynaecol, 1991. **98**(9):919–28.

1002 **Greer, F.R. et al.**, *Increasing serum calcium and magnesium concentrations in breast-fed infants: Longitudinal studies of minerals in human milk and in sera of nursing mothers and their infants*. J Pediatr, 1982. **100**(1):59–64.

1003 **Feeley, R.M. et al.**, *Calcium, phosphorus, and magnesium contents of human milk during early lactation*. J Pediatr Gastroenterol Nutr, 1983. **2**(2):262–7.

1004 **Dorea, J.G.**, *Magnesium in human milk*. J Am Coll Nutr, 2000. **19**(2):210–9.

1005 **Lipsman, S., K.G. Dewey, and B. Lonnerdal,** *Breast-feeding among teenage mothers: milk composition, infant growth, and maternal dietary intake*. J Pediatr Gastroenterol Nutr, 1985. **4**(3):426–34.

1006 **Ong, C.N., A.C. Grandjean, and R.P. Heaney,** *The mineral composition of water and its contribution to calcium and magnesium intake*, in J.B. Cotruvo and J. Bartram, eds., *Calcium and Magnesium in Drinking Water: Public Health Significance*. 2009, Geneva: World Health Organization:. p. 38–58.

1007 **Sabatier, M. et al.**, *Meal effect on magnesium bioavailability from mineral water in healthy women*. Am J Clin Nutr, 2002. **75**(1):65–71.

1008 **Hunt, S.M. and F.A. Schofield,** *Magnesium balance and protein intake level in adult human female*. Am J Clin Nutr, 1969. **22**(3):367–73.

1009 **Schwartz, R. et al.**, *Metabolic responses of adolescent boys to two levels of dietary magnesium and protein. I. Magnesium and nitrogen retention*. Am J Clin Nutr, 1973. **26**(5):510–8.

1010 **Mahalko, J.R. et al.**, *Effect of a moderate increase in dietary protein on the retention and excretion of Ca, Cu, Fe, Mg, P, and Zn by adult males*. Am J Clin Nutr, 1983. **37**(1):8–14.

1011 **Ashe, J.R., F.A. Schofield, and M.R. Gram,** *The retention of calcium, iron, phosphorus, and magnesium during pregnancy: the adequacy of prenatal diets with and without supplementation*. Am J Clin Nutr, 1979. **32**(2):286–91.

1012 **Yu, A.S.L.**, *Disorders of magnesium and phosphorus*, in **L. Goldman and D. Ausellio,** eds., *Cecil Medicine*. 2008, Philadelphia: Saunders Elsevier.

1013 American Pregnancy Association, *Magnesium*. <http://www.americanpregnancy.org/pregnancyhealth/magnesium.html> accessed 11 Jan 2013.

1014 The Antenatal Magnesium Sulphate for Neuroprotection Guideline Development Panel, *Antenatal Magnesium Sulphate Prior to Preterm Birth for Neuroprotection of the Fetus, Infant, and Child: National Clinical Practice Guidelines*. 2010, Adelaide: The University of Adelaide.

1015 **Magee, L. et al.**, *SOGC Clinical Practice Guideline. Magnesium sulphate for fetal neuroprotection*. J Obstet Gynaecol Can, 2011. **33**(5):516–29.

1016 **Peebles, D.M and A. P. Kenyon,** *Magnesium Sulphate to Prevent Cerebral Palsy Following Preterm Birth. Scientific Impact Paper No. 29*. 2011, <http://www.rcog.org.uk/files/rcog-corp/uploaded-files/SIP_No_29.pdf>.

1017 Institute of Medicine, Food and Nutrition Board, *Dietary Reference Intakes for Water, Potassium, Sodium, Chloride, and Sulfate*. 2005, Washington, DC: The National Academies Press.

1018 Khaw, K.T. and E. Barrett-Connor, *The association between blood pressure, age, and dietary sodium and potassium: a population study.* Circulation, 1988. **77**(1):53–61.

1019 Chatterjee, R. et al., *Potassium and risk of type 2 diabetes.* Expert Rev Endocrinol Metab, 2011. **6**(5):665–72.

1020 Lemann, J., Jr., J.R. Litzow, and E.J. Lennon, *The effects of chronic acid loads in normal man: further evidence for the participation of bone mineral in the defense against chronic metabolic acidosis.* J Clin Invest, 1966. **45**(10):1608–14.

1021 Forsum, E., A. Sadurskis, and J. Wager, *Resting metabolic rate and body composition of healthy Swedish women during pregnancy.* Am J Clin Nutr, 1988. **47**(6):942–7.

1022 Matsunami, K., A. Imai, and T. Tamaya, *Hypokalemia in a pregnant woman with long-term heavy cola consumption.* Int J Gynaecol Obstet, 1994. **44**(3):283–4.

1023 Appel, C.C. and T.D. Myles, *Caffeine-induced hypokalemic paralysis in pregnancy.* Obstet Gynecol, 2001. **97**(5 Pt 2):805–7.

1024 Yaguchi, M. and H. Yaguchi, *Hypokalemic myopathy due to excessive consumption of cola.* Intern Med, 2010. **49**(16):1833.

1025 Ukaonu, C., D.A. Hill, and F. Christensen, *Hypokalemic myopathy in pregnancy caused by clay ingestion.* Obstet Gynecol, 2003. **102**(5 Pt 2):1169–71.

1026 Morris, C.D. et al., *Nutrient intake and hypertensive disorders of pregnancy: evidence from a large prospective cohort.* Am J Obstet Gynecol, 2001. **184**(4):643–51.

1027 Kohrle, J. and R. Gartner, *Selenium and thyroid.* Best Pract Res Clin Endocrinol Metab, 2009. **23**(6):815–27.

1028 Arthur, J.R., R.C. McKenzie, and G.J. Beckett, *Selenium in the immune system.* J Nutr, 2003. **133**(5 Suppl 1):1457S–9S.

1029 Beck, M.A., O.A. Levander, and J. Handy, *Selenium deficiency and viral infection.* J Nutr, 2003. **133**(5 Suppl 1):1463S–7S.

1030 Mayo Medical Laboratories, Mayo Clinic, *Test ID: SEUR, selenium, random, urine. Test catalog.* <http://www.mayomedicallaboratories.com/test-catalog/Clinical+and+interpretive/60077> accessed 6 June 2013.

1031 Ashton, K. et al., *Methods of assessment of selenium status in humans: a systematic review.* Am J Clin Nutr, 2009. **89**(6):2025S–39S.

1032 Scott, R. et al., *The effect of oral selenium supplementation on human sperm motility.* Br J Urol, 1998. **82**(1):76–80.

1033 Safarinejad, M.R. and S. Safarinejad, *Efficacy of selenium and/or N-acetyl-cysteine for improving semen parameters in infertile men: a double-blind, placebo controlled, randomized study.* J Urol, 2009. **181**(2):741–51.

1034 Koller, L.D. and J.H. Exon, *The two faces of selenium-deficiency and toxicity—are similar in animals and man.* Can J Vet Res, 1986. **50**(3):297–306.

1035 Barrington, J.W. et al., *Selenium deficiency and miscarriage: a possible link?* Br J Obstet Gynaecol, 1996. **103**(2):130–2.

1036 Zachara, B.A. et al., *Blood selenium and glutathione peroxidases in miscarriage.* BJOG, 2001. **108**(3):244–7.

1037 Al-Kunani, A.S. et al., *The selenium status of women with a history of recurrent miscarriage.* BJOG, 2001. **108**(10):1094–7.

1038 Dobrzynski, W. et al., *Decreased selenium concentration in maternal and cord blood in preterm compared with term delivery.* Analyst, 1998. **123**(1):93–7.

1039 Iranpour, R. et al., *Comparison of maternal and umbilical cord blood selenium levels in term and preterm infants.* Zhongguo Dang Dai Er Ke Za Zhi, 2009. **11**(7):513–16.

1040 Buhimschi, I.A. et al., *Beneficial impact of term labor: nonenzymatic antioxidant reserve in the human fetus.* Am J Obstet Gynecol, 2003. **189**(1):181–8.

1041 Kupka, R. et al., *Selenium status, pregnancy outcomes, and mother-to-child transmission of HIV-1.* J Acquir Immune Defic Syndr, 2005. **39**(2):203–10.

1042 Baeten, J.M. et al., *Selenium deficiency is associated with shedding of HIV-1—infected cells in the female genital tract.* J Acquir Immune Defic Syndr, 2001. **26**(4):360–4.

1043 Campa, A. et al., *Mortality risk in selenium-deficient HIV-positive children.* J Acquir Immune Defic Syndr Hum Retrovirol, 1999. **20**(5):508–13.

1044 Kupka, R. et al., *Randomized, double-blind, placebo-controlled trial of selenium supplements among HIV-infected pregnant women in Tanzania: effects on maternal and child outcomes.* Am J Clin Nutr, 2008. **87**(6):1802–8.

1045 Siegfried, N. et al., *Micronutrient supplementation in pregnant women with HIV infection.* Cochrane Database Syst Rev, 2012. 3:CD009755.

1046 Mannan, S. and M.F. Picciano, *Influence of maternal selenium status on human milk selenium concentration and glutathione peroxidase activity.* Am J Clin Nutr, 1987. **46**(1):95–100.

1047 Levander, O.A., P.B. Moser, and V.C. Morris, *Dietary selenium intake and selenium concentrations of plasma, erythrocytes, and breast milk in pregnant and postpartum lactating and nonlactating women.* Am J Clin Nutr, 1987. **46**(4):694–8.

1048 Bates, C.J., *Selenium*, in B. Caballero, L. Allen, and A. Prentice, eds., *Encyclopedia of Human Nutrition.* 2005, Amsterdam: Elsevier Ltd.

1049 Goldhaber, S.B., *Trace element risk assessment: essentiality vs. toxicity.* Regul Toxicol Pharmacol, 2003. **38**(2):232–42.

1050 Stranges, S. et al., *Effects of long-term selenium supplementation on the incidence of type 2 diabetes: a randomized trial.* Ann Intern Med, 2007. **147**(4):217–23.

1051 Hellman, N.E. and J.D. Gitlin, *Ceruloplasmin metabolism and function.* Annu Rev Nutr, 2002. 22:439–58.

1052 Uauy, R., M. Olivares, and M. Gonzalez, *Essentiality of copper in humans.* Am J Clin Nutr, 1998. **67**(5 Suppl):952S–9S.

1053 Gillespie, J.M., *Keratin structure and changes with copper deficiency.* Australas J Dermatol, 1973. **14**(3):127–31.

1054 Gandhi, R. et al., *Menkes kinky hair syndrome: a rare neurodegenerative disease.* Case Rep Radiol, 2012. **2012**:684309.

1055 Milne, D.B., *Copper intake and assessment of copper status.* Am J Clin Nutr, 1998. **67** (5 Suppl):1041S–5S.

1056 Klevay, L.M., *Is the Western diet adequate in copper?* J Trace Elem Med Biol, 2011. **25**(4):204–12.

1057 Danks, D.M., *Copper deficiency in humans.* Annu Rev Nutr, 1988. 8:235–57.

1058 Failla, M.L. and R.G. Hopkins, *Is low copper status immunosuppressive?* Nutr Rev, 1998. **56**(1 Pt 2):S59–64.

1059 Uriu-Adams, J.Y. et al., *Influence of copper on early development: prenatal and postnatal considerations.* Biofactors, 2010. **36**(2):136–52.

1060 al-Rashid, R.A. and J. Spangler, *Neonatal copper deficiency.* N Engl J Med, 1971. **285**(15):841–3.

1061 Sutton, A.M. et al., *Copper deficiency in the preterm infant of very low birthweight. Four cases and a reference range for plasma copper.* Arch Dis Child, 1985. **60**(7):644–51.

1062 Seely, J.R., G.B. Humphrey, and B.J. Matter, *Copper deficiency in a premature infant fed on iron-fortified formula.* N Engl J Med, 1972. **286**(2):109–10.

1063 Committee on Copper in Drinking Water, National Research Council, *Copper in Drinking Water.* 2000, Washington, DC: The National Academies Press.

1064 Fitzgerald, D.J., *Safety guidelines for copper in water.* Am J Clin Nutr, 1998. **67**(5 Suppl):1098S–1102S.

1065 Australian National Health and Medical Research Council and the New Zealand Ministry of Health, *Nutrient reference values for Australia and New Zealand: copper.* <http://www.nrv.gov.au/nutrients/copper.htm> accessed 28 April 2013.

1066 Prasad, A.S., *Impact of the discovery of human zinc deficiency on health.* J Am Coll Nutr, 2009. **28**(3):257–65.

1067 O'Dell, B.L., *Role of zinc in plasma membrane function.* J Nutr, 2000. **130**(5S Suppl):1432S–6S.

1068 de Benoist, B. et al., *Conclusions of the Joint WHO/UNICEF/IAEA/IZiNCG Interagency Meeting on Zinc Status Indicators.* Food Nutr Bull, 2007. **28**(3 Suppl):S480–4.

1069 Hess, S.Y. et al., *Use of serum zinc concentration as an indicator of population zinc status.* Food Nutr Bull, 2007. **28**(3 Suppl):S403–29.

1070 Wessells, K.R. and K.H. Brown, *Estimating the global prevalence of zinc deficiency: results based on zinc availability in national food supplies and the prevalence of stunting.* PLoS ONE, 2012. **7**(11):e50568.

1071 Sandstrom, B. et al., *Effect of protein level and protein source on zinc absorption in humans.* J Nutr, 1989. **119**(1):48–53.

1072 Fredlund, K. et al., *Absorption of zinc and retention of calcium: dose-dependent inhibition by phytate.* J Trace Elem Med Biol, 2006. **20**(1):49–57.

1073 Wang, K. et al., *A novel member of a zinc transporter family is defective in acrodermatitis enteropathica.* Am J Hum Genet, 2002. **71**(1):66–73.

1074 MacDonald, R.S., *The role of zinc in growth and cell proliferation.* J Nutr, 2000. **130**(5S Suppl):1500S–8S.

1075 Shay, N.F. and H.F. Mangian, *Neurobiology of zinc-influenced eating behavior.* J Nutr, 2000. **130**(5S Suppl):1493S–9S.

1076 Ninh, N.X. et al., *Zinc supplementation increases growth and circulating insulin-like growth factor I (IGF-I) in growth-retarded Vietnamese children.* Am J Clin Nutr, 1996. **63**(4):514–19.

1077 Walravens, P.A., K.M. Hambidge, and D.M. Koepfer, *Zinc supplementation in infants with a nutritional pattern of failure to thrive: a double-blind, controlled study.* Pediatrics, 1989. **83**(4):532–8.

1078 Heinig, M.J. et al., *Zinc supplementation does not affect growth, morbidity, or motor development of US term breastfed infants at 4–10 mo of age.* Am J Clin Nutr, 2006. **84**(3):594–601.

1079 Mossad, S.B. et al., *Zinc gluconate lozenges for treating the common cold. A randomized, double-blind, placebo-controlled study.* Ann Intern Med, 1996. **125**(2):81–8.

1080 Yakoob, M.Y. et al., *Preventive zinc supplementation in developing countries: impact on mortality and morbidity due to diarrhea, pneumonia and malaria.* BMC Public Health, 2011. **11** (Suppl 3):S23.

1081 Sandstead, H.H., C.J. Frederickson, and J.G. Penland, *History of zinc as related to brain function.* J Nutr, 2000. **130**(2S Suppl):496S–502S.

1082 Sandstead, H.H. et al., *Zinc deficiency in pregnant rhesus monkeys: effects on behavior of infants.* Am J Clin Nutr, 1978. **31**(5):844–9.

1083 Bhatnagar, S. and S. Taneja, *Zinc and cognitive development.* Br J Nutr, 2001. **85** (Suppl 2):S139–45.

1084 Tamura, T. et al., *Effect of zinc supplementation of pregnant women on the mental and psychomotor development of their children at 5 y of age.* Am J Clin Nutr, 2003. **77**(6):1512–16.

1085 Swanson, C.A. and J.C. King, *Zinc and pregnancy outcome.* Am J Clin Nutr, 1987. **46**(5):763–71.

1086 Coyle, P., C. Cowley, and A. Rofe, *Zinc in pregnancy,* in L. Rink, ed., *Zinc in Human Health.* 2011, Amsterdam: IOS Press, pp. 305–24.

1087 Beer, W.H. et al., *Human placental transfer of zinc: normal characteristics and role of ethanol.* Alcohol Clin Exp Res, 1992. **16**(1):98–105.

1088 Fung, E.B. et al., *Zinc absorption in women during pregnancy and lactation: a longitudinal study.* Am J Clin Nutr, 1997. **66**(1):80–8.

1089 Sian, L. et al., *Zinc homeostasis during lactation in a population with a low zinc intake.* Am J Clin Nutr, 2002. **75**(1):99–103.

1090 Jameson, S., *Zinc status in pregnancy: the effect of zinc therapy on perinatal mortality, prematurity, and placental ablation.* Ann N Y Acad Sci, 1993. **678**:178–92.

1091 Hurley, L.S., *Teratogenic aspects of manganese, zinc, and copper nutrition.* Physiol Rev, 1981. **61**(2):249–95.

1092 Hanna, L.A. et al., *Zinc influences the in vitro development of peri-implantation mouse embryos.* Birth Defects Res A Clin Mol Teratol, 2003. **67**(6):414–20.

1093 Caulfield, L.E. et al., *Maternal zinc supplementation does not affect size at birth or pregnancy duration in Peru.* J Nutr, 1999. **129**(8):1563–8.

1094 Osendarp, S.J. et al., *A randomized, placebo-controlled trial of the effect of zinc supplementation during pregnancy on pregnancy outcome in Bangladeshi urban poor.* Am J Clin Nutr, 2000. **71**(1):114–19.

1095 Hafeez, A., G. Mehmood, and F. Mazhar, *Oral zinc supplementation in pregnant women and its effect on birth weight: a randomised controlled trial.* Arch Dis Child Fetal Neonatal Ed, 2005. **90**(2):F170–1.

1096 Saaka, M., J. Oosthuizen, and S. Beatty, *Effect of prenatal zinc supplementation on birthweight.* J Health Popul Nutr, 2009. **27**(5):619–31.

1097 Mahomed, K., Z. Bhutta, and P. Middleton, *Zinc supplementation for improving pregnancy and infant outcome.* Cochrane Database Syst Rev, 2007. **2**:CD000230.

1098 Mori, R. et al., *Zinc supplementation for improving pregnancy and infant outcome.* Cochrane Database Syst Rev, 2012. **7**:CD000230.

1099 Giles, E. and L.W. Doyle, *Zinc in extremely low-birthweight or very preterm infants.* NeoReviews, 2007. **8**(4):e165–e172.

1100 Fawzi, W.W. et al., *Trial of zinc supplements in relation to pregnancy outcomes, hematologic indicators, and T cell counts among HIV-1-infected women in Tanzania.* Am J Clin Nutr, 2005. **81**(1):161–7.

1101 Brown, K.H. et al., *Preventive zinc supplementation among infants, preschoolers, and older prepubertal children.* Food Nutr Bull, 2009. **30**(1 Suppl):S12–40.

1102 Hess, S.Y. and J.C. King, *Effects of maternal zinc supplementation on pregnancy and lactation outcomes.* Food Nutr Bull, 2009. **30**(1 Suppl):S60–78.

1103 Krebs, N.F. et al., *Zinc supplementation during lactation: effects on maternal status and milk zinc concentrations.* Am J Clin Nutr, 1995. **61**(5):1030–6.

1104 Walravens, P.A. et al., *Zinc supplements in breastfed infants.* Lancet, 1992. **340**(8821):683–5.

1105 Krebs, N.F. et al., *Comparison of complementary feeding strategies to meet zinc requirements of older breastfed infants.* Am J Clin Nutr, 2012. **96**(1):30–5.

1106 Heinen, F. et al., *Zinc deficiency in an exclusively breast-fed preterm infant.* Eur J Pediatr, 1995. **154**(1):71–5.

1107 Stevens, J. and L. Lubitz, *Symptomatic zinc deficiency in breast-fed term and premature infants.* J Paediatr Child Health, 1998. **34**(1):97–100.

1108 Chowanadisai, W., B. Lonnerdal, and S.L. Kelleher, *Identification of a mutation in SLC30A2 (ZnT-2) in women with low milk zinc concentration that results in transient neonatal zinc deficiency.* J Biol Chem, 2006. **281**(51):39699–707.

1109 Ackland, M.L. and A. Michalczyk, *Zinc deficiency and its inherited disorders -a review.* Genes Nutr, 2006. **1**(1):41–9.

1110 Brown, K.H. et al., *Zinc fortification of cereal flours: current recommendations and research needs.* Food Nutr Bull, 2010. **31**(1 Suppl):S62–74.

1111 O'Brien, K.O. et al., *Prenatal iron supplements impair zinc absorption in pregnant Peruvian women.* J Nutr, 2000. **130**(9):2251–5.

1112 Wood, R.J. and J.J. Zheng, *High dietary calcium intakes reduce zinc absorption and balance in humans.* Am J Clin Nutr, 1997. **65**(6):1803–9.

1113 King, J.C., *Determinants of maternal zinc status during pregnancy.* Am J Clin Nutr, 2000. **71**(5 Suppl):1334S–43S.

1114 Sandstrom, B., *Micronutrient interactions: effects on absorption and bioavailability.* Br J Nutr, 2001. **85** (Suppl 2):S181–5.

1115 Freeland-Graves, J.H. et al., *Effect of zinc supplementation on plasma high-density lipoprotein cholesterol and zinc.* Am J Clin Nutr, 1982. **35**(5):988–92.

1116 Expert Group on Vitamins and Minerals, *Risk Assessment: Zinc.* 2003, <http://multimedia.food.gov.uk/multimedia/pdfs/evm_zinc.pdf>.

1117 Saunders, A.V., W.J. Craig, and S.K. Baines, *Zinc and vegetarian diets.* MJA Open, 2012. **1**(Suppl 2):17–21.

1118 Bergheim, I. et al., *Nutritional deficiencies in German middle-class male alcohol consumers: relation to dietary intake and severity of liver disease.* Eur J Clin Nutr, 2003. **57**(3):431–8.

1119 Khan, W.U. and D.W. Sellen *Zinc supplementation in the management of diarrhoea. Biological, behavioural and contextual rationale,* in e-Library of Evidence for Nutrition Actions (eLENA) [online library]. 2011, <http://www.who.int/elena/titles/bbc/zinc_diarrhoea/en/>.

1120 Milne, D.B., R.L. Sims, and N.V. Ralston, *Manganese content of the cellular components of blood.* Clin Chem, 1990. **36**(3):450–2.

1121 Freeland-Graves, J.H. and P.H. Lin, *Plasma uptake of manganese as affected by oral loads of manganese, calcium, milk, phosphorus, copper, and zinc.* J Am Coll Nutr, 1991. **10**(1):38–43.

1122 Greger, J.L., *Dietary standards for manganese: overlap between nutritional and toxicological studies.* J Nutr, 1998. **128**(2 Suppl):368S–371S.

1123  Lutz, T.A., A. Schroff, and E. Scharrer, *Effects of calcium and sugars on intestinal manganese absorption.* Biol Trace Elem Res, 1993. **39**(2–3):221–7.

1124  Finley, J.W., P.E. Johnson, and L.K. Johnson, *Sex affects manganese absorption and retention by humans from a diet adequate in manganese.* Am J Clin Nutr, 1994. **60**(6):949–55.

1125  Friedman, B.J. et al., *Manganese balance and clinical observations in young men fed a manganese-deficient diet.* J Nutr, 1987. **117**(1):133–43.

1126  Strause, L.G. et al., *Effects of long-term dietary manganese and copper deficiency on rat skeleton.* J Nutr, 1986. **116**(1):135–41.

1127  Bolze, M.S. et al., *Influence of manganese on growth, somatomedin and glycosaminoglycan metabolism.* J Nutr, 1985. **115**(3):352–8.

1128  Clegg, M.S. et al., *The influence of manganese deficiency on serum IGF-1 and IGF binding proteins in the male rat.* Proc Soc Exp Biol Med, 1998. **219**(1):41–7.

1129  Takser, L. et al., *Manganese levels during pregnancy and at birth: relation to environmental factors and smoking in a Southwest Quebec population.* Environ Res, 2004. **95**(2):119–25.

1130  Davis, C.D. and J.L. Greger, *Longitudinal changes of manganese-dependent superoxide dismutase and other indexes of manganese and iron status in women.* Am J Clin Nutr, 1992. **55**(3):747–52.

1131  Thomson, A.B., D. Olatunbosun, and L.S. Valverg, *Interrelation of intestinal transport system for manganese and iron.* J Lab Clin Med, 1971. **78**(4):642–55.

1132  Tholin, K. et al., *Changes in blood manganese levels during pregnancy in iron supplemented and non supplemented women.* J Trace Elem Med Biol, 1995. **9**(1):13–17.

1133  Spencer, A., *Whole blood manganese levels in pregnancy and the neonate.* Nutrition, 1999. **15**(10):731–4.

1134  Fitsanakis, V.A. et al., *Manganese (Mn) and iron (Fe): interdependency of transport and regulation.* Neurotox Res, 2010. **18**(2):124–31.

1135  Garcia, S.J. et al., *Iron deficient and manganese supplemented diets alter metals and transporters in the developing rat brain.* Toxicol Sci, 2007. **95**(1):205–14.

1136  Dorner, K. et al., *Longitudinal manganese and copper balances in young infants and preterm infants fed on breast-milk and adapted cow's milk formulas.* Br J Nutr, 1989. **61**(3):559–72.

1137  Claus Henn, B. et al., *Early postnatal blood manganese levels and children's neurodevelopment.* Epidemiology, 2010. **21**(4):433–9.

1138  Williams, M. et al., *Toxicological Profile for Manganese. Agency for Toxic Substances and Disease Registry Toxicological Profiles.* 2012, Atlanta: Agency for Toxic Substances and Disease Registry.

1139  Freeland-Graves, J.H. et al., *Metabolic balance of manganese in young men consuming diets containing five levels of dietary manganese.* J Nutr, 1988. **118**(6):764–73.

1140  Cotzias, G.C. et al., *Manganese and catecholamines.* Adv Neurol, 1974. **5**:235–43.

1141  Lustig, S., S.D. Pitlik, and J.B. Rosenfeld, *Liver damage in acute self-induced hypermanganemia.* Arch Intern Med, 1982. **142**(2):405–6.

1142  Yoon, M. et al., *Physiologically based pharmacokinetic modeling of fetal and neonatal manganese exposure in humans: describing manganese homeostasis during development.* Toxicol Sci, 2011. **122**(2):297–316.

1143  Aschner, J.L. and M. Aschner, *Nutritional aspects of manganese homeostasis.* Mol Aspects Med, 2005. **26**(4–5):353–62.

1144  Erikson, K.M. et al., *Manganese neurotoxicity: a focus on the neonate.* Pharmacol Ther, 2007. **113**(2):369–77.

1145  Australian National Health and Medical Research Council and the New Zealand Ministry of Health, *Nutrient reference values for Australia and New Zealand: manganese.* <http://www.nrv.gov.au/nutrients/manganese.htm> accessed 12 May 2013.

1146  World Health Organization, *Manganese in drinking water—background document of WHO guidelines for drinking-water quality.* 2011, World Health Organization: Geneva. <http://www.who.int/water_sanitation_health/dwq/chemicals/manganese.pdf >.

1147  European Food Safety Authority, *Manganese ascorbate, manganese aspartate, manganese bisglycinate and manganese pidolate as sources of manganese added for nutritional purposes to food supplements.* EFSA Journal, 2009. **1114**:1–23.

1148  de Vrese, M. and J. Schrezenmeir, *Probiotics, prebiotics, and synbiotics.* Adv Biochem Eng Biotechnol, 2008. **111**:1–66.

1149  Conroy, M.E., H.N. Shi, and W.A. Walker, *The long-term health effects of neonatal microbial flora.* Curr Opin Allergy Clin Immunol, 2009. **9**(3):197–201.

1150  Adlerberth, I. and A.E. Wold, *Establishment of the gut microbiota in Western infants.* Acta Paediatr, 2009. **98**(2):229–38.

1151  Bode, L., *Human milk oligosaccharides: prebiotics and beyond.* Nutr Rev, 2009. **67** (Suppl 2):S183–91.

1152  Koninkx, J.F. and J.J. Malago, *The protective potency of probiotic bacteria and their microbial products against enteric infections-review.* Folia Microbiol (Praha), 2008. **53**(3):189–94.

1153  Costalos, C. et al., *The effect of a prebiotic supplemented formula on growth and stool microbiology of term infants.* Early Hum Dev, 2008. **84**(1):45–9.

1154  Strachan, D.P., *Hay fever, hygiene, and household size.* BMJ, 1989. **299**(6710): 1259–60.

1155  Lundell, A.C. et al., *Infant B cell memory differentiation and early gut bacterial colonization.* J Immunol, 2012. **188**(9):4315–22.

1156  Kalliomaki, M. and E. Isolauri, *Pandemic of atopic diseases—a lack of microbial exposure in early infancy?* Curr Drug Targets Infect Disord, 2002. **2**(3):193–9.

1157  Sanz, Y., *Gut microbiota and probiotics in maternal and infant health.* Am J Clin Nutr, 2011. **94**(6 Suppl):2000S–2005S.

1158  Kalliomaki, M. et al., *Probiotics in primary prevention of atopic disease: a randomised placebo-controlled trial.* Lancet, 2001. **357**(9262):1076–9.

1159  West, C.E. et al. *Probiotics during weaning reduce the incidence of eczema.* Pediatr Allergy Immunol, 2009. **20**(5):430–7.

1160  Chorell, E. et al., *Impact of probiotic feeding during weaning on the serum lipid profile and plasma metabolome in infants.* Br J Nutr, 2013. **110**(1):116–26.

1161  Kondo, S. et al., *Antiobesity effects of Bifidobacterium breve strain B-3 supplementation in a mouse model with high-fat diet-induced obesity.* Biosci Biotechnol Biochem, 2010. **74**(8):1656–61.

1162  Ma, X., J. Hua, and Z. Li, *Probiotics improve high fat diet-induced hepatic steatosis and insulin resistance by increasing hepatic NKT cells.* J Hepatol, 2008. **49**(5):821–30.

1163 Esteve, E., W. Ricart, and J.M. Fernandez-Real, *Gut microbiota interactions with obesity, insulin resistance and type 2 diabetes: did gut microbiote co-evolve with insulin resistance?* Curr Opin Clin Nutr Metab Care, 2011. **14**(5):483–90.

1164 Laitinen, K., T. Poussa, and E. Isolauri, *Probiotics and dietary counselling contribute to glucose regulation during and after pregnancy: a randomised controlled trial.* Br J Nutr, 2009. **101**(11):1679–87.

1165 Luoto, R. et al., *Impact of maternal probiotic-supplemented dietary counselling on pregnancy outcome and prenatal and postnatal growth: a double-blind, placebo-controlled study.* Br J Nutr, 2010. **103**(12):1792–9.

1166 Ilmonen, J. et al., *Impact of dietary counselling and probiotic intervention on maternal anthropometric measurements during and after pregnancy: a randomized placebo-controlled trial.* Clin Nutr, 2011. **30**(2):156–64.

1167 Asemi, Z. et al., *Effect of daily consumption of probiotic yoghurt on insulin resistance in pregnant women: a randomized controlled trial.* Eur J Clin Nutr, 2013. **67**(1), 71–4.

1168 Herring, S.J. et al., *Optimizing weight gain in pregnancy to prevent obesity in women and children.* Diabetes Obes Metab, 2011. **14**(3), 195–203.

1169 Hanson, M.A. and K.M. Godfrey, *Commentary: maternal constraint is a pre-eminent regulator of fetal growth.* Int J Epidemiol, 2008. **37**(2):252–4.

1170 Ounsted, M., A. Scott, and C. Ounsted, *Transmission through the female line of a mechanism constraining human fetal growth.* Int J Epidemiol, 2008. **37**(2):245–50.

1171 Rey, H. et al., *Annex: Maternal anthropometry: its predictive value for pregnancy outcome.* Bull World Health Organ, 1995. (73 Suppl):70–1.

1172 Thame, M. et al., *Body composition in pregnancies of adolescents and mature women and the relationship to birth anthropometry.* Eur J Clin Nutr, 2007. **61**(1):47–53.

1173 Mardones-Santander, F. et al., *Maternal body composition near term and birth weight.* Obstet Gynecol, 1998. **91**(6):873–7.

1174 Sebire, N.J. et al., *Maternal obesity and pregnancy outcome: a study of 287,213 pregnancies in London.* Int J Obes Relat Metab Disord, 2001. **25**(8):1175–82.

1175 Khashan, A.S. and L.C. Kenny, *The effects of maternal body mass index on pregnancy outcome.* Eur J Epidemiol, 2009. **24**(11):697–705.

1176 Liu, Y. et al., *Prepregnancy body mass index and gestational weight gain with the outcome of pregnancy: a 13-year study of 292,568 cases in China.* Arch Gynecol Obstet, 2012. **286**(4):905–11.

1177 Morton, S.B., *Maternal nutrition and fetal growth and development*, in **P.D. Gluckman and M.A. Hanson, eds.**, *Developmental Origins of Health and Disease.* 2006, Cambridge: Cambridge University Press, pp. 98–129.

1178 Yeasmin, S.F. and K. Regmi, *A qualitative study on the food habits and related beliefs of pregnant british bangladeshis.* Health Care Women Int, 2013. **34**(5):395–415.

1179 Kim, S.Y. et al., *Trends in pre-pregnancy obesity in nine states, 1993–2003.* Obesity (Silver Spring), 2007. **15**(4):986–93.

1180 Chu, S.Y., S.Y. Kim, and C.L. Bish, *Prepregnancy obesity prevalence in the United States, 2004–2005.* Matern Child Health J, 2009. **13**(5):614–20.

1181 Hauger, M.S. et al., *Prepregnancy weight status and the risk of adverse pregnancy outcome.* Acta Obstet Gynecol Scand, 2008. **87**(9):953–9.

1182 Neggers, Y.H. et al., *Maternal prepregnancy body mass index and psychomotor development in children.* Acta Obstet Gynecol Scand, 2003. **82**(3):235–40.

1183 Salihu, H.M. et al., *Low pre-pregnancy body mass index and risk of medically indicated versus spontaneous preterm singleton birth.* Eur J Obstet Gynecol Reprod Biol, 2009. **144**(2):119–23.

1184 Thangaratinam, S. et al., *Interventions to reduce or prevent obesity in pregnant women: a systematic review.* Health Technol Assess, 2012. **16**(31):iii–iv, 1–191.

1185 Kjellstrom, T., C. Hakansta, and C. Hogstedt, *Globalisation and public health-overview and a Swedish perspective.* Scand J Public Health Suppl, 2007. **70**:2–68.

1186 Hawkes, C., *Uneven dietary development: linking the policies and processes of globalization with the nutrition transition, obesity and diet-related chronic diseases.* Global Health, 2006. **2**(1):4.

1187 Reardon, T. et al., *The rise of supermarkets in Africa, Asia, and Latin America.* Am J Agric Econ, 2003. **85**(5):1140–6.

1188 Heslehurst, N. et al., *A nationally representative study of maternal obesity in England, UK: trends in incidence and demographic inequalities in 619 323 births, 1989–2007.* Int J Obes (Lond), 2010. **34**(3):420–8.

1189 Poston, L., *Developmental programming and diabetes—the human experience and insight from animal models.* Best Pract Res Clin Endocrinol Metab, 2010. **24**(4):541–52.

1190 Baeten, J.M., E.A. Bukusi, and M. Lambe, *Pregnancy complications and outcomes among overweight and obese nulliparous women.* Am J Public Health, 2001. **91**(3):436–40.

1191 O'Brien, T.E., J.G. Ray, and W.S. Chan, *Maternal body mass index and the risk of preeclampsia: a systematic overview.* Epidemiology, 2003. **14**(3):368–74.

1192 Lynch, A.M. et al., *Prepregnancy obesity and complement system activation in early pregnancy and the subsequent development of preeclampsia.* Am J Obstet Gynecol, 2012. **206**(5):428.e1–8.

1193 Walsh, S.W., *Obesity: a risk factor for preeclampsia.* Trends Endocrinol Metab, 2007. **18**(10):365–70.

1194 Knight, M., *Antenatal pulmonary embolism: risk factors, management and outcomes.* BJOG, 2008. **115**(4):453–61.

1195 Larsen, T.B. et al., *Maternal smoking, obesity, and risk of venous thromboembolism during pregnancy and the puerperium: a population-based nested case-control study.* Thromb Res, 2007. **120**(4):505–9.

1196 Usha Kiran, T.S. et al., *Outcome of pregnancy in a woman with an increased body mass index.* BJOG, 2005. **112**(6):768–72.

1197 Chu, S.Y. et al., *Maternal obesity and risk of cesarean delivery: a meta-analysis.* Obes Rev, 2007. **8**(5):385–94.

1198 Poobalan, A.S. et al., *Weight loss interventions in young people (18 to 25 year olds): a systematic review.* Obes Rev, 2010. **11**(8):580–92.

1199 Zhang, J. et al., *Poor uterine contractility in obese women.* BJOG, 2007. **114**(3):343–8.

1200 Chu, S.Y. et al., *Maternal obesity and risk of stillbirth: a metaanalysis.* Am J Obstet Gynecol, 2007. **197**(3):223–8.

1201 Torloni, M.R. et al., *Prepregnancy BMI and the risk of gestational diabetes: a systematic review of the literature with meta-analysis.* Obes Rev, 2009. **10**(2):194–203.

1202 Smith, G.C. et al., *Maternal obesity in early pregnancy and risk of spontaneous and elective preterm deliveries: a retrospective cohort study.* Am J Public Health, 2007. **97**(1):157–62.

1203 Chu, S.Y. et al., *Maternal obesity and risk of gestational diabetes mellitus*. Diabetes Care, 2007. **30**(8):2070–6.

1204 Nohr, E.A. et al., *Combined associations of prepregnancy body mass index and gestational weight gain with the outcome of pregnancy*. Am J Clin Nutr, 2008. **87**(6):1750–9.

1205 Yu, C.K., T.G. Teoh, and S. Robinson, *Obesity in pregnancy*. BJOG, 2006. **113**(10):1117–25.

1206 Tanvig, M. et al., *Pregestational body mass index is related to neonatal abdominal circumference at birth—a Danish population-based study*. BJOG, 2013. **120**(3), 320–30.

1207 Gluckman, P.D. et al., *Epigenetic mechanisms that underpin metabolic and cardiovascular diseases*. Nat Rev Endocrinol, 2009. **5**(7):401–8.

1208 Hinkle, S.N. et al., *Associations between maternal prepregnancy body mass index and child neurodevelopment at 2 years of age*. Int J Obes (Lond), 2012. **36**(10):1312–19.

1209 Basatemur, E. et al., *Maternal prepregnancy BMI and child cognition: a longitudinal cohort study*. Pediatrics, 2013. **131**(1), 56–63.

1210 Armitage, J.A., P.D. Taylor, and L. Poston, *Experimental models of developmental programming: consequences of exposure to an energy rich diet during development*. J Physiol, 2005. **565**(Pt 1):3–8.

1211 Martinez, J.A. et al., *Interplay of early-life nutritional programming on obesity, inflammation and epigenetic outcomes*. Proc Nutr Soc, 2012. **71**(2):276–83.

1212 Lillycrop, K.A., *Effect of maternal diet on the epigenome: implications for human metabolic disease*. Proc Nutr Soc, 2011. **70**(1):64–72.

1213 Desai, M. and M.G. Ross, *Fetal programming of adipose tissue: effects of intrauterine growth restriction and maternal obesity/high-fat diet*. Semin Reprod Med, 2011. **29**(3):237–45.

1214 Dietz, P.M., W.M. Callaghan, and A.J. Sharma, *High pregnancy weight gain and risk of excessive fetal growth*. Am J Obstet Gynecol, 2009. **201**(1):51.e1–6.

1215 Beyerlein, A., N. Lack, and R. von Kries, *Within-population average ranges compared with Institute of Medicine recommendations for gestational weight gain*. Obstet Gynecol, 2010. **116**(5):1111–18.

1216 Rae, A. et al., *A randomised controlled trial of dietary energy restriction in the management of obese women with gestational diabetes*. Aust N Z J Obstet Gynaecol, 2000. **40**(4):416–22.

1217 Wolff, S. et al., *A randomized trial of the effects of dietary counseling on gestational weight gain and glucose metabolism in obese pregnant women*. Int J Obes (Lond), 2008. **32**(3):495–501.

1218 Thangaratinam, S. et al., *Effects of interventions in pregnancy on maternal weight and obstetric outcomes: meta-analysis of randomised evidence*. BMJ, 2012. **344**:e2088.

1219 Oken, E. et al., *Maternal gestational weight gain and offspring weight in adolescence*. Obstet Gynecol, 2008. **112**(5):999–1006.

1220 Poston, L., L.F. Harthoorn, and E.M. van der Beek, *Obesity in pregnancy: implications for the mother and lifelong health of the child. A consensus statement*. Pediatr Res, 2011. **69**(2):175–80.

1221 Ludwig, D.S., H.L. Rouse, and J. Currie, *Pregnancy weight gain and childhood body weight: a within-family comparison*. PLoS Med, 2013. **10**(10):e1001521.

1222 Margerison-Zilko, C.E. et al., *Trimester of maternal gestational weight gain and offspring body weight at birth and age five*. Matern Child Health J, 2012. **16**(6):1215–23.

1223 Hinkle, S.N. et al., *Excess gestational weight gain is associated with child adiposity among mothers with normal and overweight prepregnancy weight status.* J Nutr, 2012. **142**(10):1851–8.

1224 von Kries, R. et al., *Late pregnancy reversal from excessive gestational weight gain lowers risk of childhood overweight—a cohort study.* Obesity (Silver Spring), 2013. **21**(6):1232–7

1225 Nehring, I., S. Lehmann, and R. von Kries, *Gestational weight gain in accordance to the IOM/NRC criteria and the risk for childhood overweight: a meta-analysis.* Pediatr Obes, 2013. **8**(3), 218–24.

1226 Yaktine, A.L. and K.M. Rasmussen, eds. *Weight Gain during Pregnancy: Reexamining the Guidelines.* 2009, Washington, DC: Institute of Medicine.

1227 Rosso, P., *A new chart to monitor weight gain during pregnancy.* Am J Clin Nutr, 1985. **41**(3):644–52.

1228 Mardones, F. and P. Rosso, *A weight gain chart for pregnant women designed in Chile.* Matern Child Nutr, 2005. **1**(2):77–90.

1229 Borberg, C. et al., *Obesity in pregnancy: the effect of dietary advice.* Diabetes Care, 1980. **3**(3):476–81.

1230 Phelan, S. et al., *Randomized trial of a behavioral intervention to prevent excessive gestational weight gain: the Fit for Delivery Study.* Am J Clin Nutr, 2011. **93**(4):772–9.

1231 Vinter, C.A. et al., *The LiP (Lifestyle in Pregnancy) study: a randomized controlled trial of lifestyle intervention in 360 obese pregnant women.* Diabetes Care, 2011. **34**(12):2502–7.

1232 Tsukamoto, H. et al., *Restricting weight gain during pregnancy in Japan: a controversial factor in reducing perinatal complications.* Eur J Obstet Gynecol Reprod Biol, 2007. **133**(1):53–9.

1233 Gluckman, P.D. et al., *Low birthweight and subsequent obesity in Japan.* Lancet, 2007. **369**(9567):1081–2.

1234 Genest, D.S. et al., *Impact of exercise training on preeclampsia: potential preventive mechanisms.* Hypertension, 2012. **60**(5):1104–9.

1235 Bergmann, A., M. Zygmunt, and J.F. Clapp, 3rd, *Running throughout pregnancy: effect on placental villous vascular volume and cell proliferation.* Placenta, 2004. **25**(8–9):694–8.

1236 Clapp, J.F., 3rd et al., *Beginning regular exercise in early pregnancy: effect on fetoplacental growth.* Am J Obstet Gynecol, 2000. **183**(6):1484–8.

1237 Jackson, M.R. et al., *The effects of maternal aerobic exercise on human placental development: placental volumetric composition and surface areas.* Placenta, 1995. **16**(2):179–91.

1238 Weissgerber, T.L., G.A. Davies, and J.M. Roberts, *Modification of angiogenic factors by regular and acute exercise during pregnancy.* J Appl Physiol, 2010. **108**(5):1217–23.

1239 Maynard, S.E. et al., *Excess placental soluble fms-like tyrosine kinase 1 (sFlt1) may contribute to endothelial dysfunction, hypertension, and proteinuria in preeclampsia.* J Clin Invest, 2003. **111**(5):649–58.

1240 FAO, *Fact sheet Pakistan: women in agriculture, environment and rural production.* <http://www.fao.org/sd/WPdirect/WPre0111.htm> accessed 1 July 2014.

1241 Rao, S. et al., *Maternal activity in relation to birth size in rural India. The Pune Maternal Nutrition Study.* Eur J Clin Nutr, 2003. **57**(4):531–42.

1242  Imdad, A. and Z.A. Bhutta, *Nutritional management of the low birth weight/preterm infant in community settings: a perspective from the developing world.* J Pediatr, 2013. **162**(3):S107–14.

1243  Gjestland, K. et al., *Do pregnant women follow exercise guidelines? Prevalence data among 3482 women, and prediction of low-back pain, pelvic girdle pain and depression.* Br J Sports Med, 2013. **47**(8):515–20.

1244  American Congress of Obstetricians and Gynecologists, *ACOG Committee opinion. Number 267, January 2002: exercise during pregnancy and the postpartum period.* Obstet Gynecol, 2002. **99**(1):171–3.

1245  Price, B.B., S.B. Amini, and K. Kappeler, *Exercise in pregnancy: effect on fitness and obstetric outcomes-a randomized trial.* Med Sci Sports Exerc, 2012. **44**(12):2263–9.

1246  Mottola, M.F. et al., *Nutrition and exercise prevent excess weight gain in overweight pregnant women.* Med Sci Sports Exerc, 2010. **42**(2):265–72.

1247  Davenport, M.H. et al., *A walking intervention improves capillary glucose control in women with gestational diabetes mellitus: a pilot study.* Appl Physiol Nutr Metab, 2008. **33**(3):511–7.

1248  Artal, R. et al., *A lifestyle intervention of weight-gain restriction: diet and exercise in obese women with gestational diabetes mellitus.* Appl Physiol Nutr Metab, 2007. **32**(3):596–601.

1249  Mudd, L.M. et al., *Health benefits of physical activity during pregnancy: an international perspective.* Med Sci Sports Exerc, 2013. **45**(2):268–77.

1250  McIntyre, H.D. et al., *Pilot study of an individualised early postpartum intervention to increase physical activity in women with previous gestational diabetes.* Int J Endocrinol, 2012. **2012**:892019.

1251  Oostdam, N. et al., *Cost-effectiveness of an exercise program during pregnancy to prevent gestational diabetes: results of an economic evaluation alongside a randomised controlled trial.* BMC Pregnancy Childbirth, 2012. **12**:64.

1252  Magnus P. et al., *Recreational physical activity and the risk of preeclampsia: a prospective cohort of Norwegian women.* Am J Epidemiol, 2008. **168**(8):952–7.

1253  Saftlas, A.F. et al., *Work, leisure-time physical activity, and risk of preeclampsia and gestational hypertension.* Am J Epidemiol, 2004. **160**(8):758–65.

1254  Sorensen, T.K. et al., *Recreational physical activity during pregnancy and risk of preeclampsia.* Hypertension, 2003. **41**(6):1273–80.

1255  Fortner, R.T. et al., *Physical activity and hypertensive disorders of pregnancy among Hispanic women.* Med Sci Sports Exerc, 2011. **43**(4):639–46.

1256  Vollebregt, K.C. et al., *Does physical activity in leisure time early in pregnancy reduce the incidence of preeclampsia or gestational hypertension?* Acta Obstet Gynecol Scand, 2010. **89**(2):261–7.

1257  Rudra, C.B. et al., *A prospective analysis of recreational physical activity and preeclampsia risk.* Med Sci Sports Exerc, 2008. **40**(9):1581–8.

1258  Tyldum, E.V., P.R. Romundstad, and S.A. Slordahl, *Pre-pregnancy physical activity and preeclampsia risk: a prospective population-based cohort study.* Acta Obstet Gynecol Scand, 2010. **89**(3):315–20.

1259  Han, S., P. Middleton, and C.A. Crowther, *Exercise for pregnant women for preventing gestational diabetes mellitus.* Cochrane Database Syst Rev, 2012. **7**:CD009021.

1260  Takito, M.Y. and M.H. Benicio, *Physical activity during pregnancy and fetal outcomes: a case-control study.* Rev Saude Publica, 2010. **44**(1):90–101.

1261 Domingues, M.R., A.J. Barros, and A. Matijasevich, *Leisure time physical activity during pregnancy and preterm birth in Brazil.* Int J Gynaecol Obstet, 2008. **103**(1):9–15.

1262 Guendelman, S. et al., *Association between preterm delivery and pre-pregnancy body mass (BMI), exercise and sleep during pregnancy among working women in southern California.* Matern Child Health J, 2013.**17**(4):723–31.

1263 Owe, K.M. et al., *Exercise during pregnancy and the gestational age distribution: a cohort study.* Med Sci Sports Exerc, 2012. **44**(6):1067–74.

1264 Jukic, A.M. et al., *A prospective study of the association between vigorous physical activity during pregnancy and length of gestation and birthweight.* Matern Child Health J, 2012. **16**(5):1031–44.

1265 van den Hove, D.L. et al., *Maternal stress-induced reduction in birth weight as a marker for adult affective state.* Front Biosci (Elite Ed), 2010. **2**:43–6.

1266 Blair, M.M. et al., *Prenatal maternal anxiety and early childhood temperament.* Stress, 2011. **14**(6):644–51.

1267 Diego, M.A. et al., *Maternal psychological distress, prenatal cortisol, and fetal weight.* Psychosom Med, 2006. **68**(5):747–53.

1268 Buss, C. et al., *Maternal pregnancy-specific anxiety is associated with child executive function at 6–9 years age.* Stress, 2011. **14**(6):665–76.

1269 Grizenko, N. et al., *Maternal stress during pregnancy, ADHD symptomatology in children and genotype: gene–environment interaction.* J Can Acad Child Adolesc Psychiatry, 2012. **21**(1):9–15.

1270 Rakhshani, A. et al., *The effects of yoga in prevention of pregnancy complications in high-risk pregnancies: a randomized controlled trial.* Prev Med, 2012. **55**(4):333–40.

1271 Babbar, S., A.C. Parks-Savage, and S.P. Chauhan, *Yoga during pregnancy: a review.* Am J Perinatol, 2012. **29**(6):459–64.

1272 Curtis, K., A. Weinrib, and J. Katz, *Systematic review of yoga for pregnant women: current status and future directions.* Evid Based Complement Alternat Med, 2012. **2012**:715942.

1273 Clapp, J.F., 3rd, *Exercise during pregnancy. A clinical update.* Clin Sports Med, 2000. **19**(2):273–86.

1274 McMurray, R.G. et al., *Recent advances in understanding maternal and fetal responses to exercise.* Med Sci Sports Exerc, 1993. **25**(12):1305–21.

1275 Gustafson, K.M. et al., *Fetal cardiac autonomic control during breathing and non-breathing epochs: the effect of maternal exercise.* Early Hum Dev, 2012. **88**(7):539–46.

1276 May, L.E. et al., *Aerobic exercise during pregnancy influences fetal cardiac autonomic control of heart rate and heart rate variability.* Early Hum Dev, 2010. **86**(4):213–17.

1277 May, L.E. et al., *Regular maternal exercise dose and fetal heart outcome.* Med Sci Sports Exerc, 2012. **44**(7):1252–8.

1278 Siebel, A.L., A.L. Carey, and B.A. Kingwell, *Can exercise training rescue the adverse cardiometabolic effects of low birth weight and prematurity?* Clin Exp Pharmacol Physiol, 2012. **39**(11):944–57.

1279 Juhl, M. et al., *Physical exercise during pregnancy and fetal growth measures: a study within the Danish National Birth Cohort.* Am J Obstet Gynecol, 2010. **202**(1): p. 63.e1–8.

1280 Leiferman, J.A. and K.R. Evenson, *The effect of regular leisure physical activity on birth outcomes.* Matern Child Health J, 2003. **7**(1):59–64.

1281 Clapp, J.F., 3rd, *Morphometric and neurodevelopmental outcome at age five years of the offspring of women who continued to exercise regularly throughout pregnancy.* J Pediatr, 1996. **129**(6):856–63.

1282 Juhl, M. et al., *Is swimming during pregnancy a safe exercise?* Epidemiology, 2010. **21**(2):253–8.

1283 Nieuwenhuijsen, M.J. et al., *Chlorination disinfection byproducts in water and their association with adverse reproductive outcomes: a review.* Occup Environ Med, 2000. **57**(2):73–85.

1284 Chu, H. and M.J. Nieuwenhuijsen, *Distribution and determinants of trihalomethane concentrations in indoor swimming pools.* Occup Environ Med, 2002. **59**(4):243–7.

1285 Clapp, J.F., 3rd and E.L. Capeless, *Neonatal morphometrics after endurance exercise during pregnancy.* Am J Obstet Gynecol, 1990. **163**(6 Pt 1):1805–11.

1286 Clapp, J.F., 3rd and S. Dickstein, *Endurance exercise and pregnancy outcome.* Med Sci Sports Exerc, 1984. **16**(6):556–62.

1287 Dwarkanath, P. et al., *The relationship between maternal physical activity during pregnancy and birth weight.* Asia Pac J Clin Nutr, 2007. **16**(4):704–10.

1288 Haakstad, L.A. and K. Bo, *Exercise in pregnant women and birth weight: a randomized controlled trial.* BMC Pregnancy Childbirth, 2011. **11**:66.

1289 Hopkins, S.A. et al., *Exercise training in pregnancy reduces offspring size without changes in maternal insulin sensitivity.* J Clin Endocrinol Metab, 2010. **95**(5):2080–8.

1290 Wolfe, L.A. and G.A. Davies, *Canadian guidelines for exercise in pregnancy.* Clin Obstet Gynecol, 2003. **46**(2):488–95.

1291 Royal College of Obstetricians and Gynaecologists, *RCOG Statement No. 4: exercise in pregnancy.* 2006, <http://www.rcog.org.uk/womens-health/clinical-guidance/exercise-pregnancy>.

1292 Shaheen, S.O. et al., *Dietary patterns in pregnancy and respiratory and atopic outcomes in childhood.* Thorax, 2009. **64**(5):411–17.

1293 Hourihane, J.O. et al., *The impact of government advice to pregnant mothers regarding peanut avoidance on the prevalence of peanut allergy in United Kingdom children at school entry.* J Allergy Clin Immunol, 2007. **119**(5):1197–202.

1294 Kramer, M.S. and R. Kakuma, *Maternal dietary antigen avoidance during pregnancy or lactation, or both, for preventing or treating atopic disease in the child.* Cochrane Database Syst Rev, 2012. **9**:CD000133.

1295 Maslova, E. et al., *Peanut and tree nut consumption during pregnancy and allergic disease in children-should mothers decrease their intake? Longitudinal evidence from the Danish National Birth Cohort.* J Allergy Clin Immunol, 2012. **130**(3):724–32.

1296 Frazier, A.L. et al., *Prospective study of peripregnancy consumption of peanuts or tree nuts by mothers and the risk of peanut or tree nut allergy in their offspring.* JAMA Pediatr, 2014. **168**(2):156–62.

1297 Selevan, S.G., C.A. Kimmel, and P. Mendola, *Identifying critical windows of exposure for children's health.* Environ Health Perspect, 2000. **108** (Suppl 3):451–5.

1298 Shenefelt, R.E., *Morphogenesis of malformations in hamsters caused by retinoic acid: relation to dose and stage at treatment.* Teratology, 1972. **5**(1):103–18.

1299 Graham, H.N., *Green tea composition, consumption, and polyphenol chemistry.* Prev Med, 1992. **21**(3):334–50.

1300 Geronikaki, A.A. and A.M. Gavalas, *Antioxidants and inflammatory disease: synthetic and natural antioxidants with anti-inflammatory activity.* Comb Chem High Throughput Screen, 2006. **9**(6):425–42.

1301 Sridharan, S., N. Archer, and N. Manning, *Premature constriction of the fetal ductus arteriosus following the maternal consumption of camomile herbal tea.* Ultrasound Obstet Gynecol, 2009. **34**(3):358–9.

1302 Roulet, M. et al., *Hepatic veno-occlusive disease in newborn infant of a woman drinking herbal tea.* J Pediatr, 1988. **112**(3):433–6.

1303 Rasenack, R. et al., *Veno-occlusive disease in a fetus caused by pyrrolizidine alkaloids of food origin.* Fetal Diagn Ther, 2003. **18**(4):223–5.

1304 Edgar, J.A., E. Roeder, and R.J. Molyneux, *Honey from plants containing pyrrolizidine alkaloids: a potential threat to health.* J Agric Food Chem, 2002. **50**(10):2719–30.

1305 Rietjens, I.M. et al., *Molecular mechanisms of toxicity of important food-borne phyto-toxins.* Mol Nutr Food Res, 2005. **49**(2):131–58.

1306 Yu, M.C. and J.M. Yuan, *Environmental factors and risk for hepatocellular carcinoma.* Gastroenterology, 2004. **127**(5 Suppl 1):S72–8.

1307 Asim, M. et al., *Role of aflatoxin B$_1$ as a risk for primary liver cancer in north Indian population.* Clin Biochem, 2011. **44**(14–5):1235–40.

1308 Liu, Y. et al., *Population attributable risk of aflatoxin-related liver cancer: systematic review and meta-analysis.* Eur J Cancer, 2012. **48**(14):2125–36.

1309 Denning, D.W. et al., *Transplacental transfer of aflatoxin in humans.* Carcinogenesis, 1990. **11**(6):1033–5.

1310 Turner, P.C. et al., *Aflatoxin exposure in utero causes growth faltering in Gambian infants.* Int J Epidemiol, 2007. **36**(5):1119–25.

1311 Dewailly, E. et al., *Inuit exposure to organochlorines through the aquatic food chain in Arctic Quebec.* Environ Health Perspect, 1993. **101**(7):618–20.

1312 Dallaire, R. et al., *Exposure to organochlorines and mercury through fish and marine mammal consumption: associations with growth and duration of gestation among Inuit newborns.* Environ Int, 2013. **54**:85–91.

1313 Grandjean, P. et al., *Neurobehavioral deficits associated with PCB in 7-year-old children prenatally exposed to seafood neurotoxicants.* Neurotoxicol Teratol, 2001. **23**(4):305–17.

1314 Harada, M., *Congenital Minamata disease: intrauterine methylmercury poisoning.* Teratology, 1978. **18**(2):285–8.

1315 Amin-Zaki, L. et al., *Intra-uterine methylmercury poisoning in Iraq.* Pediatrics, 1974. **54**(5):587–95.

1316 Strain, J.J. et al., *Associations of maternal long-chain polyunsaturated fatty acids, methyl mercury, and infant development in the Seychelles Child Development Nutrition Study.* Neurotoxicology, 2008. **29**(5):776–82.

1317 Davidson, P.W. et al., *Prenatal methyl mercury exposure from fish consumption and child development: a review of evidence and perspectives from the Seychelles Child Development Study.* Neurotoxicology, 2006. **27**(6):1106–9.

1318 Sabahi, F. et al., *Qualitative and quantitative analysis of T lymphocytes during normal human pregnancy.* Am J Reprod Immunol, 1995. **33**(5):381–93.

1319 Weinberg, E.D., *Pregnancy-associated immune suppression: risks and mechanisms.* Microb Pathog, 1987. **3**(6):393–7.

1320  Bortolussi, R., *Listeriosis: a primer.* CMAJ, 2008. **179**(8):795–7.

1321  Lopez, A. et al., *Preventing congenital toxoplasmosis.* MMWR Recomm Rep, 2000. **49**(RR-2):59–68.

1322  Dubey, J.P. et al., *High prevalence and genotypes of* Toxoplasma gondii *isolated from organic pigs in northern USA.* Vet Parasitol, 2012. **188**(1–2):14–18.

1323  Jones, J.L. and J.P. Dubey, *Foodborne toxoplasmosis.* Clin Infect Dis, 2012. **55**(6): 845–51.

1324  Athearn, P.N. et al., *Awareness and acceptance of current food safety recommendations during pregnancy.* Matern Child Health J, 2004. **8**(3):149–62.

1325  Tam, C., A. Erebara, and A. Einarson, *Food-borne illnesses during pregnancy: prevention and treatment.* Can Fam Physician, 2010. **56**(4):341–3.

1326  Frary, C.D., R.K. Johnson, and M.Q. Wang, *Food sources and intakes of caffeine in the diets of persons in the United States.* J Am Diet Assoc, 2005. **105**(1):110–13.

1327  Eteng, M.U. et al., *Caffeine and theobromine levels in selected Nigerian beverages.* Plant Foods Hum Nutr, 1999. **54**(4):337–44.

1328  Aden, U., *Methylxanthines during pregnancy and early postnatal life.* Handb Exp Pharmacol, 2011. **200**:373–89.

1329  Kirkinen, P. et al., *The effect of caffeine on placental and fetal blood flow in human pregnancy.* Am J Obstet Gynecol, 1983. **147**(8):939–42.

1330  Klebanoff, M.A. et al., *Maternal serum caffeine metabolites and small-for-gestational age birth.* Am J Epidemiol, 2002. **155**(1):32–7.

1331  Vlajinac, H.D. et al., *Effect of caffeine intake during pregnancy on birth weight.* Am J Epidemiol, 1997. **145**(4):335–8.

1332  Bracken, M.B. et al., *Association of maternal caffeine consumption with decrements in fetal growth.* Am J Epidemiol, 2003. **157**(5):456–66.

1333  Group, C.S., *Maternal caffeine intake during pregnancy and risk of fetal growth restriction: a large prospective observational study.* BMJ, 2008. **337**:a2332.

1334  Klebanoff, M.A. et al., *Maternal serum paraxanthine, a caffeine metabolite, and the risk of spontaneous abortion.* N Engl J Med, 1999. **341**(22):1639–44.

1335  Cnattingius, S. et al., *Caffeine intake and the risk of first-trimester spontaneous abortion.* N Engl J Med, 2000. **343**(25):1839–45.

1336  Wisborg, K. et al., *Maternal consumption of coffee during pregnancy and stillbirth and infant death in first year of life: prospective study.* BMJ, 2003. **326**:420.

1337  Barr, H.M. and A.P. Streissguth, *Caffeine use during pregnancy and child outcome: a 7-year prospective study.* Neurotoxicol Teratol, 1991. **13**(4):441–8.

1338  Miles, L. and R. Foxen, *New guidelines on caffeine in pregnancy.* Nutr Bulletin, 2009. **34**(2):203–6.

1339  Santos, I.S., A. Matijasevich, and M.R. Domingues, *Maternal caffeine consumption and infant nighttime waking: prospective cohort study.* Pediatrics, 2012. **129**(5):860–8.

1340  Lane, J.D. et al., *Menstrual cycle effects on caffeine elimination in the human female.* Eur J Clin Pharmacol, 1992. **43**(5):543–6.

1341  Jensen, T.K. et al., *Caffeine intake and fecundability: a follow-up study among 430 Danish couples planning their first pregnancy.* Reprod Toxicol, 1998. **12**(3):289–95.

1342  Brent, R.L., M.S. Christian, and R.M. Diener, *Evaluation of the reproductive and developmental risks of caffeine.* Birth Defects Res B Dev Reprod Toxicol, 2011. **92**(2):152–87.

1343 American Congress of Obstetricians and Gynecologists (ACOG), *Committee Opinion No. 575: exposure to toxic environmental agents.* Fertil Steril, 2013. **100**(4):931–4.

1344 Dissanayake, V. and T.B. Erickson, *Ball and chain: the global burden of lead poisoning.* Clin Toxicol (Phila), 2012. **50**(6):528–31.

1345 Gardella, C., *Lead exposure in pregnancy: a review of the literature and argument for routine prenatal screening.* Obstet Gynecol Surv, 2001. **56**(4):231–8.

1346 Li, Y. et al., *Monitoring of lead load and its effect on neonatal behavioral neurological assessment scores in Guiyu, an electronic waste recycling town in China.* J Environ Monit, 2008. **10**(10):1233–8.

1347 Emory, E. et al., *Maternal blood lead effects on infant intelligence at age 7 months.* Am J Obstet Gynecol, 2003. **188**(4):S26–32.

1348 Canfield, R.L. et al., *Intellectual impairment in children with blood lead concentrations below 10 microg per deciliter.* N Engl J Med, 2003. **348**(16):1517–26.

1349 Hertz-Picciotto, I. et al., *Patterns and determinants of blood lead during pregnancy.* Am J Epidemiol, 2000. **152**(9):829–37.

1350 Johnson, M.A., *High calcium intake blunts pregnancy-induced increases in maternal blood lead.* Nutr Rev, 2001. **59**(5):152–6.

1351 Ettinger, A.S. et al., *Effect of calcium supplementation on blood lead levels in pregnancy: a randomized placebo-controlled trial.* Environ Health Perspect, 2009. **117**(1):26–31.

1352 Ettinger, A.S., H. Hu, and M. Hernandez-Avila, *Dietary calcium supplementation to lower blood lead levels in pregnancy and lactation.* J Nutr Biochem, 2007. **18**(3):172–8.

1353 Ettinger, A.S. et al., *Influence of maternal bone lead burden and calcium intake on levels of lead in breast milk over the course of lactation.* Am J Epidemiol, 2006. **163**(1):48–56.

1354 Gulson, B.L. et al., *Blood lead changes during pregnancy and postpartum with calcium supplementation.* Environ Health Perspect, 2004. **112**(15):1499–507.

1355 Simon, J.A. and E.S. Hudes, *Relationship of ascorbic acid to blood lead levels.* JAMA, 1999. **281**(24):2289–93.

1356 Lee, D.H. et al., *Graded associations of blood lead and urinary cadmium concentrations with oxidative-stress-related markers in the U.S. population: results from the third National Health and Nutrition Examination Survey.* Environ Health Perspect, 2006. **114**(3):350–4.

1357 CDC, *Lead: pregnant women.* <http://www.cdc.gov/nceh/lead/tips/pregnant.htm> accessed 7 May 2013.

1358 Weidner, I.S. et al., *Cryptorchidism and hypospadias in sons of gardeners and farmers.* Environ Health Perspect, 1998. **106**(12):793–6.

1359 Kristensen, P. et al., *Birth defects among offspring of Norwegian farmers, 1967–1991.* Epidemiology, 1997. **8**(5):537–44.

1360 Andersen, H.R. et al., *Impaired reproductive development in sons of women occupationally exposed to pesticides during pregnancy.* Environ Health Perspect, 2008. **116**(4):566–72.

1361 Nilsson, E.E. et al., *Transgenerational epigenetic effects of the endocrine disruptor vinclozolin on pregnancies and female adult onset disease.* Reproduction, 2008. **135**(5):713–21.

1362 Eskenazi, B. et al., *In utero exposure to dichlorodiphenyltrichloroethane (DDT) and dichlorodiphenyldichloroethylene (DDE) and neurodevelopment among young Mexican American children.* Pediatrics, 2006. **118**(1):233–41.

1363 **Ribas-Fito, N. et al.**, *In utero exposure to background concentrations of DDT and cognitive functioning among preschoolers*. Am J Epidemiol, 2006. **164**(10):955–62.

1364 **Wohlfahrt-Veje, C. et al.**, *Lower birth weight and increased body fat at school age in children prenatally exposed to modern pesticides: a prospective study*. Environ Health, 2011. **10**(1):79.

1365 **Young, J.G. et al.**, *Association between in utero organophosphate pesticide exposure and abnormal reflexes in neonates*. Neurotoxicology, 2005. **26**(2):199–209.

1366 **Whyatt, R.M. et al.**, *Contemporary-use pesticides in personal air samples during pregnancy and blood samples at delivery among urban minority mothers and newborns*. Environ Health Perspect, 2003. **111**(5):749–56.

1367 US Environmental Protection Agency, *Basic information about atrazine in drinking water. Water: basic information about regulated drinking water contaminants*. <http://www.epa.gov/tri/> accessed 31 May 2013.

1368 European Commission, Health & Consumer Protection Directorate-General, *Review report for the active substance atrazine*. 2003, <http://ec.europa.eu/food/plant/protection/evaluation/existactive/list_atrazine.pdf>.

1369 **Mattix, K.D., P.D. Winchester, and L.R. Scherer**, *Incidence of abdominal wall defects is related to surface water atrazine and nitrate levels*. J Pediatr Surg, 2007. **42**(6):947–9.

1370 **Waller, S.A. et al.**, *Agricultural-related chemical exposures, season of conception, and risk of gastroschisis in Washington State*. Am J Obstet Gynecol, 2010. **202**(3):241.e1–6.

1371 **Agopian, A.J. et al.**, *Maternal residential atrazine exposure and gastroschisis by maternal age*. Matern Child Health J, 2013. **17**(10), 1768–75.

1372 **Munger, R. et al.**, *Intrauterine growth retardation in Iowa communities with herbicide-contaminated drinking water supplies*. Environ Health Perspect, 1997. **105**(3):308–14.

1373 **Savitz, D.A. et al.**, *Male pesticide exposure and pregnancy outcome*. Am J Epidemiol, 1997. **146**(12):1025–36.

1374 **Arbuckle, T.E., Z. Lin, and L.S. Mery**, *An exploratory analysis of the effect of pesticide exposure on the risk of spontaneous abortion in an Ontario farm population*. Environ Health Perspect, 2001. **109**(8):851–7.

1375 **Castro, D.J. et al.**, *Lymphoma and lung cancer in offspring born to pregnant mice dosed with dibenzo[a,l]pyrene: the importance of in utero vs. lactational exposure*. Toxicol Appl Pharmacol, 2008. **233**(3):454–8.

1376 **Bocskay, K.A. et al.**, *Chromosomal aberrations in cord blood are associated with prenatal exposure to carcinogenic polycyclic aromatic hydrocarbons*. Cancer Epidemiol Biomarkers Prev, 2005. **14**(2):506–11.

1377 **Sanyal, M.K. et al.**, *Augmentation of polynuclear aromatic hydrocarbon metabolism of human placental tissues of first-trimester pregnancy by cigarette smoke exposure*. Am J Obstet Gynecol, 1993. **168**(5):1587–97.

1378 Agency for Toxic Substances and Disease Registry, *Toxicological profile for polycyclic aromatic hydrocarbons*. 1995, <http://www.atsdr.cdc.gov/toxprofiles/tp.asp?id=122&tid=25>.

1379 **Choi, H. et al.**, *International studies of prenatal exposure to polycyclic aromatic hydrocarbons and fetal growth*. Environ Health Perspect, 2006. **114**(11):1744–50.

1380 **Perera, F.P. et al.**, *Effect of prenatal exposure to airborne polycyclic aromatic hydrocarbons on neurodevelopment in the first 3 years of life among inner-city children*. Environ Health Perspect, 2006. **114**(8):1287–92.

1381 **Perera, F.P. et al.**, *Prenatal airborne polycyclic aromatic hydrocarbon exposure and child IQ at age 5 years.* Pediatrics, 2009. **124**(2):e195–202.

1382 **Choi, H. et al.**, *Fetal window of vulnerability to airborne polycyclic aromatic hydrocarbons on proportional intrauterine growth restriction.* PLoS ONE, 2012. **7**(4):e35464.

1383 **Cordier, S. et al.**, *Parental exposure to polycyclic aromatic hydrocarbons and the risk of childhood brain tumors: The SEARCH International Childhood Brain Tumor Study.* Am J Epidemiol, 2004. **159**(12):1109–16.

1384 **Lupo, P.J. et al.**, *Maternal occupational exposure to polycyclic aromatic hydrocarbons: effects on gastroschisis among offspring in the National Birth Defects Prevention Study.* Environ Health Perspect, 2012. **120**(6):910–15.

1385 **vom Saal, F.S. et al.**, *A physiologically based approach to the study of bisphenol A and other estrogenic chemicals on the size of reproductive organs, daily sperm production, and behavior.* Toxicol Ind Health, 1998. **14**(1–2):239–60.

1386 **Veiga-Lopez, A. et al.**, *Developmental programming: gestational bisphenol-A treatment alters trajectory of fetal ovarian gene expression.* Endocrinology, 2013. **154**(5):1873–84.

1387 **Howdeshell, K.L. et al.**, *Exposure to bisphenol A advances puberty.* Nature, 1999. **401**(6755):763–4.

1388 **Lee, M.H. et al.**, *Enhanced interleukin-4 production in CD4 + T cells and elevated immunoglobulin E levels in antigen-primed mice by bisphenol A and nonylphenol, endocrine disruptors: involvement of nuclear factor-AT and Ca2 +.* Immunology, 2003. **109**(1):76–86.

1389 **Tian, X., M. Takamoto, and K. Sugane**, *Bisphenol A promotes IL-4 production by Th2 cells.* Int Arch Allergy Immunol, 2003. **132**(3):240–7.

1390 **Yan, H., M. Takamoto, and K. Sugane**, *Exposure to Bisphenol A prenatally or in adulthood promotes T(H)2 cytokine production associated with reduction of CD4CD25 regulatory T cells.* Environ Health Perspect, 2008. **116**(4):514–19.

1391 **Donohue, K.M. et al.**, *Prenatal and postnatal bisphenol A exposure and asthma development among inner-city children.* J Allergy Clin Immunol, 2013. **131**(3):736–42.

1392 **Schonfelder, G. et al.**, *Parent bisphenol A accumulation in the human maternal-fetal-placental unit.* Environ Health Perspect, 2002. **110**(11):A703–7.

1393 **Yamamoto, T. and A. Yasuhara**, *Quantities of bisphenol a leached from plastic waste samples.* Chemosphere, 1999. **38**(11):2569–76.

1394 **Braun, J.M. et al.**, *Prenatal bisphenol A exposure and early childhood behavior.* Environ Health Perspect, 2009. **117**(12):1945–52.

1395 Agency for Toxic Substances and Disease Registry, *Priority list of hazardous substances.* <http://www.atsdr.cdc.gov/SPL/index.html> accessed 1 July 2014.

1396 **Kozul-Horvath, C.D. et al.**, *Effects of low-dose drinking water arsenic on mouse fetal and postnatal growth and development.* PLoS ONE, 2012. **7**(5):e38249.

1397 **Nickson, R. et al.**, *Arsenic poisoning of Bangladesh groundwater.* Nature, 1998. **395**(6700):338.

1398 **Rahman, A. et al.**, *Arsenic exposure during pregnancy and size at birth: a prospective cohort study in Bangladesh.* Am J Epidemiol, 2009. **169**(3):304–12.

1399 **Ahmad, S.A. et al.**, *Arsenic in drinking water and pregnancy outcomes.* Environ Health Perspect, 2001. **109**(6):629–31.

1400 **Gilbert-Diamond, D. et al.**, *Rice consumption contributes to arsenic exposure in US women.* Proc Natl Acad Sci U S A, 2011. **108**(51):20656–60.

1401 Thompson, J. and J. Bannigan, *Cadmium: toxic effects on the reproductive system and the embryo.* Reprod Toxicol, 2008. **25**(3):304–15.

1402 Kippler, M. et al., *Maternal cadmium exposure during pregnancy and size at birth: a prospective cohort study.* Environ Health Perspect, 2012. **120**(2):284–9.

1403 Lappe, M. and N. Chalfin, *Identifying toxic risks before and during pregnancy: a decision tree and action plan. A report to the March of Dimes.* 2002, <http://www.environmentalcommons.org/cetos/articles/MoDFinalReport.pdf>.

1404 Jarup, L. and A. Akesson, *Current status of cadmium as an environmental health problem.* Toxicol Appl Pharmacol, 2009. **238**(3):201–8.

1405 Faroon, O. et al., *Toxicological profile for cadmium. Agency for Toxic Substances and Disease Registry (ATSDR) Toxicological Profiles.* 2012, Atlanta: Agency for Toxic Substances and Disease Registry.

1406 Lauder, J.M. and U.B. Schambra, *Morphogenetic roles of acetylcholine.* Environ Health Perspect, 1999. **107** (Suppl 1):65–9.

1407 O'Leary, C.M. et al., *Prenatal alcohol exposure and risk of birth defects.* Pediatrics, 2010. **126**(4):e843–50.

1408 Hutchinson, D. et al., *Alcohol use in pregnancy: prevalence and predictors in the Longitudinal Study of Australian Children.* Drug Alcohol Rev, 2013. **32**(5):475–82.

1409 O'Leary, C.M. and C. Bower, *Guidelines for pregnancy: what's an acceptable risk, and how is the evidence (finally) shaping up?* Drug Alcohol Rev, 2012. **31**(2):170–83.

1410 Australian National Health and Medical Research Council, *Australian Guidelines to Reduce Health Risks from Drinking Alcohol.* 2009, Canberra: Commonwealth of Australia.

1411 Royal College of Obstetricians and Gynaecologists, *Alcohol and pregnancy: information for you.* 2006, <http://www.rcog.org.uk/files/rcog-corp/Alcohol%20and%20Pregnancy.pdf>.

1412 Kesmodel, U.S. et al., *The effect of different alcohol drinking patterns in early to mid pregnancy on the child's intelligence, attention, and executive function.* BJOG, 2012. **119**(10):1180–90.

1413 Kelly, Y. et al., *Light drinking versus abstinence in pregnancy—behavioural and cognitive outcomes in 7-year-old children: a longitudinal cohort study.* BJOG, 2013. **120**(11):1340–7.

1414 Shea, A.K. and M. Steiner, *Cigarette smoking during pregnancy.* Nicotine Tob Res, 2008. **10**(2):267–78.

1415 Morrow, R.J., J.W. Ritchie, and S.B. Bull, *Maternal cigarette smoking: the effects on umbilical and uterine blood flow velocity.* Am J Obstet Gynecol, 1988. **159**(5):1069–71.

1416 Kramer, M.S., *Determinants of low birth weight: methodological assessment and meta-analysis.* Bull World Health Organ, 1987. **65**(5):663–737.

1417 Kallen, K., *Maternal smoking during pregnancy and infant head circumference at birth.* Early Hum Dev, 2000. **58**(3):197–204.

1418 Raatikainen, K., P. Huurinainen, and S. Heinonen, *Smoking in early gestation or through pregnancy: a decision crucial to pregnancy outcome.* Prev Med, 2007. **44**(1):59–63.

1419 Hammoud, A.O. et al., *Smoking in pregnancy revisited: findings from a large population-based study.* Am J Obstet Gynecol, 2005. **192**(6):1856–62; discussion, 1862–3.

1420 Aliyu, M.H. et al., *Prenatal smoking among adolescents and risk of fetal demise before and during labor.* J Pediatr Adolesc Gynecol, 2010. **23**(3):129–35.

1421 Mattsson, K. et al., *Maternal smoking during pregnancy and daughters' risk of gestational diabetes and obesity*. Diabetologia, 2013. **56**(8):1689–95.

1422 Suzuki, K. et al., *Differences in the effect of maternal smoking during pregnancy for childhood overweight before and after 5 years of age*. J Obstet Gynaecol Res, 2013. **39**(5):914–21.

1423 Lumley, J. et al., *Interventions for promoting smoking cessation during pregnancy*. Cochrane Database Syst Rev, 2009. 3:CD001055.

1424 Geissler, P.W. et al., *Perceptions of soil-eating and anaemia among pregnant women on the Kenyan coast*. Soc Sci Med, 1999. **48**(8):1069–79.

1425 Edwards, C.H. et al., *Pica in an urban environment*. J Nutr, 1994. **124**(6 Suppl): 954S–62S.

1426 Corbett, R.W., C. Ryan, and S.P. Weinrich, *Pica in pregnancy: does it affect pregnancy outcomes?* MCN Am J Matern Child Nurs, 2003. **28**(3):183–9; quiz, 190–1.

1427 Young, S.L., *Pica in pregnancy: new ideas about an old condition*. Annu Rev Nutr, 2010. **30**:403–22.

1428 Danford, D.E., *Pica and nutrition*. Annu Rev Nutr, 1982. **2**:303–22.

1429 Hambidge, K.M. and A. Silverman, *Pica with rapid improvement after dietary zinc supplementation*. Arch Dis Child, 1973. **48**(7):567–8.

1430 Jackson, W.C. and J.P. Martin, *Amylophagia presenting as gestational diabetes*. Arch Fam Med, 2000. **9**(7):649–52.

1431 Barton, J.R., C.A. Riely, and B.M. Sibai, *Baking powder pica mimicking preeclampsia*. Am J Obstet Gynecol, 1992. **167**(1):98–9.

1432 Luoba, A.I. et al., *Earth-eating and reinfection with intestinal helminths among pregnant and lactating women in western Kenya*. Trop Med Int Health, 2005. **10**(3): 220–7.

1433 Guinee, V.F., *Pica and lead poisoning*. Nutr Rev, 1971. **29**(12):267–9.

1434 Thihalolipavan, S., B.M. Candalla, and J. Ehrlich, *Examining pica in NYC pregnant women with elevated blood lead levels*. Matern Child Health J, 2013. **17**(1):49–55.

1435 Pearl, M. and L.M. Boxt, *Radiographic findings in congenital lead poisoning*. Radiology, 1980. **136**(1):83–4.

1436 Lakudzala, D.D. and J.J. Khonje, *Nutritive potential of some 'edible' soils in Blantyre city, Malawi*. Malawi Med J, 2011. **23**(2):38–42.

1437 Li, D.K., L. Liu, and R. Odouli, *Exposure to non-steroidal anti-inflammatory drugs during pregnancy and risk of miscarriage: population based cohort study*. BMJ, 2003. **327**(7411):368.

1438 Nakhai-Pour, H.R. et al., *Use of nonaspirin nonsteroidal anti-inflammatory drugs during pregnancy and the risk of spontaneous abortion*. CMAJ, 2011. **183**(15):1713–20.

1439 Edwards, D.R. et al., *Periconceptional over-the-counter nonsteroidal anti-inflammatory drug exposure and risk for spontaneous abortion*. Obstet Gynecol, 2012. **120**(1): 113–22.

1440 Van Marter, L.J. et al., *Persistent pulmonary hypertension of the newborn and smoking and aspirin and nonsteroidal antiinflammatory drug consumption during pregnancy*. Pediatrics, 1996. **97**(5):658–63.

1441 Alano, M.A. et al., *Analysis of nonsteroidal antiinflammatory drugs in meconium and its relation to persistent pulmonary hypertension of the newborn*. Pediatrics, 2001. **107**(3):519–23.

1442 Philips, J.B., 3rd and R.K. Lyrene, *Prostaglandins, related compounds, and the perinatal pulmonary circulation.* Clin Perinatol, 1984. **11**(3):565–79.

1443 Van Marter, L.J. et al., *Nonsteroidal antiinflammatory drugs in late pregnancy and persistent pulmonary hypertension of the newborn.* Pediatrics, 2013. **131**(1):79–87.

1444 Shaheen, S.O. et al., *Prenatal paracetamol exposure and risk of asthma and elevated immunoglobulin E in childhood.* Clin Exp Allergy, 2005. **35**(1):18–25.

1445 Shaheen, S.O. et al., *Prenatal paracetamol exposure and asthma: further evidence against confounding.* Int J Epidemiol, 2010. **39**(3):790–4.

1446 Eyers, S. et al., *Paracetamol in pregnancy and the risk of wheezing in offspring: a systematic review and meta-analysis.* Clin Exp Allergy, 2011. **41**(4):482–9.

1447 Dworski, R., *Oxidant stress in asthma.* Thorax, 2000. **55** (Suppl 2):S51–3.

1448 Fogarty, A. and G. Davey, *Paracetamol, antioxidants and asthma.* Clin Exp Allergy, 2005. **35**(6):700–2.

1449 Eneli, I. et al., *Acetaminophen and the risk of asthma: the epidemiologic and pathophysiologic evidence.* Chest, 2005. **127**(2):604–12.

1450 Etminan, M. et al., *Acetaminophen use and the risk of asthma in children and adults: a systematic review and metaanalysis.* Chest, 2009. **136**(5):1316–23.

1451 Brandlistuen, R.E. et al., *Prenatal paracetamol exposure and child neurodevelopment: a sibling-controlled cohort study.* Int J Epidemiol, 2013. **42**(6):1702–13.

1452 Kurepa, D. et al., *Elevated acetoacetate and monocyte chemotactic protein-1 levels in cord blood of infants of diabetic mothers.* Neonatology, 2012. **102**(3):163–8.

1453 Churchill, J.A. and H.W. Berendes, *Intelligence of children whose mothers had acetonuria during pregnancy, in Perinatal Factors Affecting Human Development. Proceedings of the Special Session held during the Eighth Meeting of the PAHO Advisory Committee on Medical Research.* 1969, Washington, DC: PAHO.

1454 Metzger, B.E. et al., *'Accelerated starvation' and the skipped breakfast in late normal pregnancy.* Lancet, 1982. **1**(8272):588–92.

1455 Felig, P., *Maternal and fetal fuel homeostasis in human pregnancy.* Am J Clin Nutr, 1973. **26**(9):998–1005.

1456 Rudolf, M.C. and R.S. Sherwin, *Maternal ketosis and its effects on the fetus.* Clin Endocrinol Metab, 1983. **12**(2):413–28.

1457 Dikensoy, E. et al., *Effect of fasting during Ramadan on fetal development and maternal health.* J Obstet Gynaecol Res, 2008. **34**(4):494–8.

1458 Dikensoy, E. et al., *The effect of Ramadan fasting on maternal serum lipids, cortisol levels and fetal development.* Arch Gynecol Obstet, 2009. **279**(2):119–23.

1459 Ozturk, E. et al., *Effect of Ramadan fasting on maternal oxidative stress during the second trimester: a preliminary study.* J Obstet Gynaecol Res, 2011. **37**(7):729–33.

1460 Hizli, D. et al., *Impact of maternal fasting during Ramadan on fetal Doppler parameters, maternal lipid levels and neonatal outcomes.* J Matern Fetal Neonatal Med, 2012. **25**(7):975–7.

1461 Gale, C.R. et al., *Maternal diet during pregnancy and carotid intima-media thickness in children.* Arterioscler Thromb Vasc Biol, 2006. **26**(8):1877–82.

1462 Herrick, K. et al., *Maternal consumption of a high-meat, low-carbohydrate diet in late pregnancy: relation to adult cortisol concentrations in the offspring.* J Clin Endocrinol Metab, 2003. **88**(8):3554–60.

1463 Godfrey, K.M. et al., *Epigenetic gene promoter methylation at birth is associated with child's later adiposity.* Diabetes, 2011. **60**(5):1528–34.

1464 Royal College of Obstetricians and Gynaecologists, *Chemical exposures during pregnancy: dealing with potential, but unproven, risks to child health.* 2013. <http://www.rcog.org.uk/files/rcog-corp/5.6.13ChemicalExposures.pdf>.

1465 Witorsch, R.J. and J.A. Thomas, *Personal care products and endocrine disruption: a critical review of the literature.* Crit Rev Toxicol, 2010. **40** (Suppl 3):1–30.

1466 Cosmetic Ingredient Review Expert Panel, C.I.R.E., *Annual review of cosmetic ingredient safety assessments—2002/2003.* Int J Toxicol, 2005. **24** (Suppl 1):1–102.

1467 Bozzo, P., A. Chua-Gocheco, and A. Einarson, *Safety of skin care products during pregnancy.* Can Fam Physician, 2011. **57**(6):665–7.

1468 Holly, E.A. et al., *West Coast study of childhood brain tumours and maternal use of hair-colouring products.* Paediatr Perinat Epidemiol, 2002. **16**(3):226–35.

1469 McCall, E.E., A.F. Olshan, and J.L. Daniels, *Maternal hair dye use and risk of neuroblastoma in offspring.* Cancer Causes Control, 2005. **16**(6):743–8.

1470 Chen, H.L. et al., *Interactive effects between CYP1A1 genotypes and environmental polychlorinated dibenzo-p-dioxins and dibenzofurans exposures on liver function profile.* J Toxicol Environ Health A, 2006. **69**(3–4):269–81.

1471 Hueber-Becker, F. et al., *Occupational exposure of hairdressers to [14C]-paraphenylenediamine-containing oxidative hair dyes: a mass balance study.* Food Chem Toxicol, 2007. **45**(1):160–9.

1472 Bergman, Å. et al., eds., *State of the Science of Endocrine Disrupting Chemicals 2012.* 2013, Geneva: World Health Organization.

1473 Katz, S.H., M.L. Hediger, and L.A. Valleroy, *Traditional maize processing techniques in the new world.* Science, 1974. **184**(4138):765–73.

1474 Beck, W., *Aboriginal preparation of cycas seeds in Australia.* Econ. Bot., 1992. **46**(2):133–47.

1475 Whiting, M.G., *Toxicity of cycads.* Econ. Bot., 1963. **17**(4): p. 270–302.

1476 Wilson, W. and D.L. Dufour, *Why 'bitter' cassava? Productivity of 'bitter' and 'sweet' cassava in a Tukanoan Indian settlement in the northwestern Amazon.* Econ. Bot., 2002. **56**(1):49–57.

1477 Billing, J. and P.W. Sherman, *Antimicrobial functions of spices: why some like it hot.* Q Rev Biol, 1998. **73**(1):3–49.

1478 Mukhopadhyay, S. and A. Sarkar, *Pregnancy-related food habits among women of rural Sikkim, India.* Public Health Nutr, 2009. **12**(12):2317–22.

1479 Meyer-Rochow, V.B., *Food taboos: their origins and purposes.* J Ethnobiol Ethnomed, 2009. **5**:18.

1480 Henrich, J. and N. Henrich, *The evolution of cultural adaptations: Fijian food taboos protect against dangerous marine toxins.* Proc Biol Sci, 2010. **277**(1701): 3715–24.

1481 Choudhry, U.K., *Traditional practices of women from India: pregnancy, childbirth, and newborn care.* J Obstet Gynecol Neonatal Nurs, 1997. **26**(5):533–9.

1482 *A Handbook of Korea.* 1987, Seoul: International Publishing House.

1483 Brems, S. and A. Berg, *Eating down during Pregnancy: Nutrition, Obstetric and Cultural Considerations in the Third World.* 1989, Geneva: ACC/SCN.

1484  Karim, R. et al., *Determinants of food consumption during pregnancy in rural Bangldesh: examination of evaluative data from the Bangladesh Integrated Nutrition Project. Discussion Paper No. 11.* 2002. <http://www.nutrition.tufts.edu/documents/fpan/wp11-food_consumption.pdf>.

1485  Painter, R.C., T.J. Roseboom, and O.P. Bleker, *Prenatal exposure to the Dutch famine and disease in later life: an overview.* Reprod Toxicol, 2005. **20**(3):345–52.

1486  Li, Y. et al., *Exposure to the Chinese famine in early life and the risk of hyperglycemia and type 2 diabetes in adulthood.* Diabetes, 2010. **59**(10):2400–6.

1487  Malhotra, A. et al., *Metabolic changes in Asian Muslim pregnant mothers observing the Ramadan fast in Britain.* Br J Nutr, 1989. **61**(3):663–72.

1488  Prentice, A.M. et al., *Metabolic consequences of fasting during Ramadan in pregnant and lactating women.* Hum Nutr Clin Nutr, 1983. **37**(4):283–94.

1489  Almond, D. and B. Mazumder, *Health capital and the prenatal environment: the effect of maternal fasting during pregnancy.* Am Econ J Appl Econ, 2011. **3**(4):56–85.

1490  Alwasel, S.H. et al., *Changes in placental size during Ramadan.* Placenta, 2010. **31**(7):607–10.

1491  Chee, C.Y. et al., *Confinement and other psychosocial factors in perinatal depression: a transcultural study in Singapore.* J Affect Disord, 2005. **89**(1–3):157–66.

1492  Kaewsarn, P., W. Moyle, and D. Creedy, *Traditional postpartum practices among Thai women.* J Adv Nurs, 2003. **41**(4):358–66.

1493  Kim-Godwin, Y.S., *Postpartum beliefs and practices among non-Western cultures.* MCN Am J Matern Child Nurs, 2003. **28**(2):74–8; quiz, 79–80.

1494  Chan, S.M. et al., *Special postpartum dietary practices of Hong Kong Chinese women.* Eur J Clin Nutr, 2000. **54**(10):797–802.

1495  Kartchner, R. and L. Callister, *Giving birth. Voices of Chinese women.* J Holist Nurs, 2003. **21**(2):100–16.

1496  Leung, S.K., D. Arthur, and I.M. Martinson, *Perceived stress and support of the Chinese postpartum ritual 'doing the month'.* Health Care Women Int, 2005. **26**(3):212–24.

1497  Brathwaite, A.C. and C.C. Williams, *Childbirth experiences of professional Chinese Canadian women.* J Obstet Gynecol Neonatal Nurs, 2004. **33**(6):748–55.

1498  Callister, L.C., *Doing the Month: Chinese Postpartum Practices.* Global Health and Nursing, 2006. **31**(6):390.

1499  Chu, C.M., *Postnatal experience and health needs of Chinese migrant women in Brisbane, Australia.* Ethn Health, 2005. **10**(1):33–56.

1500  Matthey, S., P. Panasetis, and B. Barnett, *Adherence to cultural practices following childbirth in migrant Chinese women and relation to postpartum mood.* Health Care Women Int, 2002. **23**(6–7):567–75.

1501  Semega-Janneh, I.J. et al., *Promoting breastfeeding in rural Gambia: combining traditional and modern knowledge.* Health Policy Plan, 2001. **16**(2):199–205.

1502  Rogers, N.L. et al., *Colostrum avoidance, prelacteal feeding and late breast-feeding initiation in rural Northern Ethiopia.* Public Health Nutr, 2011. **14**(11):2029–36.

1503  Dixon, G., *Colostrum avoidance and early infant feeding in Asian societies.* Asia Pac J Clin Nutr, 1992. **1**(4):225–9.

1504  Geckil, E., T. Sahin, and E. Ege, *Traditional postpartum practices of women and infants and the factors influencing such practices in South Eastern Turkey.* Midwifery, 2009. **25**(1):62–71.

1505  Ayaz, S. and S.Y. Efe, *Potentially harmful traditional practices during pregnancy and postpartum.* Eur J Contracept Reprod Health Care, 2008. **13**(3):282–8.

1506  Hall, H.G., D.L. Griffiths, and L.G. McKenna, *The use of complementary and alternative medicine by pregnant women: a literature review.* Midwifery, 2011. **27**(6):817–24.

1507  Dugoua, J.J., *Herbal medicines and pregnancy.* J Popul Ther Clin Pharmacol, 2010. **17**(3):e370–8.

1508  Chen, F.P. et al., *Use frequency of traditional Chinese medicine in Taiwan.* BMC Health Serv Res, 2007. **7**:26.

1509  Yeh, H.Y. et al., *Use of traditional Chinese medicine among pregnant women in Taiwan.* Int J Gynaecol Obstet, 2009. **107**(2):147–50.

1510  Chuang, C.H. et al., *Chinese herbal medicine use in Taiwan during pregnancy and the postpartum period: a population-based cohort study.* Int J Nurs Stud, 2009. **46**(6): 787–95.

1511  Vutyavanich, T., T. Kraisarin, and R. Ruangsri, *Ginger for nausea and vomiting in pregnancy: randomized, double-masked, placebo-controlled trial.* Obstet Gynecol, 2001. **97**(4):577–82.

1512  Willetts, K.E., A. Ekangaki, and J.A. Eden, *Effect of a ginger extract on pregnancy-induced nausea: a randomised controlled trial.* Aust N Z J Obstet Gynaecol, 2003. **43**(2):139–44.

1513  Keating, A. and R.A. Chez, *Ginger syrup as an antiemetic in early pregnancy.* Altern Ther Health Med, 2002. **8**(5):89–91.

1514  Tiran, D., *Ginger to reduce nausea and vomiting during pregnancy: evidence of effectiveness is not the same as proof of safety.* Complement Ther Clin Pract, 2012. **18**(1):22–5.

1515  Finnish Food Safety Authority Evira, *Warning label to be added on food supplements containing ginger as well as on ginger tea, and corresponding drink powders.* 24 Sep 2010. <http://www.evira.fi/portal/en/food> accessed 1 July 2014.

1516  Jacobsgaard, H., *[The pharmacists request that pregnant women consult physicians prior to GraviFrisk use].* Ugeskr Laeger, 2008. **170**(10):867.

1517  Born, D. and M.L. Barron, *Herb use in pregnancy: what nurses should know.* MCN Am J Matern Child Nurs, 2005. **30**(3):201–6; quiz, 207–8.

1518  Dante, G. et al., *Herb remedies during pregnancy: a systematic review of controlled clinical trials.* J Matern Fetal Neonatal Med, 2013. **26**(3):306–12.

1519  Wing, D.A. et al., *Daily cranberry juice for the prevention of asymptomatic bacteriuria in pregnancy: a randomized, controlled pilot study.* J Urol, 2008. **180**(4):1367–72.

1520  Jepson, R.G., G. Williams, and J.C. Craig, *Cranberries for preventing urinary tract infections.* Cochrane Database Syst Rev, 2012. **10**:CD001321.

1521  Freda, M.C. and E.T. Patterson, *Preterm Labor and Birth: Prevention and Nursing Management, Third Edition.* 2003, White Plains: March of Dimes.

1522  Chatterjee, S.S. et al., *Hyperforin as a possible antidepressant component of hypericum extracts.* Life Sci, 1998. **63**(6):499–510.

1523  Chatterjee, S.S. et al., *Antidepressant activity of hypericum perforatum and hyperforin: the neglected possibility.* Pharmacopsychiatry, 1998. **31** (Suppl 1):7–15.

1524  Parsons, M., M. Simpson, and T. Ponton, *Raspberry leaf and its effect on labour: safety and efficacy.* Aust Coll Midwives Inc J, 1999. **12**(3):20–5.

1525  Simpson, M. et al., *Raspberry leaf in pregnancy: its safety and efficacy in labor.* J Midwifery Womens Health, 2001. **46**(2):51–9.

1526  Holst, L., S. Haavik, and H. Nordeng, *Raspberry leaf—should it be recommended to pregnant women?* Complement Ther Clin Pract, 2009. **15**(4):204–8.

1527  Garry, D. et al., *Use of castor oil in pregnancies at term.* Altern Ther Health Med, 2000. **6**(1):77–9.

1528  Jones, T.K. and B.M. Lawson, *Profound neonatal congestive heart failure caused by maternal consumption of blue cohosh herbal medication.* J Pediatr, 1998. **132**(3 Pt 1): 550–2.

1529  Finkel, R.S. and K.M. Zarlengo, *Blue cohosh and perinatal stroke.* N Engl J Med, 2004. **351**(3):302–3.

1530  Gunn, T.R. and I.M. Wright, *The use of black and blue cohosh in labour.* N Z Med J, 1996. **109**(1032):410–11.

1531  Teixeira, J.M., N.M. Fisk, and V. Glover, *Association between maternal anxiety in pregnancy and increased uterine artery resistance index: cohort based study.* BMJ, 1999. **318**(7177):153–7.

1532  Myers, R.E., *Maternal psychological stress and fetal asphyxia: a study in the monkey.* Am J Obstet Gynecol, 1975. **122**(1):47–59.

1533  Morishima, H.O., H. Pedersen, and M. Finster, *The influence of maternal psychological stress on the fetus.* Am J Obstet Gynecol, 1978. **131**(3):286–90.

1534  Wortsman, J., *Role of epinephrine in acute stress.* Endocrinol Metab Clin North Am, 2002. **31**(1):79–106.

1535  Habib, K.E., P.W. Gold, and G.P. Chrousos, *Neuroendocrinology of stress.* Endocrinol Metab Clin North Am, 2001. **30**(3):695–728; vii–viii.

1536  Ulrich-Lai, Y.M. and J.P. Herman, *Neural regulation of endocrine and autonomic stress responses.* Nat Rev Neurosci, 2009. **10**(6):397–409.

1537  Shams, M. et al., *11Beta-hydroxysteroid dehydrogenase type 2 in human pregnancy and reduced expression in intrauterine growth restriction.* Hum Reprod, 1998. **13**(4): 799–804.

1538  Dy, J. et al., *Placental 11beta-hydroxysteroid dehydrogenase type 2 is reduced in pregnancies complicated with idiopathic intrauterine growth restriction: evidence that this is associated with an attenuated ratio of cortisone to cortisol in the umbilical artery.* Placenta, 2008. **29**(2):193–200.

1539  Phillips, D.I. et al., *Elevated plasma cortisol concentrations: a link between low birth weight and the insulin resistance syndrome?* J Clin Endocrinol Metab, 1998. **83**(3):757–60.

1540  Jones, A. et al., *Fetal growth and the adrenocortical response to psychological stress.* J Clin Endocrinol Metab, 2006. **91**(5):1868–71.

1541  Cottrell, E.C. and J.R. Seckl, *Prenatal stress, glucocorticoids and the programming of adult disease.* Front Behav Neurosci, 2009. **3**:19.

1542  Csemiczky, G., B.M. Landgren, and A. Collins, *The influence of stress and state anxiety on the outcome of IVF-treatment: psychological and endocrinological assessment of Swedish women entering IVF-treatment.* Acta Obstet Gynecol Scand, 2000. **79**(2): 113–18.

1543  Boivin, J., E. Griffiths, and C.A. Venetis, *Emotional distress in infertile women and failure of assisted reproductive technologies: meta-analysis of prospective psychosocial studies.* BMJ, 2011. **342**:d223.

1544  Dole, N. et al., *Maternal stress and preterm birth.* Am J Epidemiol, 2003. **157**(1):14–24.

1545  Hedegaard, M. et al., *Do stressful life events affect duration of gestation and risk of pre-term delivery?* Epidemiology, 1996. **7**(4):339–45.

1546  Lobel, M., C. Dunkel-Schetter, and S.C. Scrimshaw, *Prenatal maternal stress and pre-maturity: a prospective study of socioeconomically disadvantaged women.* Health Psychol, 1992. **11**(1):32–40.

1547  Bryce, R.L., F.J. Stanley, and J.B. Garner, *Randomized controlled trial of antenatal social support to prevent preterm birth.* Br J Obstet Gynaecol, 1991. **98**(10):1001–8.

1548  Villar, J. et al., *A randomized trial of psychosocial support during high-risk pregnancies. The Latin American Network for Perinatal and Reproductive Research.* N Engl J Med, 1992. **327**(18):1266–71.

1549  Ohlsson, A., P.S. Shah, and L.B.W.b., Knowledge Synthesis Group of Determinants of Preterm, *Effects of the September 11, 2001 disaster on pregnancy outcomes: a system-atic review.* Acta Obstet Gynecol Scand, 2011. **90**(1):6–18.

1550  Harris, A. and J. Seckl, *Glucocorticoids, prenatal stress and the programming of disease.* Horm Behav, 2011. **59**(3):279–89.

1551  Phillips, D.I., *Programming of the stress response: a fundamental mechanism underly-ing the long-term effects of the fetal environment?* J Intern Med, 2007. **261**(5):453–60.

1552  Entringer, S. et al., *Prenatal exposure to maternal psychosocial stress and HPA axis reg-ulation in young adults.* Horm Behav, 2009. **55**(2):292–8.

1553  O'Connor, T.G. et al., *Maternal antenatal anxiety and behavioural/emotional prob-lems in children: a test of a programming hypothesis.* J Child Psychol Psychiatry, 2003. **44**(7):1025–36.

1554  Van den Bergh, B.R. et al., *Antenatal maternal anxiety and stress and the neurobehav-ioural development of the fetus and child: links and possible mechanisms. A review.* Neurosci Biobehav Rev, 2005. **29**(2):237–58.

1555  O'Connor, T.G. et al., *Maternal antenatal anxiety and children's behavioural/emotional problems at 4 years. Report from the Avon Longitudinal Study of Pa7rents and Children.* Br J Psychiatry, 2002. **180**:502–8.

1556  Kraszpulski, M., P.A. Dickerson, and A.K. Salm, *Prenatal stress affects the develop-mental trajectory of the rat amygdala.* Stress, 2006. **9**(2):85–95.

1557  De Bellis, M.D. et al., *A pilot study of amygdala volumes in pediatric generalized anxi-ety disorder.* Biol Psychiatry, 2000. **48**(1):51–7.

1558  Buss, C. et al., *Maternal cortisol over the course of pregnancy and subsequent child amygdala and hippocampus volumes and affective problems.* Proc Natl Acad Sci U S A, 2012. **109**(20):E1312–9.

1559  Kinney, D.K. et al., *Autism prevalence following prenatal exposure to hurricanes and tropical storms in Louisiana.* J Autism Dev Disord, 2008. **38**(3):481–8.

1560  Ronald, A., C.E. Pennell, and A.J. Whitehouse, *Prenatal maternal stress associated with ADHD and autistic traits in early childhood.* Front Psychol, 2010. **1**:223.

1561  Class, Q.A. et al., *Offspring psychopathology following preconception, prenatal and postnatal maternal bereavement stress.* Psychol Med, 2014. **44**(1):71–84.

1562  Rai, D. et al., *Prenatal and early life exposure to stressful life events and risk of autism spectrum disorders: population-based studies in Sweden and England.* PLoS ONE, 2012. **7**(6):e38893.

1563 Hansen, D., H.C. Lou, and J. Olsen, *Serious life events and congenital malformations: a national study with complete follow-up.* Lancet, 2000. **356**(9233):875–80.

1564 Catalani, A. et al., *Maternal corticosterone during lactation permanently affects brain corticosteroid receptors, stress response and behaviour in rat progeny.* Neuroscience, 2000. **100**(2):319–25.

1565 Glynn, L.M. et al., *Postnatal maternal cortisol levels predict temperament in healthy breastfed infants.* Early Hum Dev, 2007. **83**(10):675–81.

1566 Grey, K.R. et al., *Human milk cortisol is associated with infant temperament.* Psycho-neuroendocrinology, 2013. **38**(7):1178–85.

1567 James, W.H., *Evidence that mammalian sex ratios at birth are partially controlled by parental hormone levels around the time of conception.* J Endocrinol, 2008. **198**(1):3–15.

1568 Lyster, W.R., *Altered sex ratio after the London smog of 1952 and the Brisbane flood of 1965.* J Obstet Gynaecol Br Commonw, 1974. **81**(8):626–31.

1569 Fukuda, M. et al., *Decline in sex ratio at birth after Kobe earthquake.* Hum Reprod, 1998. **13**(8):2321–2.

1570 Graffelman, J. and R.F. Hoekstra, *A statistical analysis of the effect of warfare on the human secondary sex ratio.* Hum Biol, 2000. **72**(3):433–45.

1571 Zorn, B. et al., *Decline in sex ratio at birth after 10-day war in Slovenia: brief communication.* Hum Reprod, 2002. **17**(12):3173–7.

1572 Catalano, R.A., *Sex ratios in the two Germanies: a test of the economic stress hypothesis.* Hum Reprod, 2003. **18**(9):1972–5.

1573 Catalano, R.A. and T. Bruckner, *Economic antecedents of the Swedish sex ratio.* Soc Sci Med, 2005. **60**(3):537–43.

1574 Bruckner, T.A., R. Catalano, and J. Ahern, *Male fetal loss in the U.S. following the terrorist attacks of September 11, 2001.* BMC Public Health, 2010. **10**:273.

1575 Fukuda, M. et al., *Kobe earthquake and reduced sperm motility.* Hum Reprod, 1996. **11**(6):1244–6.

1576 Oates, M.R., *Adverse effects of maternal antenatal anxiety on children: causal effect or developmental continuum?* Br J Psychiatry, 2002. **180**:478–9.

1577 Heron, J. et al., *The course of anxiety and depression through pregnancy and the postpartum in a community sample.* J Affect Disord, 2004. **80**(1):65–73.

1578 Dulitzki, M. et al., *Effect of very advanced maternal age on pregnancy outcome and rate of cesarean delivery.* Obstet Gynecol, 1998. **92**(6):935–9.

1579 Luke, B. and M.B. Brown, *Elevated risks of pregnancy complications and adverse outcomes with increasing maternal age.* Hum Reprod, 2007. **22**(5):1264–72.

1580 Hedley, A.A. et al., *Prevalence of overweight and obesity among US children, adolescents, and adults, 1999–2002.* JAMA, 2004. **291**(23):2847–50.

1581 Conti, N. et al., *Uterine fibroids affect pregnancy outcome in women over 30 years old: role of other risk factors.* J Matern Fetal Neonatal Med, 2013. **26**(6):584–7.

1582 van Katwijk, C. and L.L. Peeters, *Clinical aspects of pregnancy after the age of 35 years: a review of the literature.* Hum Reprod Update, 1998. **4**(2):185–94.

1583 Jacobsson, B., L. Ladfors, and I. Milsom, *Advanced maternal age and adverse perinatal outcome.* Obstet Gynecol, 2004. **104**(4):727–33.

1584 Temmerman, M. et al., *Delayed childbearing and maternal mortality.* Eur J Obstet Gynecol Reprod Biol, 2004. **114**(1):19–22.

1585 Hollier, L.M. et al., *Maternal age and malformations in singleton births.* Obstet Gynecol, 2000. **96**(5 Pt 1):701–6.

1586 Baird, P.A., A.D. Sadovnick, and I.M. Yee, *Maternal age and birth defects: a population study.* Lancet, 1991. **337**(8740):527–30.

1587 Pradat, P., *Epidemiology of major congenital heart defects in Sweden, 1981–1986.* J Epidemiol Community Health, 1992. **46**(3):211–15.

1588 Cleary-Goldman, J. et al., *Impact of maternal age on obstetric outcome.* Obstet Gynecol, 2005. **105**(5 Pt 1):983–90.

1589 Friede, A. et al., *Older maternal age and infant mortality in the United States.* Obstet Gynecol, 1988. **72**(2):152–7.

1590 Yoon, P.W. et al., *Advanced maternal age and the risk of Down syndrome characterized by the meiotic stage of chromosomal error: a population-based study.* Am J Hum Genet, 1996. **58**(3):628–33.

1591 Snijders, R.J. et al., *Maternal age- and gestation-specific risk for trisomy 21.* Ultrasound Obstet Gynecol, 1999. **13**(3):167–70.

1592 Allen, E.G. et al., *Maternal age and risk for trisomy 21 assessed by the origin of chromosome nondisjunction: a report from the Atlanta and National Down Syndrome Projects.* Hum Genet, 2009. **125**(1):41–52.

1593 Hytten, F.E., *Clinical and chemical studies in human lactation. VIII. Relationship of the age, physique, and nutritional status of the mother to the yield and composition of her milk.* Br Med J, 1954. **2**(4892):844–5.

1594 Hausman Kedem, M. et al., *The effect of advanced maternal age upon human milk fat content.* Breastfeed Med, 2013. **8**(1):116–19.

1595 Makinson, C., *The health consequences of teenage fertility.* Fam Plann Perspect, 1985. **17**(3):132–9.

1596 Fraser, A.M., J.E. Brockert, and R.H. Ward, *Association of young maternal age with adverse reproductive outcomes.* N Engl J Med, 1995. **332**(17):1113–17.

1597 Naeye, R.L., *Teenaged and pre-teenaged pregnancies: consequences of the fetal-maternal competition for nutrients.* Pediatrics, 1981. **67**(1):146–50.

1598 Scholl, T.O. et al., *Maternal growth during pregnancy and the competition for nutrients.* Am J Clin Nutr, 1994. **60**(2):183–8.

1599 Croen, L.A. and G.M. Shaw, *Young maternal age and congenital malformations: a population-based study.* Am J Public Health, 1995. **85**(5):710–13.

1600 Sipsma, H.L. et al., *Breastfeeding behavior among adolescents: initiation, duration, and exclusivity.* J Adolesc Health, 2013. **53**(3):394–400.

1601 Sowers, M.F. et al., *Bone loss in adolescent and adult pregnant women.* Obstet Gynecol, 2000. **96**(2):189–93.

1602 Bezerra, F.F. et al., *Bone mass is recovered from lactation to postweaning in adolescent mothers with low calcium intakes.* Am J Clin Nutr, 2004. **80**(5):1322–6.

1603 Chantry, C.J., P. Auinger, and R.S. Byrd, *Lactation among adolescent mothers and subsequent bone mineral density.* Arch Pediatr Adolesc Med, 2004. **158**(7): 650–6.

1604 Chan, G.M. et al., *Effects of increased dietary calcium intake upon the calcium and bone mineral status of lactating adolescent and adult women.* Am J Clin Nutr, 1987. **46**(2):319–23.

1605 Diogenes, M.E. et al., *Effect of calcium plus vitamin D supplementation during pregnancy in Brazilian adolescent mothers: a randomized, placebo-controlled trial.* Am J Clin Nutr, 2013. **98**(1):82–91.

1606 Baccetti, B. et al., *Insulin-dependent diabetes in men is associated with hypothalamo-pituitary derangement and with impairment in semen quality.* Hum Reprod, 2002. **17**(10):2673–7.

1607 Agbaje, I.M. et al., *Insulin dependant diabetes mellitus: implications for male reproductive function.* Hum Reprod, 2007. **22**(7):1871–7.

1608 Handelsman, D.J. et al., *Testicular function and glycemic control in diabetic men. A controlled study.* Andrologia, 1985. **17**(5):488–96.

1609 Hammiche, F. et al., *Body mass index and central adiposity are associated with sperm quality in men of subfertile couples.* Hum Reprod, 2012. **27**(8):2365–72.

1610 Jensen, T.K. et al., *Body mass index in relation to semen quality and reproductive hormones among 1,558 Danish men.* Fertil Steril, 2004. **82**(4):863–70.

1611 MacDonald, A.A. et al., *The impact of body mass index on semen parameters and reproductive hormones in human males: a systematic review with meta-analysis.* Hum Reprod Update, 2010. **16**(3):293–311.

1612 Colaci, D.S. et al., *Men's body mass index in relation to embryo quality and clinical outcomes in couples undergoing in vitro fertilization.* Fertil Steril, 2012. **98**(5):1193–9.e1.

1613 Boxmeer, J.C. et al., *Low folate in seminal plasma is associated with increased sperm DNA damage.* Fertil Steril, 2009. **92**(2):548–56.

1614 Young, S.S. et al., *The association of folate, zinc and antioxidant intake with sperm aneuploidy in healthy non-smoking men.* Hum Reprod, 2008. **23**(5):1014–22.

1615 Wallock, L.M. et al., *Low seminal plasma folate concentrations are associated with low sperm density and count in male smokers and nonsmokers.* Fertil Steril, 2001. **75**(2):252–9.

1616 Lambrot, R. et al., *Low paternal dietary folate alters the mouse sperm epigenome and is associated with negative pregnancy outcomes.* Nat Commun, 2013. **4**:2889.

1617 Dissanayake, D. et al., *Relationship between seminal plasma zinc and semen quality in a subfertile population.* J Hum Reprod Sci, 2010. **3**(3):124–8.

1618 Colagar, A.H., E.T. Marzony, and M.J. Chaichi, *Zinc levels in seminal plasma are associated with sperm quality in fertile and infertile men.* Nutr Res, 2009. **29**(2):82–8.

1619 Bjorndahl, L. and U. Kvist, *Human sperm chromatin stabilization: a proposed model including zinc bridges.* Mol Hum Reprod, 2010. **16**(1):23–9.

1620 Wong, W.Y. et al., *Effects of folic acid and zinc sulfate on male factor subfertility: a double-blind, randomized, placebo-controlled trial.* Fertil Steril, 2002. 77(3):491–8.

1621 Garcia, P.C. et al., *Could zinc prevent reproductive alterations caused by cigarette smoke in male rats?* Reprod Fertil Dev, 2012. **24**(4):559–67.

1622 Aitken, R.J., *Free radicals, lipid peroxidation and sperm function.* Reprod Fertil Dev, 1995. **7**(4):659–68.

1623 Rolf, C. et al., *Antioxidant treatment of patients with asthenozoospermia or moderate oligoasthenozoospermia with high-dose vitamin C and vitamin E: a randomized, placebo-controlled, double-blind study.* Hum Reprod, 1999. **14**(4):1028–33.

1624 Tremellen, K., *Oxidative stress and male infertility—a clinical perspective.* Hum Reprod Update, 2008. **14**(3):243–58.

1625 Zini, A., M. San Gabriel, and A. Baazeem, *Antioxidants and sperm DNA damage: a clinical perspective.* J Assist Reprod Genet, 2009. **26**(8):427–32.

1626 Gharagozloo, P. and R.J. Aitken, *The role of sperm oxidative stress in male infertility and the significance of oral antioxidant therapy.* Hum Reprod, 2011. **26**(7): 1628–40.

1627 Gaskins, A.J. et al., *Dietary patterns and semen quality in young men.* Hum Reprod, 2012. **27**(10):2899–907.

1628 Eslamian, G. et al., *Intake of food groups and idiopathic asthenozoospermia: a case-control study.* Hum Reprod, 2012. **27**(11):3328–36.

1629 Afeiche, M. et al., *Dairy food intake in relation to semen quality and reproductive hormone levels among physically active young men.* Hum Reprod, 2013. **28**(8):2265–75.

1630 International Labour Organization, *Male and female reproductive health hazards in the workplace.* <http://actrav.itcilo.org/actrav-english/telearn/osh/rep/remain.htm> accessed 1 July 2014.

1631 Petrelli, G. and A. Mantovani, *Environmental risk factors and male fertility and reproduction.* Contraception, 2002. **65**(4):297–300.

1632 Colt, J.S. and A. Blair, *Parental occupational exposures and risk of childhood cancer.* Environ Health Perspect, 1998. **106** (Suppl 3):909–25.

1633 Close, C.E., P.L. Roberts, and R.E. Berger, *Cigarettes, alcohol and marijuana are related to pyospermia in infertile men.* J Urol, 1990. **144**(4):900–3.

1634 Meri, Z.B. et al., *Does cigarette smoking affect seminal fluid parameters? A comparative study.* Oman Med J, 2013. **28**(1):12–5.

1635 Shen, H.M., S.E. Chia, and C.N. Ong, *Evaluation of oxidative DNA damage in human sperm and its association with male infertility.* J Androl, 1999. **20**(6):718–23.

1636 Viloria, T. et al., *Cigarette smoking affects specific sperm oxidative defenses but does not cause oxidative DNA damage in infertile men.* Fertil Steril, 2010. **94**(2):631–7.

1637 Fraga, C.G. et al., *Smoking and low antioxidant levels increase oxidative damage to sperm DNA.* Mutat Res, 1996. **351**(2):199–203.

1638 Shen, H.M. et al., *Detection of oxidative DNA damage in human sperm and the association with cigarette smoking.* Reprod Toxicol, 1997. **11**(5):675–80.

1639 Hales, B.F. and B. Robaire, *Paternal exposure to drugs and environmental chemicals: effects on progeny outcome.* J Androl, 2001. **22**(6):927–36.

1640 Yazigi, R.A., R.R. Odem, and K.L. Polakoski, *Demonstration of specific binding of cocaine to human spermatozoa.* JAMA, 1991. **266**(14):1956–9.

1641 Brackett, B.G. et al., *Uptake of heterologous genome by mammalian spermatozoa and its transfer to ova through fertilization.* Proc Natl Acad Sci U S A, 1971. **68**(2):353–7.

1642 Torres-Calleja, J. et al., *Effect of androgenic anabolic steroids on sperm quality and serum hormone levels in adult male bodybuilders.* Life Sci, 2001. **68**(15):1769–74.

1643 Dunphy, B.C., C.L. Barratt, and I.D. Cooke, *Male alcohol consumption and fecundity in couples attending an infertility clinic.* Andrologia, 1991. **23**(3):219–21.

1644 Curtis, K.M., D.A. Savitz, and T.E. Arbuckle, *Effects of cigarette smoking, caffeine consumption, and alcohol intake on fecundability.* Am J Epidemiol, 1997. **146**(1): 32–41.

1645 de Jong, A.M. et al., *Effect of alcohol intake and cigarette smoking on sperm parameters and pregnancy.* Andrologia, 2014. **46**(2):112–17.

1646 Gomathi, C. et al., *Effect of chronic alcoholism on semen—studies on lipid profiles.* Int J Androl, 1993. **16**(3):175–81.

1647 Goverde, H.J. et al., *Semen quality and frequency of smoking and alcohol consumption—an explorative study.* Int J Fertil Menopausal Stud, 1995. **40**(3):135–8.

1648 Donnelly, G.P. et al., *Direct effect of alcohol on the motility and morphology of human spermatozoa.* Andrologia, 1999. **31**(1):43–7.

1649 Muthusami, K.R. and P. Chinnaswamy, *Effect of chronic alcoholism on male fertility hormones and semen quality.* Fertil Steril, 2005. **84**(4):919–24.

1650 Joo, K.J. et al., *The effects of smoking and alcohol intake on sperm quality: light and transmission electron microscopy findings.* J Int Med Res, 2012. **40**(6):2327–35.

1651 Vicari, E. et al., *A case of reversible azoospermia following withdrawal from alcohol consumption.* J Endocrinol Invest, 2002. **25**(5):473–6.

1652 Sermondade, N. et al., *Progressive alcohol-induced sperm alterations leading to spermatogenic arrest, which was reversed after alcohol withdrawal.* Reprod Biomed Online, 2010. **20**(3):324–7.

1653 Nudell, D.M., M.M. Monoski, and L.I. Lipshultz, *Common medications and drugs: how they affect male fertility.* Urol Clin North Am, 2002. **29**(4):965–73.

1654 Zhang, J. et al., *A case-control study of paternal smoking and birth defects.* Int J Epidemiol, 1992. **21**(2):273–8.

1655 McCowan, L.M. et al., *Paternal contribution to small for gestational age babies: a multicenter prospective study.* Obesity (Silver Spring), 2011. **19**(5):1035–9.

1656 Davey Smith, G. et al., *Is there an intrauterine influence on obesity? Evidence from parent child associations in the Avon Longitudinal Study of Parents and Children (ALSPAC).* Arch Dis Child, 2007. **92**(10):876–80.

1657 Pembrey, M.E. et al., *Sex-specific, male-line transgenerational responses in humans.* Eur J Hum Genet, 2006. **14**(2):159–66.

1658 Ng, S.F. et al., *Chronic high-fat diet in fathers programs beta-cell dysfunction in female rat offspring.* Nature, 2010. **467**(7318):963–6.

1659 Fullston, T. et al., *Paternal obesity initiates metabolic disturbances in two generations of mice with incomplete penetrance to the F2 generation and alters the transcriptional profile of testis and sperm microRNA content.* FASEB J, 2013. **27**(10):4226–43.

1660 Kong, A. et al., *Rate of de novo mutations and the importance of father's age to disease risk.* Nature, 2012. **488**(7412):471–5.

1661 De Souza, E., E. Alberman, and J.K. Morris, *Down syndrome and paternal age, a new analysis of case-control data collected in the 1960s.* Am J Med Genet A, 2009. **149A**(6): 1205–8.

1662 Erickson, J.D. and T.O. Bjerkedal, *Down syndrome associated with father's age in Norway.* J Med Genet, 1981. **18**(1):22–8.

1663 Stene, E., J. Stene, and S. Stengel-Rutkowski, *A reanalysis of the New York State prenatal diagnosis data on Down's syndrome and paternal age effects.* Hum Genet, 1987. **77**(4):299–302.

1664 Fisch, H. et al., *The influence of paternal age on down syndrome.* J Urol, 2003. **169**(6): 2275–8.

1665 Malaspina, D. et al., *Advancing paternal age and the risk of schizophrenia.* Arch Gen Psychiatry, 2001. **58**(4):361–7.

1666 Malaspina, D., *Paternal factors and schizophrenia risk: de novo mutations and imprinting.* Schizophr Bull, 2001. **27**(3):379–93.

1667 Momand, J.R., G. Xu, and C.A. Walter, *The paternal age effect: a multifaceted phenomenon.* Biol Reprod, 2013. **88**(4):108.

1668 McIntosh, G.C., A.F. Olshan, and P.A. Baird, *Paternal age and the risk of birth defects in offspring.* Epidemiology, 1995. **6**(3):282–8.

1669 Malaspina, D. et al., *Paternal age and intelligence: implications for age-related genomic changes in male germ cells.* Psychiatr Genet, 2005. **15**(2):117–25.

1670 Tai, T.Y. et al., *A case-control study on risk factors for Type 1 diabetes in Taipei City.* Diabetes Res Clin Pract, 1998. **42**(3):197–203.

1671 Min, Y.I., A. Correa-Villasenor, and P.A. Stewart, *Parental occupational lead exposure and low birth weight.* Am J Ind Med, 1996. **30**(5):569–78.

1672 Shah, P.S. and Knowledge Synthesis Group on determinants of preterm/low birthweight, *Paternal factors and low birthweight, preterm, and small for gestational age births: a systematic review.* Am J Obstet Gynecol, 2010. **202**(2):103–23.

1673 Milham, S. and E.M. Ossiander, *Low proportion of male births and low birth weight of sons of flour mill worker fathers.* Am J Ind Med, 2008. **51**(2):157–8.

1674 Potashnik, G. and A. Porath, *Dibromochloropropane (DBCP): a 17-year reassessment of testicular function and reproductive performance.* J Occup Environ Med, 1995. **37**(11):1287–92.

1675 Callaway, L.K., M.J. O'Callaghan, and H.D. McIntyre, *Barriers to addressing overweight and obesity before conception.* Med J Aust, 2009. **191**(8):425–8.

1676 Cordier, S. et al., *Paternal exposure to mercury and spontaneous abortions.* Br J Ind Med, 1991. **48**(6):375–81.

1677 Temple, R.C., V.J. Aldridge, and H.R. Murphy, *Prepregnancy care and pregnancy outcomes in women with type 1 diabetes.* Diabetes Care, 2006. **29**(8):1744–9.

1678 National Collaborating Centre for Women's and Children's Health, National Institute for Health and Clinical Excellence. *Diabetes in pregnancy: management of diabetes and its complications from pre-conception to the postnatal period. NICE guidelines [CG63].* 2008. <http://www.nice.org.uk/guidance/CG63>.

1679 Hanson, L.A. et al., *The transfer of immunity from mother to child.* Ann N Y Acad Sci, 2003. **987**:199–206.

1680 Ip, S. et al., *Breastfeeding and maternal and infant health outcomes in developed countries.* Evid Rep Technol Assess (Full Rep), 2007(153):1–186.

1681 Owen, C.G., P.H. Whincup, and D.G. Cook, *Breast-feeding and cardiovascular risk factors and outcomes in later life: evidence from epidemiological studies.* Proc Nutr Soc, 2011. **70**(4):478–84.

1682 Dewey, K.G., *Growth characteristics of breast-fed compared to formula-fed infants.* Biol Neonate, 1998. **74**(2):94–105.

1683 Agostoni, C. et al., *Growth patterns of breast fed and formula fed infants in the first 12 months of life: an Italian study.* Arch Dis Child, 1999. **81**(5):395–9.

1684 Arenz, S. et al., *Breast-feeding and childhood obesity—a systematic review.* Int J Obes Relat Metab Disord, 2004. **28**(10):1247–56.

1685 Owen, C.G. et al., *Effect of infant feeding on the risk of obesity across the life course: a quantitative review of published evidence.* Pediatrics, 2005. **115**(5):1367–77.

1686 Baker, J.L. et al., *Breastfeeding reduces postpartum weight retention*. Am J Clin Nutr, 2008. **88**(6):1543–51.

1687 Collaborative Group on Hormonal Factors in Breast Cancer, *Breast cancer and breast-feeding: collaborative reanalysis of individual data from 47 epidemiological studies in 30 countries, including 50302 women with breast cancer and 96973 women without the disease*. Lancet, 2002. **360**(9328):187–95.

1688 Rea, M.F., *[Benefits of breastfeeding and women's health]*. J Pediatr (Rio J), 2004. **80** (5 Suppl): S142–6.

1689 Allen, J. and D. Hector, *Benefits of breastfeeding*. N S W Public Health Bull, 2005. **16**(3–4):42–6.

1690 Lawrence, R.M., *Circumstances when breastfeeding is contraindicated*. Pediatr Clin North Am, 2013. **60**(1):295–318.

1691 Butte, N.F. and J.C. King, *Energy requirements during pregnancy and lactation*. Public Health Nutr, 2005. 8(7A):1010–27.

1692 Lovelady, C.A. et al., *The effect of weight loss in overweight, lactating women on the growth of their infants*. N Engl J Med, 2000. **342**(7):449–53.

1693 Allen, L.H., *Lactation: dietary requirements*, in B. Caballero, L. Allen, and A. Prentice, eds., *Encyclopedia of Nutrition*. 2013, Elsevier, pp. 54–9.

1694 Chappell, J.E., M.T. Clandinin, and C. Kearney-Volpe, *Trans fatty acids in human milk lipids: influence of maternal diet and weight loss*. Am J Clin Nutr, 1985. **42**(1): 49–56.

1695 Markhus, M.W. et al., *Low omega-3 index in pregnancy is a possible biological risk factor for postpartum depression*. PLoS ONE, 2013. **8**(7):e67617.

1696 Fidler, N. et al., *Docosahexaenoic acid transfer into human milk after dietary supplementation: a randomized clinical trial*. J Lipid Res, 2000. **41**(9):1376–83.

1697 van Goor, S.A. et al., *Human milk arachidonic acid and docosahexaenoic acid contents increase following supplementation during pregnancy and lactation*. Prostaglandins Leukot Essent Fatty Acids, 2009. **80**(1):65–9.

1698 Lapillonne, A. and C.L. Jensen, *Reevaluation of the DHA requirement for the premature infant*. Prostaglandins Leukot Essent Fatty Acids, 2009. **81**(2–3):143–50.

1699 Lapillonne, A. et al., *Lipid needs of preterm infants: updated recommendations*. J Pediatr, 2013. **162**(3 Suppl):S37–47.

1700 Committee on Nutritional Status during Pregnancy and Lactation, Institute of Medicine, *Nutrition during Lactation*. 1991, Washington, DC: The National Academies Press.

1701 Martin-Sosa, S. et al., *Sialyloligosaccharides in human and bovine milk and in infant formulas: variations with the progression of lactation*. J Dairy Sci, 2003. **86**(1):52–9.

1702 Barger-Lux, M.J. et al., *Vitamin D and its major metabolites: serum levels after graded oral dosing in healthy men*. Osteoporos Int, 1998. **8**(3):222–30.

1703 Braegger, C. et al., *Vitamin D in the healthy European paediatric population*. J Pediatr Gastroenterol Nutr, 2013. **56**(6):692–701.

1704 Emmett, P.M. and I.S. Rogers, *Properties of human milk and their relationship with maternal nutrition*. Early Hum Dev, 1997. 49 (Suppl):S7–28.

1705 McMillan, J.A., S.A. Landaw, and F.A. Oski, *Iron sufficiency in breast-fed infants and the availability of iron from human milk*. Pediatrics, 1976. **58**(5):686–91.

1706 Donangelo, C.M. and J.C. King, *Maternal zinc intakes and homeostatic adjustments during pregnancy and lactation.* Nutrients, 2012. **4**(7):782–98.

1707 Lovelady, C.A. et al., *The effects of dieting on food and nutrient intake of lactating women.* J Am Diet Assoc, 2006. **106**(6):908–12.

1708 Chao, H.H. et al., *Arsenic, cadmium, lead, and aluminium concentrations in human milk at early stages of lactation.* Pediatr Neonatol, 2014. **55**(2):127–34.

1709 Ho, E. et al., *Alcohol and breast feeding: calculation of time to zero level in milk.* Biol Neonate, 2001. **80**(3):219–22.

1710 Astley, S.J. and R.E. Little, *Maternal marijuana use during lactation and infant development at one year.* Neurotoxicol Teratol, 1990. **12**(2):161–8.

1711 Campolongo, P. et al., *Developmental exposure to cannabinoids causes subtle and enduring neurofunctional alterations.* Int Rev Neurobiol, 2009. **85**:117–33.

1712 Mennella, J.A., L.M. Yourshaw, and L.K. Morgan, *Breastfeeding and smoking: short-term effects on infant feeding and sleep.* Pediatrics, 2007. **120**(3):497–502.

1713 Laurberg, P. et al., *Iodine nutrition in breast-fed infants is impaired by maternal smoking.* J Clin Endocrinol Metab, 2004. **89**(1):181–7.

1714 Haberg, S.E. et al., *Effects of pre- and postnatal exposure to parental smoking on early childhood respiratory health.* Am J Epidemiol, 2007. **166**(6):679–86.

1715 Kharasch, S.J. et al., *Unsuspected cocaine exposure in young children.* Am J Dis Child, 1991. **145**(2):204–6.

1716 Hendrick, V. et al., *Use of sertraline, paroxetine and fluvoxamine by nursing women.* Br J Psychiatry, 2001. **179**:163–6.

1717 Berle, J.O. et al., *Breastfeeding during maternal antidepressant treatment with serotonin reuptake inhibitors: infant exposure, clinical symptoms, and cytochrome p450 genotypes.* J Clin Psychiatry, 2004. **65**(9):1228–34.

1718 Rowe, H., T. Baker, and T.W. Hale, *Maternal medication, drug use, and breastfeeding.* Pediatr Clin North Am, 2013. **60**(1):275–94.

1719 Beardmore, K.S., J.M. Morris, and E.D. Gallery, *Excretion of antihypertensive medication into human breast milk: a systematic review.* Hypertens Pregnancy, 2002. **21**(1):85–95.

1720 Niebyl, J.R., *Antibiotics and other anti-infective agents in pregnancy and lactation.* Am J Perinatol, 2003. **20**(8):405–14.

1721 Mactal-Haaf, C., M. Hoffman, and A. Kuchta, Use of anti-infective agents during lactation, Part 3: antivirals, antifungals, and urinary antiseptics. J Hum Lact, 2001. **17**(2):160–6.

1722 Njoku, J.C., D. Gumeel, and E.D. Hermsen, *Antifungal therapy in pregnancy and breastfeeding.* Curr Fungal Infect Rep, 2010. **4**(2):62–9.

1723 Dinsdale, E.C. and W.E. Ward, *Early exposure to soy isoflavones and effects on reproductive health: a review of human and animal studies.* Nutrients, 2010. **2**(11):1156–87.

1724 Dennison, B.A. et al., *Rapid infant weight gain predicts childhood overweight.* Obesity (Silver Spring), 2006. **14**(3):491–9.

1725 Cunnane, S.C. et al., *Breast-fed infants achieve a higher rate of brain and whole body docosahexaenoate accumulation than formula-fed infants not consuming dietary docosahexaenoate.* Lipids, 2000. **35**(1):105–11.

1726  Jorgensen, M.H. et al., *Visual acuity and erythrocyte docosahexaenoic acid status in breast-fed and formula-fed term infants during the first four months of life.* Lipids, 1996. **31**(1):99–105.

1727  Hoffman, D.R., J.A. Boettcher, and D.A. Diersen-Schade, *Toward optimizing vision and cognition in term infants by dietary docosahexaenoic and arachidonic acid supplementation: a review of randomized controlled trials.* Prostaglandins Leukot Essent Fatty Acids, 2009. **81**(2–3):151–8.

1728  Martinez, J.A. and M.P. Ballew, *Infant formulas.* Pediatr Rev, 2011. **32**(5):179–89; quiz, 189.

1729  Rassin, D.K., J.A. Sturman, and G.E. Guall, *Taurine and other free amino acids in milk of man and other mammals.* Early Hum Dev, 1978. **2**(1):1–13.

1730  Koletzko, B. et al., *Compositional requirements of follow-up formula for use in infancy: recommendations of an international expert group coordinated by the Early Nutrition Academy.* Ann Nutr Metab, 2013. **62**(1):44–54.

1731  Host, A. et al., *Dietary prevention of allergic diseases in infants and small children.* Pediatr Allergy Immunol, 2008. **19**(1):1–4.

1732  Prescott, S.L. et al., *The importance of early complementary feeding in the development of oral tolerance: concerns and controversies.* Pediatr Allergy Immunol, 2008. **19**(5): 375–80.

1733  Zutavern, A. et al., *Timing of solid food introduction in relation to eczema, asthma, allergic rhinitis, and food and inhalant sensitization at the age of 6 years: results from the prospective birth cohort study LISA.* Pediatrics, 2008. **121**(1):e44–52.

1734  Ivarsson, A. et al., *Breast-feeding protects against celiac disease.* Am J Clin Nutr, 2002. **75**(5):914–21.

1735  EFSA Panel on Dietetic Products, Nutrition and Allergies, *Scientific Opinion on the appropriate age for introduction of complementary feeding of infants.* EFSA Journal, 2009. **7**(12):1423–42.

1736  Butte, N.F. et al., *Energy expenditure and deposition of breast-fed and formula-fed infants during early infancy.* Pediatr Res, 1990. **28**(6):631–40.

1737  Agostoni, C., E. Riva, and M. Giovannini, *Dietary fiber in weaning foods of young children.* Pediatrics, 1995. **96**(5 Pt 2):1002–5.

# Index

Notes: Page numbers suffixed with 't' refer to details in table, 'f' in figures, and 'b' in boxes.

**A**
AA *see* arachidonic acid (AA)
AAP *see* American Academy of Pediatrics (AAP)
abdominal circumference, fetal growth measures 15
abortion, spontaneous *see* spontaneous abortion
accelerated starvation 245
ACE (angiotensin-converting enzyme) inhibitors 301
acetaminophen *see* paracetamol (acetaminophen)
acetylcholine 104
acetyl-CoA-carboxylases 77
ACOG *see* American Congress of Obstetricians and Gynecologists (ACOG)
acrodermatitis enteropathica 199–200
acute lower respiratory tract infections 199
acute otitis media 293
acyclovir 302
adequate intake (AI) 30, 30t
 *see also specific nutrients*
ADHD *see* attention deficit hyperactivity disorder (ADHD)
adiposity
 fetal 16–17
 of infant/child 113, 216
 maternal diet 246
 maternal fructose 36
 paternal 266, 270
 pesticide exposure 237
 prebiotics/probiotics 211
 pre-pregnancy obesity 216
 protein intake 34
 vitamin D recommendations 111
 *see also* obesity; overweight
adolescent pregnancies 263–4
 calcium deficiency 299
 calcium intake guidelines 143, 145–6, 148, 149, 150
 cigarette smoking 242
 copper intake guidelines 194
 general health 13–14
 iodine intake guidelines 159
 iron deficiency 165
 iron intake guidelines 170, 171
 magnesium in breastmilk 180

magnesium intake guidelines 186
manganese intake guidelines 206
micronutrients 263
preconception lifestyle 13
vitamin A intake guidelines 54
vitamin $B_1$ (thiamine) intake guidelines 60
vitamin $B_3$ (niacin) intake guidelines 70
vitamin $B_7$ (biotin) intake guidelines 79
vitamin $B_{12}$ (cobalamin) intake guidelines 99
vitamin E intake guidelines 136
vitamin K intake guidelines 125
zinc deficiency 201
adrenaline *see* epinephrine (adrenaline)
adrenocorticotrophic hormone 257
aflatoxins 229
Africa
 calcium deficiency 141, 147
 colostrum withholding 251
 contaminated grains 229
 eating down 250
 food restriction during pregnancy 250
 gestational weight gain 219
 iodine deficiency 158
 iron deficiency 164
 iron supplements 166
 magnesium deficiency 175
 maternal stress 258
 pica 243
 prelacteal feeds 251
 riboflavin deficiency 63, 65
 vitamin A intakes 290
 vitamin $B_6$ (pyridoxine) 75
 vitamin $B_9$ (folate) intake guidelines 90
 vitamin D 119
 vitamin D supplements 118
 zinc deficiency 197, 291
age effects *see* maternal age effects
Agency for Toxic Substances and Disease Registry Priority List of Hazardous Substances 240
AI *see* adequate intake (AI)
AIDS
 selenium deficiency 189
 vitamin $B_1$ (thiamine) deficiency 58
 *see also* HIV infection
ALA *see* alpha-linolenic acid (ALA)

alcohol intake  11, 241–2
  birth defects  241
  breastfeeding  300–1
  diabetes mellitus control  285
  early pregnancy  288
  iron  173
  magnesium  174
  paternal intake  266, 267, 269–70, 273
  pre-conception  277
  recommendations  247
  selenium  188
  vitamin A  52, 53
  vitamin $B_1$ (thiamine)  58
  vitamin $B_3$ (niacin)  68
  vitamin $B_9$ (folate)  83, 93
  vitamin $B_{12}$ (cobalamin)  95
  zinc  197, 198, 201
allergies/allergens
  antioxidants  129, 139
  avoidance  227, 307
  bisphenol A  239
  exposure during weaning  307
  infant formula  302
  peanut/food allergens  227
  polyunsaturated fatty acids  44
  weaning foods  307
almond oil  253
aloe  253
alpha-carotene  47
alpha-linolenic acid (ALA)  40
  essentiality  6
  infant formula  305
alpha-tocopherol  134–5
American Academy of Pediatrics (AAP)
  iron intake for infants  172, 173
  vitamin $B_2$ (riboflavin)  66
  vitamin D supplements  120
  vitamin K  125, 297
American Congress of Obstetricians and
    Gynecologists (ACOG)
  exercise  222, 225
  iron intake in pregnancy  171
  vitamin $B_6$ (pyridoxine) supplements  73
  vitamin D  119, 282
  vitamin D supplements  120
American Pregnancy Association
  calcium  150
  magnesium  182
  predatory fish consumption  230
American Thyroid Association  160–1
amino acid(s)
  conditionally essential  5–6, 6t
  deficiency  5–6
  essential  6t
  metabolism, vitamin $B_9$ (folate)  81
  transport  33
  see also specific amino acids
aminoglycosides  301–2

amylophagia  243
anaemia
  copper deficiency  193
  iron deficiency  162
  iron supplementation  167
  vitamin A supplementation  51
  vitamin $B_6$ (pyridoxine)  73
  vitamin $B_9$ (folate)  83, 87
  vitamin $B_{12}$ (cobalamin)  96, 98
analgesic drugs  244–5
  during breastfeeding  301
  see also specific drugs
angiotensin-converting enzyme (ACE)
    inhibitors  301
anorexia  59, 149, 197
  calcium excess  149
  vitamin $B_1$ (thiamine)  59
  zinc deficiency  197
antenatal depression  42
anticoagulant effects, ginger  254
anticonvulsant drugs
  vitamin $B_9$ (folate)  83, 92
  vitamin K deficiency  92, 123
antidepressant drugs, during
    breastfeeding  301
antifungal agents, during breastfeeding  302
antihypertensive drugs, during
    breastfeeding  301
anti-infective drugs, during
    breastfeeding  301–2
anti-inflammatory cytokines, exercise effects  221
antioxidant enzymes  127
  manganese  204
  selenium  187
antioxidants  127–40
  allergies/allergens  129, 139
  asthma  129
  copper-dependent oxidases  193
  gestational hypertension  140
  herbal teas  228
  hypertension  128
  male fertility  267–8
  manganese  205
  selenium  186, 188
  see also vitamin C (ascorbic acid); vitamin E;
      specific antioxidants
apnoea, recurrent  193
apolipoprotein E gene polymorphisms  124
appetite
  fetal effects on  18–19
  magnesium deficiency  175
  regulation of  7–8
  vitamin D excess  175
  zinc deficiency  197
apple juice, arsenic in  240
arachidonic acid (AA)  40
  allergy effects  44
  growth and development  42

infant formulas 305
  sources 41
arsenic 240
  exposure during breastfeeding 300
ascorbic acid *see* vitamin C (ascorbic acid)
Asia
  arsenic exposure 240
  calcium deficiency 141, 147, 148
  contaminated grain 229
  eating down 250, 251
  food restriction during pregnancy 250
  gestational diabetes mellitus 9, 289
  gestational weight gain 219
  iodine deficiency 154, 159
  iron deficiency 164
  iron supplements 166
  prelacteal feeds 251
  riboflavin deficiency 63
  vitamin B$_1$ (thiamine) deficiency 58
  vitamin B$_{12}$ (cobalamin) deficiency 96
  vitamin D deficiency 112, 119
  vitamin K deficiency 124
  Westernization of diet 129
  zinc deficiency 197, 291
aspirin 244, 254
asthma
  antioxidants 129
  bisphenol A 239
  maternal vitamin B$_9$ (folate supplements) 90
  oxidative stress effects 129
  paracetamol 244–5, 292
  vitamin D deficiency 109
  vitamin D excess 113
Atherosclerosis Risk in Communities
    Study 175–6
atherosclerosis, vitamin E 134
atopic disorders
  allergen avoidance 227, 307
  polyunsaturated fatty acids 44
  prebiotics/probiotics 210
  probiotics 210
  vitamin B$_6$ (folate) 90
  weaning foods 307
atrazine 237–8
attention activity, zinc deficiency 198
attention deficit hyperactivity disorder (ADHD)
  iodine 154
  maternal stress 223, 259
Australia
  alcohol intake studies 241
  food labelling 31–2
  iodine recommendations 159
  iron recommendations 172
  macronutrient intake guidelines 38, 38t
  magnesium supplements 182
  manganese intake guidelines 206–7
  polyunsaturated fatty acids 41, 44
  vitamin A intake guidelines 56

vitamin B$_9$ (folate) supplements 85
vitamin C (ascorbic acid) intake
    guidelines 134
vitamin D supplements 120
vitamin E intake guidelines 136–7
vitamin E recommendations 136
Australian National Health and Medical
    Research Council
  alcohol intake 241
  copper intake guidelines 194
  iodine intake guidelines 159
  iron intake during breastfeeding 172
autism
  maternal stress 259
  vitamin B$_9$ (folate) deficiency 86
autoimmune thyroid disease 157
Avon Longitudinal Study of Parents and
    Children
  parental BMI 270
  swimming pool risks 224
Ayurvedic herbal remedies 229
  preconception exposure 284

**B**
*Bacillus* infections, geophagia 244
balanced diets 6–7
basal metabolic processes
  nutrition 5
  vitamin B$_6$ (pyridoxine) 71
Beckwith–Wiedemann syndrome 22
behavioural intervention programmes,
    gestational weight gain management 219
behavioural problems
  iron deficiency 165
  maternal stress 258–9
  vitamin B$_9$ (folate) deficiency 86
  zinc deficiency 197–8
  *see also* attention deficit hyperactivity
    disorder (ADHD)
benzene 272
benzodiazepines, during breastfeeding 301
benzyl peroxide 246
beriberi 58
beta-blockers 301
beta-carotene 47
  as antioxidant 130
  sources 52
beta-cryptoxanthin 47
betaine 87, 102
Biafra civil war famine 250
*Bifidobacterium lactis* B12 211
  *see also* probiotics
biotin *see* vitamin B$_7$ (biotin)
birth
  preterm *see* preterm birth/labour
  *see* labour
Birth Cohort Linked Birth and Infant Death
    Data 261

birth defects
  adolescent pregnancies 264
  alcohol consumption 241
  choline 104
  hair dyes/skin care products 246
  herbicides 237
  maternal age effects 262–3
  paternal cigarette smoking 270
  paternal exposures 268–9, 272
  pollutants 285
  skin-care products 246
  teratogens 124, 228
  vitamin A deficiency 49, 50, 281
  vitamin A excess 53, 56, 288
  vitamin B$_7$ (biotin) deficiency 78
  vitamin B$_9$ (folate) 85–6, 278
  vitamin B$_{12}$ (cobalamin) 97–8
  vitamin K deficiency 124
  *see also* congenital abnormalities; neural
      tube defects (NTDs)
birthweight
  adolescent pregnancies 263–4
  cigarette smoking 242
  Dutch Hunger Winter (1944–1945) 10
  extreme exercise effects 225
  homocysteine levels 97
  hyper-homocystinaemia 72
  hypertension 165
  increase in 293
  iodine deficiency 154
  iron deficiency 164–5
  magnesium effects 177
  maternal age effects 261
  maternal stress 258
  moderate exercise effects 223
  paternal factors 270–1
  protein intake 34–5
  vitamin A 49
  vitamin A deficiency 51
  vitamin B$_9$ (folate) 85
  vitamin D deficiency 111, 113–14
  vitamin E deficiency 135
  vitamin K deficiency 124
  zinc 198
bisphenol A (BPA) 239–40
Bitot spots 48
bleeding *see* haemorrhages
blood clotting, vitamin K 122
blood loss *see* haemorrhages
blood pressure
  exercise effects 221, 222
  fibre intake 36–7
  herbal remedies 255
  high *see* hypertension
  low carbohydrate diets 25, 35–6
  low, magnesium deficiency 176
  magnesium 176, 177, 179
  maternal calcium intake 146
  potassium 184, 185, 186
  protein intake 35
  unbalanced diets 246
blue cohosh 255
BMC *see* bone mineral content (BMC)
BMD *see* bone mineral density (BMD)
BMI *see* body mass index (BMI)
body composition 17–18
  metabolic control 8
  pre-conception 215–16
body coverings, vitamin D deficiency 13
body mass index (BMI)
  maternal pre-conception
      bodyweight 277
  paternal factors 266, 270
  postnatal growth 17
bodyweight *see* weight
bodyweight, pre-conception *see* pre-conception
      bodyweight
bone
  calcium 141
  loss 110, 142–3, 176, 264
  magnesium 174
  maternal breastfeeding benefits 293
  vitamin D 107
bone fracture, calcium deficiency 147
bone growth, manganese 204
bone health
  copper deficiency 193
  vitamin D deficiency 111
bone mineral content (BMC)
  calcium intake 143
  formula feeding 147
bone mineral density (BMD) 179
  calcium 143–4, 147, 298–9
  magnesium 179
  vitamin D 116
BPA (bisphenol A) 239–40
brain development 73–4
  choline 102–4
  environmental effects 24
  epinephrine (adrenaline) 73–4
  glucose 5
  iodine deficiency 154
  manganese excess 206, 208
  maternal stress 259
  polyunsaturated fatty acids 40, 43
  timing of 23–4
  vitamin B$_6$ (pyridoxine) 73
  vitamin B$_{12}$ (cobalamin) 73
  *see also* cerebral cortex development;
      neurodevelopment
breakfast 245–6
breastfeeding 293–310
  adolescent pregnancies 264
  alcohol consumption 300–1
  alcohol intake 300–1
  benefits 293–4

cigarette smoking 300–1
cocaine 300–1
developing countries 293
dieting during 299–300
drugs 300–1
environmental contaminants 300
hypertension reduction 293
malnutrition 294
maternal age effects 263
maternal nutrition 294–9
   *see also specific nutrients/micronutrients*
maternal stress 302
maternal weight loss 294
prescribed drugs 301–2
   *see also specific drugs*
recommended intakes 279–81t, 294
breast milk composition
aflatoxin contamination 229
calcium 146–7, 151, 235
changes in 306–7
choline 104–5, 106
copper 192, 193
environmental toxins 300
flavour learning 309
glucocorticoids 259
IgA antibodies 294
infant formulas *vs.*, 293
iodine 155, 157, 159, 160, 299
iron 165, 166, 172, 298
lactoferrin 294
magnesium 180, 182
manganese 205, 208
marijuana 300
maternal dietary effects 295
micronutrients 296
polyunsaturated fatty acids 41–2, 44, 295
potassium 185–6
prebiotics/probiotics 209
prescribed drugs 301
probiotic organisms 209
protein 295–6
selenium 189–90
vitamin A 51, 54, 297
vitamin B$_1$ (thiamine) 59–60
vitamin B$_2$ (riboflavin) 64–5
vitamin B$_3$ (niacin) 68
vitamin B$_6$ (pyridoxine) 74, 76
vitamin B$_7$ (biotin) 79
vitamin B$_{12}$ (cobalamin) 97, 98, 100, 298
vitamin C (ascorbic acid) 132
vitamin D 116–17, 120, 296
vitamin E 136
vitamin K 123, 297
zinc 199–200, 201–2, 203, 299
breech presentation, caffeine 233
British Dietetic Association 307
brown rice, arsenic 240
Buddhism, food taboos 250

**C**
cadmium 240–1
breastfeeding 300
caesarian delivery, obesity pre-conception 216
caffeine 233–4
potassium loss 185
pre-conception intake guidelines 285
calciferol *see* vitamin D
calcitonin 142
calcitriol *see* 1,25-hydroxyvitamin D
   (calcitriol)
calcium 141–51
absorption *see* calcium absorption
adolescent pregnancies 143, 145–6, 148,
   149, 150
bone mineral density 143–4, 147, 298–9
bone turnover 142–3
breastfeeding 146–7, 298–9
breast milk composition 146–7, 151
Canadian recommendations 149
clinical trials 143–4
dairy products 149, 150–1
deficiency *see* calcium deficiency
deposition in vitamin D excess 118
excess *see* calcium excess
functions 141–2
   *see also specific functions*
high urine levels 149
hypertension 144, 145, 146
infant formulas 303t
intake guidelines 149–51
iron absorption inhibition 168
lead effects 146, 235
low blood levels 174
magnesium 174
middle/late pregnancy 290–1
pre-conception intake guidelines 282
pre-eclampsia 144, 145, 151
in pregnancy 142–6
preterm delivery 145–6
recommended dietary allowance 148, 150b,
   279t
sources 148–9
status indicators 142
supplements *see* calcium supplements
upper intake level 149, 150b
weaning 147
zinc absorption 200–1
calcium absorption
infant formulas 147, 151
phytates 6
vitamin D deficiency 108
calcium channel blockers (CCBs) 301
calcium deficiency 174
adolescent pregnancies 299
Africa 141, 147
Asia 141, 148
fibre 148–9

calcium deficiency (*continued*)
  Gambia 144
  hypertension 142
  magnesium deficiency with 174
  malnutrition 142
  pregnancy-induced hypertension (PIH) 145
  prevalence 147–8
  vitamin D deficiency 147
calcium economy 146
calcium excess 149
  Ethiopia 145
calcium supplements
  breast milk composition 235
  China 144
  clinical trials 143–4
  Gambia 144, 146
  India 144
calories from fat, labelling 31
calories (kcal) per serving, labelling 31
Camden Study, adolescent pregnancies 263
Canada
  calcium deficiency 148
  calcium recommendations 149
  exercise guidelines 225
  food labelling 31
  iron excess 169
  iron intake guidelines 172
  iron supplements 167
  magnesium intake guidelines 182
  Motherisk programme 232
  vitamin $B_3$ (niacin) 70
  vitamin $B_9$ (folate) recommendations 84, 90, 92
  vitamin $B_9$ (folate) supplements 85, 89
  vitamin $B_{12}$ (cobalamin) recommendations 98, 105
carbapenems 301–2
carbohydrate(s) 35–6
  breastfeeding requirements 296
  daily intake guidelines 37, 38
  dairy products 35
  infant formulas 305
  recommended dietary allowance 279t
  transport 33
carbohydrate metabolism
  magnesium deficiency 175
  metabolic interactions 7
  vitamin $B_1$ (thiamine) 57
cardiovascular disease
  exercise 221
  fructose intake 36
  of infant, maternal obesity 216
  magnesium deficiency 176
  maternal age effects 262
  weaning timing 307
L-carnitine 304t
carotenoids 127, 130
cassava 248

castor oil 255
catecholamines
  caffeine 233
  maternal stress 257
cat litter trays 231
central nervous system (CNS)
  iron intake in pregnancy 171
  myelination, iodine deficiency 154
  vitamin $B_6$ 75
  vitamin $B_{12}$ (cobalamin) 92, 94
  *see also* brain development; neurodevelopment
cephalosporins 301–2
ceramide 102
cerebral cortex development
  alcohol intake 241
  iodine deficiency 154
  *see also* brain development
cerebral palsy 178
ceruloplasmin 192, 193
chamomile 253
cheeses *see* dairy products
cheilosis 64
chemotherapy, male fertility 269
childhood diarrhoea, zinc 199
China
  calcium supplemements 144
  cigarette smoking 270
  great famine (1959–1961) 10
  herbal medicine guidelines 284
  herbal remedies 229
  iodine deficiency 154, 158
  iodine excess 158, 159
  magnesium supplements 177
  postpartum dietary practices 251
  postpartum food practices 251
  prelacteal feeds 251
  selenium deficiency 187
  under-nutrition 10
  vitamin $B_9$ (folate) deficiency 86
  vitamin $B_9$ (folate) supplementation 85
chloride, infant formulas 303t
chlorine disinfection, swimming pools 224
cholecalciferol *see* vitamin $D_3$ (cholecalciferol)
choline 102–6
  birth defects 104
  brain development 102–4
  breastfeeding 104–5
  breast milk composition 104–5, 106
  cognitive development 102, 104
  deficiency 103
  epigenetic mechanisms 105
  functions 102
  homocysteine interactions 103–4
  infant formulas 104, 303t
  intake guidelines 105–6
  neural development 104
  neural tube defects 104

pre-eclampsia 104
in pregnancy 103–4
recommended dietary allowance 280t
sources 105
status indicators 102–3
upper intake level, 106b
vitamin B₉ (folate) interactions 87–8, 102, 103–4
chromium, paternal factors 272
chronic hypercortisolaemia 257
chronic lung disease, vitamin A deficiency 51
chylomicrons, vitamin K 124
cigarette smoking 238–9, 242
breastfeeding 300–1
cadmium 240–1
China 270
Germany 242
gestational diabetes mellitus 242
iron deficiency 164
male fertility 273
micronutrients 300
paternal factors 266, 269, 270
pre-conception guidelines 285
vitamin B₁₂ (cobalamin) deficiency 95
vitamin C (ascorbic acid) 133
*see also* polycyclic aromatic hydrocarbons (PAH)
clay eating *see* geophagia
cleft lip, vitamin B₉ (folate) deficiency 86
cleft palate 228
*Clostridium,* geophagia 244
clothing styles, vitamin D synthesis 115
club foot 262
cobalamin *see* vitamin B₁₂ (cobalamin)
cocaine
breastfeeding 300–1
male fertility 269
coeliac disease 197
cofactors, vitamin B₁₂ (cobalamin) 94
cognitive development 228
choline 102, 104
iodine deficiency 154, 156
iron deficiency 165
lead effects 235
manganese deficiency 205
maternal obesity 216
maternal stress effects 259
paternal age 271
pollutants 234
polycyclic aromatic hydrocarbons 238
polyunsaturated fatty acids 43
pre-pregnancy obesity 216
problems 154
vitamin B₁₂ (cobalamin)–vitamin B₆ (pyridoxine) interactions 96
zinc deficiency 197–8
cohosh, blue 255
cold foods, India 249t, 250

colostrum
cultural withholding 251
maternal age effects 263
vitamin A 51
combustion products 268–9
complementary foods 306–10, 308t
introduction of 309–10
complementary remedies *see* herbal remedies
conception 258
conditionally essential amino acids 5–6, 6t
confinement diets 251
Confucianism, food taboos 250
congenital abnormalities 216
*see also* birth defects
congenital hypothyroidism 154
connective tissue, copper 192
constipation, iron excess 169
copper 192–5
adolescent pregnancies 194
breastfeeding 193
breast milk composition 192, 193
deficiency *see* copper deficiency
epinephrine (adrenaline) 191
excess 193
functions 192
infant feeding 193
infant formulas 303t
intake guidelines 194–5
in pregnancy 193
recommended dietary allowance 19b, 194–5, 194b, 280t
sources 194
status indicators 192
upper intake level 194, 194b
copper deficiency 192–3
iron supplementation 169–70
zinc excess 201
copper-dependent oxidases 193
copper/zinc superoxide dismutase 192
cortisol 257
Cosmetic Ingredient Review Expert Panel 246
coumarin anticoagulants 124
cranberry juice 253
urinary tract infections 254
craniofacial malformations 228
paternal age 271
vitamin A 281
*see also* birth defects
craniotabes 110
Crohn's disease 68, 174, 175, 197
crown-rump length 15
cultural/traditional practices 12, 248–52
exercise 221–2
food taboos 248–9
immigrants 248
Korea 250
malnutrition 248–9
postpartum practices 251

cultural/traditional practices (*continued*)
  processing techniques 248
  under-nutrition 219
  vitamin D synthesis 115
  *see also specific cultures*
cycads 248
cyclophosphamide 269
cysteine 71
cytochrome C oxidase 192
cytochrome P450 enzymes 47
cytosine–guanine dinucleotide (CpG) sites 21

**D**
dairy products
  calcium source 148, 149, 150–1
  carbohydrate sources 35
  contamination 11, 231, 232
  iodine 157
  lack of intake 63, 64, 147–8
  male fertility 268
  manganese 206
  potassium 185
  pre-conception intake 282
  protein source 34
  selenium 190
  semen quality 268
  vitamin A 290
  vitamin $B_2$ (riboflavin) 63, 64, 65, 66
  vitamin $B_3$ (niacin) 69
  vitamin $B_7$ (biotin) 78
  vitamin $B_{12}$ (cobalamin) 99
  vitamin D 115, 282
  vitamin K 124
  zinc 200
Danish National Birth Cohort
  moderate exercise effects 223–4
  swimming pool risks 224
  vitamin C/E supplement trials 138
dark skin, vitamin D synthesis 114–15
DDT (dichloro-diphenyl-
    trichloroethane) 236–7
deaf–mutism 154
delivery *see* labour
5-deoxyadenosylcobalamin 94
depression
  herbal remedies 254–5
  postpartum *see* postpartum depression
dermatitis
  herbal remedies 255
  vitamin $B_2$ (riboflavin) deficiency 64
  vitamin $B_3$ (niacin) excess 69
developed countries
  vitamin $B_1$ (thiamine) breastfeeding/
    infancy 59
  vitamin $B_2$ (riboflavin) deficiency 65
developing countries
  breastfeeding 293
  developmental mismatch 25

exercise 221–2
pica 243
under-nutrition 10
vitamin A deficiency 50
vitamin $B_2$ (riboflavin) deficiency 63
development 3–14
  biological control 4
  environmental effects 4, 15–18
  macronutrient profile 33–4
  mismatch 24–5
  non-automatic processes 3–5
  nutritional needs 4
  plasticity *see* developmental plasticity
  polyunsaturated fatty acids effects 42–3
  pre-conception behaviour effects 23
  range of micronutrient values 4
  timetable of 23–4
  vitamin A deficiency 49
  vitamin $B_9$ (folate) deficiency 86
  *see also* fetal growth; growth
developmental plasticity 18–25
  critical periods 22–4
  definition 18–19
  environmental effects 19–20
  *see also* epigenetics
  evolutionary biology 19
  ubiquity 19
DHA *see* docosahexaenoic acid (DHA)
diabetes mellitus
  alcohol consumption 285
  developmental mismatch 25
  fibre 36–7
  first-born infants 19
  macrosomia 7
  magnesium 174
  maternal age effects 261, 262, 264
  paternal factors 266, 270–1
  pre-conception guidelines 285–6
  type 1 *see* diabetes mellitus type 1
  type 2 *see* diabetes mellitus type 2
  vitamin $B_1$ (niacin) deficiency 68
  vitamin $B_6$ (pyridoxine) deficiency 72
  *see also* gestational diabetes mellitus (GDM)
diabetes mellitus type 1
  oxidative stress 128
  paternal age 271
  poor control effects 286
  pre-eclampsia 128
  vitamin $B_6$ (pyridoxine) deficiency 72
  vitamin D deficiency 109
diabetes mellitus type 2
  fetal developmental plasticity 19
  fibre 37
  fructose intake 36
  gestational diabetes mellitus 9
  iron excess 169
  magnesium deficiency 175
  modern sedentary lifestyle 222

paternal age 272
potassium deficiency 185
risk of 9
selenium 190
weaning 307
diacylglycerol 102
diaphragmatic hernia 262
diarrhoea
  iron excess 169
  vitamin A absorption 52
  zinc 199
dibromochloropropane 272
dichloro-diphenyl-trichloroethane
  (DDT) 236–7
diclofenac 244
diet
  adiposity 246
  balanced 6–7
  barriers to 12
  breast milk composition 295
  confinement 251
  developmental mismatch 25
  eczema 227
  effects on child's diet 34
  high-fibre 148–9
  middle/late pregnancy 289–91
  pre-eclampsia 12, 17
  vitamin D 115
dietary advice
  maternal age 264
  pre-conception period 277
dietary reference intake (DRI) 29–30
  *see also specific nutrients*
dietary reference value (DRV)
  definition 29
  *see also specific nutrients*
diet-induced obesity 35
dieting 250–1
  glucose intolerance 250
dieting (planned weight loss) 250–1
  labour 289
dioxins 268
diseases/disorders, developmental origins
  3–4
diuretic drugs 197
DNA
  acetylation 20
  chemical alterations 20
  choline 105
  coiling 22
  instability, vitamin B$_3$ (niacin) deficiency 67
  methylation *see* DNA methylation
  polycyclic aromatic hydrocarbon
    damage 238–9
  repair *see* DNA repair
  structure 22
  synthesis *see* DNA synthesis
  ubiquitation 20

DNA methylation 20, 22
  vitamin B$_9$ (folate) 81
DNA repair
  nicotinamide adenine dinucleotide 67
  parental age 271
DNA synthesis
  vitamin B$_9$ (folate) 81
  vitamin B$_{12}$ (cobalamin) 94
  vitamin B$_{12}$ (cobalamin)–vitamin B$_6$
    (pyridoxine) interactions 96
docosahexaenoic acid (DHA) 40
  allergy effects 44
  breastfeeding requirements 295
  cognitive development 43
  essentiality 6
  infant formulas 305
  intake guidelines 45
  levels during pregnancy 41
  levels in breast milk 42
  maternal mental health 42
  preterm infants 295
  sources 41
'doing the month' 251
dopamine 74
dose–response studies, vitamin B$_9$ (folate)
  deficiency 83
Down syndrome *see* trisomy 21 (Down's
  syndrome)
drinking water
  magnesium 180
  manganese 206
drugs *see* prescription drugs
drugs of abuse, paternal factors 269–70
Dutch Hunger Winter (1944–1945) 10
dyskinesias 206

E
EAR *see* estimated average requirement
  (EAR)
Early Childhood Longitudinal Study - Birth
  Cohort 217
early development 3
early pregnancy guidelines 287–9
eating down
  Africa 250
  Asia 250, 251
echinacea 253
eczema
  dietary effects 44, 227
  oxidative stress 129
  polyunsaturated fatty acids 44
  prebiotics/probiotics 209, 210
  vitamin D 112, 113
egg(s) 232t
  iodine 157
  *Salmonella enterica* infection 231
egg whites 77
egg yolks 78

eicosapentaenoic acid (EPA) 40
  intake guidelines 45
  maternal mental health 42
  sources 41
emotional problems in infants 259
endocrine disruption by pesticides 236
Endocrine Society
  iodine intake 160
  vitamin D breastfeeding requirements
    296–7
  vitamin D intake guidelines 119, 120, 282
endometrial cancer 293
endothelial cell proliferation 221
energy balance 9–10
  during breastfeeding 294–6
  daily dietary reference values 34
energy density, infant formulas 304–5
energy intake
  during breastfeeding 299
  early pregnancy 287
  gestational weight gain management 219
energy transfer, iron-containing enzymes 162
environment
  brain development effects 24
  developmental plasticity 19–20
  see also epigenetics
  development, effects on 4, 15–18
  paternal factors 266, 268–9
environmental contaminants 300
enzymes
  vitamin $B_2$ (riboflavin) deficiency 63–4
  vitamin $B_6$ (pyridoxine) 71
  zinc 196
  see also specific enzymes
EPA see eicosapentaenoic acid (EPA)
epigenetics 20–2
  animals 23
  choline 105
  definition 20
  egg quality 23
  functions of 22
  obesity pre-conception 216
  parental imprinting 21–2
  spermatogenesis 23
epinephrine (adrenaline)
  copper metabolism 191
  fetal brain development 73–4
  maternal stress 257
  vitamin $B_6$ (pyridoxine) 73–4
ergocalciferol see vitamin $D_2$ (ergocalciferol)
erythrocyte(s)
  formation 94
  manganese 204
erythrocyte dismutase 192
erythrocyte glutathione reductase 63
erythrocyte thiamine pyrophosphate 58, 58t
Escherichia coli septicaemia 170
essential amino acids 6t

essential fatty acids
  pre-conception intake guidelines 283–4
  transport 33
essential nutrients 5
estimated average requirement (EAR) 30t
  definition 29–30
Ethiopia
  calcium excess 145
  iodine deficiency 158
  postpartum food practices 251
ethnicity
  calcium requirements 141
  vitamin D deficiency 112
  vitamin D intake guidelines 119
  see also specific ethnicities
ethylene dichloride 268
Europe
  herbal remedies 254, 256
  iodine deficiency 158
  iodine supplements 155, 166
  iron supplements in infant formula 173
  organochlorine chemicals 230
  selenium recommendations 190
  vitamin A recommendations 56
  vitamin $B_6$ (pyridoxine)
    recommendations 76
  vitamin K recommendations 124
European Commission 76
European Community Committee on
    Food 172
European Food Safety Authority
  manganese intake guidelines 207
  polyunsaturated fatty acids intake
    guidelines 45
European Scientific Committee
  vitamin $B_{12}$ (cobalamin) excess 89
  vitamin $B_{12}$ (cobalamin) supplements 93
European Society of Paediatric
    Gastroenterology and Nutrition
  infant formula components 302
  iron in infant formulas 306
  vitamin D supplements 120, 297
EURRECA (EURopean micronutrient
    RECcommendations Aligned) 172–3
evolutionary biology 19
exercise 12–13, 221–6
  benefits 222
  blood pressure 221, 222
  during breastfeeding 299
  cultural factors 221–2
  extreme exercise 225
  gestational diabetes mellitus 222
  guidelines 225–6
  importance of 10–11
  long-term effects 224
  middle/late pregnancy 289
  moderate exercise effects 223–4
  physiological changes 221

pre-conception behaviour  284
pre-eclampsia  221, 222, 226
preterm birth/labour  223, 225
risks  224–5

**F**
factor II (prothrombin)  122
  vitamin K  123
factor VII  122
factor IX  122
factor X  122
FAD (flavin adenine dinucleotide)
  synthetase  62
famines  250
fasting  250–1
fat(s)
  daily intake guidelines  39
  deposition  9–10
  diet  35
  gestational diabetes mellitus  35
  vitamin E  135
  *see also specific fats*
fatty acid desaturase gene  40
fatty acids
  breastfeeding requirements  295
  essential *see* essential fatty acids
  fetal heart development  9
  infant formulas  305
  monosaturated  210
  polyunsaturated *see* polyunsaturated fatty
    acids (PUFAs)
  synthesis  94
FDA (Food Standards Agency) (UK)  201
femoral length  15
fennel  253
ferritin  162, 163
fetal breathing movements  23
fetal death  234
fetal growth  16f
  first pregnancy  16
  gender differences  15
  head size constraints  16–17
  maternal constraint processes  16
  maternal reduction of  17
  measures of  15
  multiple conceptions  15–16
  polyunsaturated fatty acids effects  42–3
  population differences  15
  protein  34
  restriction  25, 128, 233
  vitamin A  49
  *see also* development
fetal heart development
  fatty acids  9
  glucose  9
  timing of  23
fetal heart rate  223
fetal hepatic veno-occlusive disease  229

fetal hyperinsulinaemia  216
fetal hypoxic–ischaemic encephalopathy  178
fetal metabolic health, paternal factors  270–1
fetal mortality, iodine deficiency  153–4
fetal warfarin syndrome  124
fibre  36–7
  benefits  36–7
  blood pressure  37
  calcium deficiency  148–9
  guideline daily amounts  32
  importance  33–4
  intake guidelines  34, 37–9
  labelling  31
  middle/late pregnancy  290
  pre-eclampsia  37
  sources  36
  in weaning  307–8
Finland
  herbal remedies  254
  prebiotics/probiotics  211
First and Second Trimester Evaluation of Risk
  trial  262
first-born infants
  disease risks  19
  fetal growth  16
fish diets
  allergy development  44
  cultural/traditional practices  249
flavin adenine dinucleotide (FAD)
  synthetase  62
flavin mononucleotide (FMN)  62
flavocoenzymes  62
flavonoids *see* polyphenols (flavonoids)
flavoprotein gene mutations  62
flavour learning  309–10
flour mills  272
flour refining  181
fluconazole  302
fluoride
  infant formulas  304t
  recommended dietary allowance  280t
fluoxetine  301
FMN (flavin mononucleotide)  62
folate *see* vitamin B$_9$ (folate)
follow-up formulas  306
food(s)
  cultural/traditional taboos  248–9
  fortification *see* supplementation
  information problems  227–8
  intake guidelines  247
  labelling *see* food labelling
  preferences in weaning  309–10
  risks  11, 228–41, 232t
  sensitization  307
  *see also specific foods*
food and drinks industry  14
foodbourne infections  230–2
  *see also specific infections*

food labelling 30–2
  Australia 31–2
  Canada 31
  New Zealand 31–2
  UK 31–2
  US 31
Food Standards Agency (FDA) (UK) 201
free radicals 127
fructose 36
  daily intake guidelines 39
  diabetes mellitus type 2, 36
fruits
  pre-conception intake guidelines 286t
  washing/peeling 231
fungal mycotoxins 11

**G**
gallbladder disease 36
Gambia
  calcium deficiency 144
  calcium supplements 144, 146
  under-nutrition 10
  vitamin B$_2$ deficiency 64
gamma-aminobutyric acid (GABA) 73–4
gamma-tocopherols 134–5
gastrointestinal disorders
  breastfeeding benefits 293
  copper excess 193
  fibre intake 37
  infections 52
  potassium excess 184
  vitamin B$_{12}$ (cobalamin) deficiency 95
  vitamin C (ascorbic acid) excess 132
  zinc excess 201
gastroschisis 237–8
GDA (guideline daily amounts) 32
GDM see gestational diabetes mellitus (GDM)
gender
  fetal growth differences 15
  maternal stress 260
  sex ratio 260
gene(s) 20–1
  regulatory mechanisms 21, 21f
  see also DNA; specific genes
Generation R study 84
genetic disorders, parental age 271
genotype 20
geographic effects
  calcium deficiency 147
  iodine deficiency 155, 158
  see also specific countries
geophagia 242–3, 243–4
  potassium loss 185
German E Commission 254
Germany
  cigarette smoking 242
  gestational weight gain 217
germ cell tumours, hair dyes 247

germline mutations, parental age 271
gestational diabetes mellitus (GDM) 9
  amylophagia 243
  Asia 9, 289
  cigarette smoking 242
  diabetes mellitus type 2 development 9
  energy balance 10
  exercise 222
  fat intake 35
  fibre intake 37
  incidence 9
  iron deficiency 164, 166
  magnesium 176–7
  maternal age effects 262
  nutrient transport effects 33, 34
  overweight children 16
  oxidative stress 128
  pathology 9
  pre-pregnancy obesity 216
  probiotics 210–11
  vitamin D deficiency 113
  see also diabetes mellitus
gestational hypertension
  antioxidants 140
  carotenoids 130
  iron deficiency 166
  vitamin B$_9$ (folate) in 84
  vitamin C/D supplementation trials 137–8
  zinc 199
gestational length, iron deficiency 164–5
gestational weight gain 216–19
  active management 219
  Africa 219
  Asia 219
  breastfeeding effects 294
  Germany 217
  guidelines 218, 220
  middle/late pregnancy 289
  offspring obesity 217–18
  pre-eclampsia 217, 219
GH (growth hormone) 8
GI (glycaemic index) 35–6
ginger 253–4
glossitis 64
glucagon 7
glucocorticoids 257
  breast milk composition 259
gluconeogenesis 7
glucose
  blood level controls 7
  brain development 5
  diet 35–6
  fetal heart development 9
  high levels see hyperglycaemia
  infant formulas 305
  low blood levels 245
  magnesium effects 175
  maternal constraint processes 16

monitoring in middle/late pregnancy 289
prebiotics/probiotics 210–11
transport 33
vitamin D effects 107, 109
glucose intolerance
Dutch Hunger Winter (1944–1945) 10
fat levels 35
fructose intake 36
maternal 9
potassium deficiency 184
protein levels 34
glutamine synthase 204
glutathione peroxidase(s) 188
breast milk 189–90
selenium 187
glycaemic index (GI) 35–6
glycerophosphocholine 104
glycine 5–6
glycolic acid 246
grains
contamination 229
pre-conception intake guidelines 286t
grape juice 240
GraviFrisk™ 254
Great Leap Forward famine 250
green tea 228–9
groundwater contamination, arsenic 240
growth 15–17
functions 18
intrauterine restriction *see* intrauterine
growth restriction
nutrient needs 5
uneven rate 15, 16f
zinc deficiency 197
*see also* fetal growth; postnatal growth
growth charts 15
growth hormone (GH) 8
guideline daily amounts (GDA) 32
guidelines for pregnancy 287–92
early pregnancy 287–9
late pregnancy 289–91
middle pregnancy 289–91
*see also specific nutrients*
gut microbiota 209–10
vitamin B₇ (biotin) synthesis 78

**H**
haem iron 168
haemoglobin 162
haemorrhages
at birth 164
intracranial 123
iron deficiency 164
maternal 164
haemorrhagic disease of the newborn
(HDN) 123
haemosiderin 162
hair dyes 246–7

haptocorrin 94
hard water 180
harvest season, Gambia 10
HDN (haemorrhagic disease of the
newborn) 123
head circumference
cigarette smoking 242
fetal growth measures 15
vitamin D supplements 116
head volume, fetal growth measures 15
Health Canada
calcium 149
iron supplementation during pregnancy 167
health literacy 25
Health Professionals Follow-up Study 175
health promotion initiatives 13
hearing impairment 154
heartburn, iron excess 169
heart development *see* fetal heart development
heart disease
developmental mismatch 25
fetal developmental plasticity 19
magnesium deficiency 175
socioeconomics 25
heavy metals 300
height, gestational weight gain 218
helminth infections 243
heme biosynthesis 63
heparin 143
hepatic gluconeogenesis 7
hepatoxicity *see* liver
hepcidin 162
iron status 163
herbal remedies 253–6
blood pressure 255
depression 254–5
Europe 254, 256
Finland 254
indications 253–5
intake guidelines 255–6, 284
labour aids 255
middle/late pregnancy 291–2
morning sickness 253–4
skin conditions 255
urinary tract infections 254
*see also specific remedies*
herbal tea 228–9
herbicides 237–8
exposure during breastfeeding 300
hernia, diaphragmatic 262
herpes simplex infection 294
hexachlorobenzene 229–30
high blood pressure *see* hypertension
high-density lipoprotein (HDL) cholesterol 67
high-fibre diets 148–9
high-risk groups, vitamin D deficiency 111–12
hippocampal cholinergic system 104
histamine 74

histones 22
    methylation 105
    modification 20
HIV infection
    breastfeeding contraindications 294
    selenium deficiency 189
    vitamin A deficiency 50
    vitamin $B_1$ (thiamine) deficiency 58
    zinc 199
    *see also* AIDS
holotranscobalamin 95
homocysteine 81
    associated defects 97
    choline interactions 103–4
    metabolism 82f, 96
    vitamin $B_6$ (pyridoxine) 71
    vitamin $B_{12}$ (cobalamin) interactions 87
    vitamin $B_{12}$ (cobalamin) status 95
    vitamin $B_{12}$ (cobalamin) vitamin $B_6$
        (pyridoxine) interactions 96
homocysteine–methionine metabolism 81
honey 229
'hot foods' 249t, 250
human T-cell lymphotropic viruses (HTLVs)
    infections 294
hungry season, Gambia 10
hydrocephalus 228
hydrogen peroxide 246
hydroquinone 246
3-hydroxyisovalerate 77
1,25-hydroxyvitamin D (calcitriol) 107
    calcium 142
    degradation 147
    magnesium deficiency 174
    *see also* vitamin D
hygiene, breastfeeding 293
hygiene hypothesis 210
hypercalcaemia 149
hypercalciuria 149
hypercortisolaemia, chronic 257
hyperglycaemia 9, 16, 25, 128
    fetal abnormalities 9
    normal pregnancy 9
    obesity pre-conception 216
hyper-homocystinaemia 72
hypericin 254–5
*Hypericum perforatum* (St John's Wort) 254–5
hyperinsulinaemia, fetal 216
hyperkalaemia 184
hyperketonaemia 245
hyperlipidaemia, vitamin E 135
hypermagnesaemia 181
hyperparathyroidism, secondary 108
hypertension
    antioxidants 128
    birthweight 165
    breastfeeding benefits 293
    calcium 142, 144, 145, 146

iron deficiency 164, 166
iron supplements 170
magnesium deficiency 175–6, 182
maternal age effects 261, 262, 264, 265
non-steroidal anti-inflammatory drugs 244
during pregnancy *see* gestational
        hypertension
pregnancy-induced *see* pregnancy-induced
        hypertension (PIH)
vitamin D deficiency 109
hypervitaminosis A 53
hypocalcaemia 174
hypoglycaemia 7, 245
hypokalaemia 184
hypotension, magnesium deficiency 176
hypothalamic–pituitary–adrenal (HPA)
    axis 257
hypothyroidism
    congenital 154
    iodine deficiency 153
    neonatal 159

**I**
IBD (inflammatory bowel disease) 72
ibuprofen 244
idiopathic spontaneous abortion 188
IgA antibodies
    breast milk 294
immigrants 248
immune system
    copper deficiency 193
    oxidative stress 129
    probiotics 210
    selenium 187
    vitamin $B_7$ (biotin) deficiency 78
    vitamin D 107, 109
    zinc 197, 199
immunoglobulin A (IgA) antibodies
    breast milk 294
implantation, timing of 23
India
    calcium deficiency 148
    calcium supplements 144
    food taboos 249t, 250
    herbal medicine 229, 284
    magnesium supplements 177
    postpartum food practices 251
    prelacteal feeds 251
    vitamin A deficiency 49
    vitamin A supplements 56, 290
    vitamin $B_{12}$ (coblamin) supplements 96–7
    vitamin D deficiency 112
infant behaviour 74
infant feeding, zinc 199–200
infant formulas 302–6
    allergies/allergens 302
    breast milk *vs.*, 293
    calcium absorption 147, 151

carbohydrates 305
choline 104
energy density 304–5
essential components/composition 302–6
  *see also specific components*
fatty acids 305
follow-up formulas 306
glucose 305
iodine 157, 161
iron 170, 172, 306
manganese 205
micronutrients 300, 302, 303–4t
  *see also specific micronutrients*
niacin supplementation 69
oligosaccharides 296
patient guidance 294
prebiotics/probiotics 210
protein 305
protein hydrolase 302
soy formulas 302
vitamin $B_1$ (thiamine) deficient 59–60
vitamin D supplements 115, 120
vitamin K supplements 123
infant growth patterns, maternal
  pre-conception bodyweight 215
infantile scurvy 132
infant mortality 261
  iodine deficiency 153–4
infection(s)
  excess iron 170
  foodbourne 230–2
  obesity pre-conception 216
  paternal factors 266
  reduction by breastfeeding 293
  selenium deficiency 189
  vitamin A deficiency 48–9
  vitamin D deficiency 113
  zinc 196, 197
  *see also specific infections*
infertility
  caffeine 233
  vitamin A deficiency 48
  vitamin D 114
inflammatory bowel disease (IBD) 72
Institute of Medicine (IOM)
  calcium 149, 150b
  calorie intake 37
  choline 105, 106b
  copper 194, 194b
  dietary reference intakes 29
  gestational weight gain 216–17, 218, 218b
  iodine 159, 160b
  iodine when breastfeeding 299
  iron 170–1, 171b
  magnesium 181, 182b
  manganese 206–7, 207b
  middle/late pregnancy 289
  potassium 185–6, 186b

selenium 190, 191b
vitamin A 54, 55b
vitamin $B_1$ (thiamine) 60, 61b
vitamin $B_2$ (riboflavin) 65–6, 66b
vitamin $B_3$ (niacin) 69–70, 69b
vitamin $B_6$ (pyridoxine) 75, 76b, 297–8
vitamin $B_7$ (biotin) 79, 79b
vitamin $B_{12}$ (cobalamin) 89, 91–2, 91b,
  99–100, 100b
vitamin C (ascorbic acid) 133, 133b
vitamin D 109, 118–19, 118b, 120, 282, 296
vitamin E 136, 137b
vitamin K, 125b
zinc 201–2, 202b
insulin 7
insulin-dependent diabetes mellitus *see*
  diabetes mellitus type 1
insulin-independent diabetes mellitus *see*
  diabetes mellitus type 2
insulin insensitivity 221
  fructose intake 36
  vitamin D deficiency 109
  *see also* diabetes mellitus
insulin resistance
  development in pregnancy 8
  iron excess 169
  magnesium 176–7
  normal pregnancy 9
  *see also* diabetes mellitus; gestational
    diabetes mellitus (GDM)
INTAPP group 138
International Association of the Diabetes and
  Pregnancy Study Groups 9
International Council for the Council of Iodine
  Deficiency Disorders 159–60, 161
intracranial haemorrhage 123
intrapartum period 166
intrauterine growth restriction
  cigarette smoking 242
  herbicides 238
  vitamin $B_{12}$ (cobalamin) vitamin $B_6$
    (pyridoxine) interactions 96–7
  zinc 198
intrinsic factor 94
  receptors 97
in vitro fertilization
  vitamin $B_6$ (pyridoxine) pre-conception 73
  vitamin D 114
iodine 152–61
  adolescent pregnancies 159
  availability concerns 158
  breastfeeding 155, 299
  breast milk composition 155, 157, 159, 160,
    299
  deficiency *see* iodine deficiency
  early pregnancy 289
  excess 158–9
  functions 152

iodine (*continued*)
  infant formulas 157, 161, 304t
  intake guidelines 159–61
  iron deficiency 165
  pre-conception intake guidelines 283
  recommended dietary allowance 159–60,
    160b, 280t
  recommended nutrient intake 160
  sources 157
  status indicators 152–3
  supplementation 153–4, 155–7
  upper intake level 158, 160b
iodine deficiency 153–5, 156–7
  Africa 158
  Asia 154, 159
  attention deficit hyperactivity disorder 154
  cerebral cortex development 154
  China 154, 158
  cognitive development 154, 156
  Ethiopia 158
  Europe 158
  interventional studies 156 7
  Turkey 158
iodothyronine deiodinases 187
IOM *see* Institute of Medicine (IOM)
ion channels 174
ionizing radiation exposure 268
iron 162–73
  alcohol consumption 173
  breast milk composition 165, 166, 172, 298
  complementary foods 309
  copper deficiency with 193
  deficiency *see* iron deficiency
  excess 169–70
  functions 162
  guidelines *see* iron intake guidelines
  homeostasis 162–3
  infant formulas 170, 172
  lead protection 235
  metabolism 168–9
  mobilization 51
  pica 243
  in pregnancy 163–4
  sources 168–9
  status 163
  supplements *see* iron supplements
  zinc absorption 200–1
iron deficiency 163, 164–6
  adolescent pregnancies 165
  Africa 164
  Asia 164
  behavioural problems 165
  birthweight 164–5
  causes 164
  gestational diabetes mellitus 164, 166
  gestational hypertension 166
  gestational length 164–5
  high-risk groups 165–6

  hypertension 164
  manganese 205, 206
  micronutrients 167
  neurobehaviour 165
iron intake guidelines 168–9, 170–3
  adolescent pregnancies 170, 171
  Australia 172
  during breastfeeding 172
  breastfeeding requirements 298
  Canada 172
  early pregnancy 287, 288–9
  infant formulas 304t, 306
  infant requirements 166
  infants 172–3
  middle/late pregnancy 291
  pre-conception guidelines 282
  in pregnancy 171–2
  recommended dietary allowance 168–9,
    171b, 280t
  tolerable upper levels 173
  upper intake level, 171b 173
  in weaning 307, 309
iron supplements 166–8
  Africa 166
  Asia 166
  hypertension 170
  in infant formula, Europe 173
  New Zealand 170
isotretinoin 246
Israel 59–60

**K**
keratomalacia 48
Keshan disease 187
ketosis 245
  maternal 245
kidneys
  developmental mismatch 24
  magnesium excess 181
  zinc deficiency 197
KOALA Birth Cohort study 90
Korea
  cultural food practices 250
  iodine excess 159
  postpartum dietary practices 251
Krebs cycle 7

**L**
LA *see* linoleic acid (LA)
labelling *see* food labelling
labour
  breech presentation 233
  dieting during pregnancy 289
  exposure risks 11
  fear of 17
  herbal remedies 255
  'hot foods' 250
  induction 216

magnesium 176, 178, 179
maternal age 261
obstruction risk 17
pre-pregnancy obesity 216
preterm *see* preterm birth/labour
stress management 223
timing, moderate exercise effects 223
lactation *see* breastfeeding
*Lactobacillus rhamnosus,* 211
*see also* probiotics
lactoferrin 294
lactogen 8
lactogen-dependent recruitment of intrinsic
factor receptors 97
lactose 296
intolerance 63
large for gestational age (LGA) 10
late pregnancy guidelines 289–91
lead 234–5
calcium intake 146
exposure during breastfeeding 300
paternal factors 272
precautionary advice 235, 236b
learning capacity 154
lecithin 105
Leigh syndrome 62
LGA (large for gestational age) 10
life-course approach 25–6
Lifestyle in Pregnancy Study 219
lifestyle risk factors 227–47
guidelines 247
*see also specific risk factors*
linoleic acid (LA) 40
alpha-linolenic acid ratio 40
growth and development 42
levels in breast milk 41–2
sources 41
lipid metabolism
fructose intake 36
vitamin B$_6$ (pyridoxine) 71
lipid transport 33
liquorice 253
*Listeria monocytogenes* infection
(listeriosis) 230–1
unpasteurized cheese 11
liver 232t
avoidance guidelines 56
choline deficiency 103
choline synthesis 102
excess vitamin A 228
risks 228
vitamin A excess 52–3
vitamin B$_3$ (niacin) excess 69
vitamin B$_7$ (biotin) 78
vitamin B$_9$ (folate) deficiency 83
vitamin B$_{12}$ (cobalamin) 95
low birthweight, Dutch Hunger Winter
(1944–1945) 10

low-carbohydrate diets 245–6
blood pressure 25, 35–6
low-density lipoprotein (LDL) cholesterol
67
lower respiratory tract infections, acute 199
lowest recommended nutrient intake
(LRNI) 30t
definition 30
lung disease, chronic 51
lysyl oxidase 192

**M**
macronutrients 33–9
balanced diets 7
breastfeeding requirements 294–6
pregnancy requirements 33–7
requirements 34, 37–9
transfer to fetus 33
*see also specific nutrients*
magnesium 174–83
alcohol consumption 174
alcohol intake 174
birthweight 177
blood pressure 176, 177, 179
bone mineral density 179
breast milk composition 180, 182
deficiency *see* magnesium deficiency
excess 181
functions 174
glucose, effects on 175
infant formulas 304t
insulin resistance 176–7
intake guidelines *see* magnesium intake
guidelines
labour 176
metabolic disturbances 176–7
muscle cramps 179
neuroprotection 177
pre-eclampsia 177, 179, 181
in pregnancy 176–9
pregnancy-induced hypertension 177
preterm birth/labour 177, 181
skeletal development 179
sources 180–1
status indicators 175
supplements *see* magnesium supplements
magnesium deficiency 175–6
with calcium deficiency 174
diabetes mellitus type 2 175
gestational diabetes mellitus 176–7
heart disease 175
hypertension 175–6, 182
magnesium intake guidelines 181–3
adolescent pregnancies 186
Canada 182
recommended dietary allowance 181–2,
182b, 280t
upper intake level 182, 182b

magnesium supplements 179
  Australia 182
  China 177
  India 177
  labour 178, 179
  preterm birth/labour 177, 178
  South Africa 178
magnetic resonance imaging (MRI) 205
malabsorption
  vitamin B$_6$ (pyridoxine) deficiency 72
  vitamin B$_9$ (folate) deficiency 83
malaria-endemic areas, pre-pregnancy iron
    supplementation 166–7
male fertility
  antioxidants 267–8
  guidelines 272–3
  micronutrients 267
  zinc 202
  see also paternal factors
malnutrition
  body composition 17
  breastfeeding 294
  cadmium exposure 240
  calcium deficiency 142
  copper deficiency 192
  cultural practices 248–9
  vitamin A excess 53
  vitamin E deficiency 134
  zinc deficiency 196–7
manganese 204–8
  antioxidants 127, 205
  brain development 206, 208
  breast milk composition 208
  dairy products 206
  excess 206
  functions 204
  infant formulas 205, 304t
  intake guidelines see manganese intake
    guidelines
  in pregnancy 205
  sources 206
  status indicators 204–5
manganese deficiency 204
  cognitive development 205
manganese intake guidelines 206–8
  adolescent pregnancies 206
  Australia 206
  New Zealand 206
  recommended dietary allowance 206, 280t
  upper intake level, 207b
marijuana 270
  breast milk composition 300
maternal age effects
  birth defects 262–3
  birthweight 261
  breastfeeding 263
  colostrum 263
  gestational diabetes mellitus 261, 262

guidelines 264–5
  hypertension 261, 262, 265
  infant death 261
  labour 261
  maternal morbidity 262
  maternal mortality 262
  neonatal mortality 262–3
  obesity 261
  overweight 261
  pre-eclampsia 262
  pregnancy-induced hypertension 262
  thromboembolism 262
  uterine fibroids 261
maternal factors 241–2
  age see maternal age effects
  constraint of fetal growth 16
  diet see diet
  haemorrhage 164
  ketosis 245
  mental health 42
  morbidity/mortality 262
  pre-conception bodyweight see pre-
    conception bodyweight
  stress see maternal stress
maternal stress 257–60
  Africa 258
  attention deficit hyperactivity disorder 223,
    259
  autism 259
  birthweight 258
  brain development 259
  breastfeeding 259, 302
  cognitive development 259
  conception 258
  epinephrine (adrenaline) 257
  offspring behavioural patterns 258–9
  offspring sex ratio 260
  in pregnancy 257–8
  pregnancy outcomes 258–9
  preterm birth/labour 258
  risk recommendations 247–8
  under-nutrition 257
  USA 258
  yoga 222
meat, undercooked see undercooked meats
Medical Birth Registry (Sweden) 84
Medical Research Council Vitamin
    Study 85–6
Mediterranean diet 73, 76
megaloblastic (pernicious) anaemia 96
  vitamin B$_9$ (folate) deficiency 81
membrane phospholipids, choline 103
menaquinone (vitamin K$_2$) 124
mental health, maternal 42
mercury
  exposure during breastfeeding 300
  oily fish 45
  predatory fish 229–30

messenger RNA (mRNA) 21
metabolic control 7–9
  body composition 8
  body weight 8
  development of 9
  evolutionary biology 19
metabolic disturbances
  of infant, maternal obesity 216
  magnesium 176–7
  vitamin B$_1$ (thiamine) deficiency 59
metabolic syndrome 36
methionine synthase 87
methionine synthesis 87–8
methylation cycle, vitamin B$_9$
  (folate) 81
methylation of DNA 20
methylcobalamin 94
methylenetetrahydrofolate reductase
  (MTHFR) 62, 87
methylmalonic acid 95
methylmalonyl coenzyme A mutase 94
methylmercury 230
5-methyl tetrahydrofolate 62
micronutrients
  adolescent pregnancies 263
  balanced diets 7
  breastfeeding requirements 296
  breast milk composition 296
  cigarette smoking 300
  in development 4
  dose/response relations 7
  early pregnancy 287–9
  functions 5
  infant formulas 300, 302, 303–4t
  intake recommendations 4
  iron deficiency effects 167
  male fertility 267
  middle/late pregnancy 289–91
  other food component effects 6
  paternal factors 267
  recommended dietary allowance 287
  recommended dietary intakes 287
  supplement inconsistency 29
  see also specific micronutrients
micro-ophthalmia 228
micro-organism synthesis 209–10
  essential vitamins 209
  vitamin B$_9$ (folate) 81
  vitamin B$_{12}$ (cobalamin) 98–9
microRNAs 21
middle-income countries 10
middle pregnancy guidelines 289–91
miscarriage see spontaneous abortion
mitochondrial beta-oxidation 64
moderate exercise effects 223–4
modern sedentary lifestyle 222
monosaturated fatty acids 210
morbidity, maternal 262

morning sickness
  herbal remedies 253–4
  potassium loss 185
  vitamin B$_6$ (pyridoxine) supplements 73
mortality
  infant see infant mortality
  iodine deficiency 153–4
  neonatal 262–3
mother–infant bonding, breastfeeding
  benefits 293
Motherisk programme (Canada) 232
motor abnormalities 154
motor development 198
mould-ripened soft cheeses 232t
  Listeria monocytogenes infection 231
MRI (magnetic resonance imaging) 205
mRNA (messenger RNA) 21
MTHFR (methylenetetrahydrofolate
  reductase) 62, 87
MTHFR gene 86, 87, 104–5
mucosal epithelium 49
mucosal uptake 197
multiple conceptions
  calcium intake 143
  fetal growth 15–16
  iron deficiency 165–6
multivitamin supplements 116
muscle contraction 184
muscle cramps 179
musculoskeletal system 57
  lead accumulation 234
  magnesium 179
  vitamin D 110
  see also bone
mycotoxins, grains 229
myelination 71
myoglobin 162
myoinositol 304t
myxedermatous cretinism 154

**N**
N1-methyl-2-pyridone-5-carboxamide 68
N1-methyl-nicotinamide 67
Na/K-ATPase 174
naproxen 244
National Center for Health Statistics 261
National Health and Nutrition Examination
  Survey
  vitamin B$_6$ (pyridoxine) 75
  vitamin E deficiency 134
National Infant Mortality Surveillance
  Project 262
National Institute for Clinical Excellence (NICE)
  antioxidants 140
  cigarette smoking 242
  magnesium intake guidelines 182
  vitamin B$_{12}$ (cobalamin) supplements 92–3
  vitamin D 118

National Prevention of Cancer Trial 190
Native Americans 248
nausea and vomiting
  iron excess 169
  pregnancy-induced *see* morning sickness
  vitamin B$_6$ (pyridoxine) 73
  *see also* vomiting
neonatal hypothyroidism 159
neonatal mortality 262–3
neonatal pulmonary hypertension 229
neonatal respiratory insufficiency 50
nerve impulses, potassium 184
nervous system
  atrophy 197–8
  magnesium effects 177
  vitamin B$_1$ (thiamine) 57
  vitamin B$_{12}$ (cobalamin) 94
  vitamin D deficiency 109
  *see also* neurodevelopment
neural tube defects (NTDs)
  choline 104
  genetics 87
  maternal obesity 281
  pathogenesis 228
  pre-conception ionizing radiation 285
  prior history 278, 281
  toxicant exposure 228
  vitamin B$_9$ (folate) 7, 83, 84, 85–6, 87, 88–9, 90–1, 92, 93, 278
  vitamin B$_{12}$ (cobalamin) deficiency 97
  *see also* birth defects
neurobehavioural development
  iron deficiency 165
  zinc 196
neuroblastoma 247
neurodevelopment 104
  iodine deficiency 154–5
  lead effects 234
  maternal exercise effects 224
  vitamin B$_9$ (folate) 86
  zinc deficiency 197–8
  *see also* brain development
neuroendocrine control 18
neuromuscular system
  caffeine effects 233
  hyperexcitability, magnesium deficiency 175
neuropsychological behaviour
  manganese excess 206
  zinc deficiency 198
neurotoxicity 236
neurotransmitters 71, 73–4
New Zealand
  food labelling 31–2
  iodine recommendations 159
  iron supplementation 170
  manganese intake guidelines 206–7
  vitamin C (ascorbic acid) 134
  vitamin D recommendations 120

vitamin E intake guidelines 136–7
New Zealand Ministry of Health
  copper intake guidelines 194
  iodine 159
niacin *see* vitamin B$_3$ (niacin)
NICE *see* National Institute for Clinical Excellence (NICE)
nicotinamide 67
  *see also* vitamin B$_3$ (niacin)
nicotinamide adenine dinucleotide (NAD) 67
nicotinamide adenine dinucleotide phosphate (NADP) 67
nicotinic acid 67
  *see also* vitamin B$_3$ (niacin)
Nigeria famine (1967-1970) 10
*N*-methyl-D-aspartate (NMDA) receptor 73
  magnesium effects 178
nocturnal muscle cramps 179
non-automatic development 3–5
non-coding RNAs 21
non-haem iron 168
nonsteroidal anti-inflammatory drugs (NSAIDs) 244
  during breastfeeding 301
  hypertension 244
  middle/late pregnancy 292
norepinephrine (noradrenaline)
  maternal stress 257
  vitamin B$_6$ (pyridoxine) 73–4
NSAIDs *see* nonsteroidal anti-inflammatory drugs (NSAIDs)
NTDs *see* neural tube defects (NTDs)
nucleotide biosynthesis 81
Nurses Health Study
  iron excess 169
  magnesium deficiency 175
nutrient(s)
  availability in balanced diets 6
  deficiencies 243
  dietary reference intakes 29–30
  intake guidelines 29–32, 31t
  labelling 31
  weaning requirements 307–8
  *see also* macronutrients; micronutrients; *specific nutrients*
nutrition 5–10
  basal metabolic processes 5
  definition of 5
  development effects 4
  essential *vs.* non-essential components 5–6
  needs of 5
  pre-conception behaviour 278–84
nutritional status, maternal age 264
Nutrition Facts panel 31
nutrition information panel (NIP) 31–2

**O**

obesity
  breastfeeding  295, 299
  cigarette smoking  242
  developmental mismatch  25
  energy balance  9
  energy intake guidelines  39
  excessive food intake  7
  fetal developmental plasticity  19
  fibre intake  37
  fructose intake  36
  maternal age effects  261
  maternal pre-conception bodyweight  277
  modern sedentary lifestyle  222
  neural tube defects  281
  omega-6 to omega-3 polyunsaturated fatty
     acids ratio  43
  paternal factors  266
  pre-conception  216, 284
  with under-nutrition  9
  vitamin $B_9$ (folate) deficiency  83–4
  vitamin D  111
  weaning timing  307
  *see also* adiposity; overweight
obstruction risk during labour  17
occupational exposures  268–9
oedema  193
oily fish
  contaminants  45
  visual development  43
oligosaccharides  296
omega-3 polyunsaturated fatty acids
  allergy development  44
  beneficial effects  40
  fish eating risk *vs.,*  230
  growth and development  42–3
  intake guidelines  37
  pre-conception intake guidelines  283–4
  recommended dietary allowance  279t
  sources  41
omega-6 polyunsaturated fatty acids
  effects  40
  intake guidelines  37
  pre-adipocyte development  43
  pre-conception intake guidelines  283–4
  recommended dietary allowance  279t
  sources  41
omega-6 to omega-3 polyunsaturated fatty acid
    ratio  40, 41
  allergy development  44
  obesity  43
omnivory  5
oral contraceptives  255
organochlorine chemicals  230
organogenesis  228
organ size  18
orofacial clefts  86
osteomalacia

calcium deficiency  147
  vitamin D deficiency  109
osteopenia  110
osteoporosis
  magnesium deficiency  176
  vitamin K deficiency  122
outcome of pregnancy, maternal stress  258–9
ovarian cancer  293
over-nutrition, energy balance  9–10
over-the-counter drugs  244–5
  *see also specific drugs*
overweight
  breastfeeding  295, 299
  energy balance  9, 10
  energy intake guidelines  39
  iron deficiency  166
  magnesium deficiency  175
  maternal age effects  261
  vitamin D deficiency  113–14
  *see also* adiposity; obesity
ovum quality  23
oxalic acid  148
oxidase metalloenzymes  192
oxidation–reduction reactions  192
oxidative metabolism  62
oxidative stress  127
  asthma  129
  diabetes mellitus type  1, 128
  eczema  129
  exercise effects  221
  fetal growth restriction  128
  gestational diabetes mellitus  128
  hyperketonaemia  245
  immune system  129
  pre-eclampsia  128
oxygen transport, in pregnancy  163

**P**

PAF (platelet activating factor)  102
pagophagia  243
PAH *see* polycyclic aromatic hydrocarbons
  (PAH)
painkillers *see* analgesic drugs
Paleoliothic diet  245–6
Pan American Health Organization  309
pantothenic acid (vitamin $B_5$)  303t
paracetamol (acetaminophen)  244–5
  asthma  244–5, 292
  during breastfeeding  301
  middle/late pregnancy  292
parathyroid hormone (PTH)
  calcitonin *vs.,*  142
  calcium absorption  109–10
  secondary excess  108
parental factors
  age  271
  definition  20
  high-fat diets  270–1

parental factors (*continued*)
  see also maternal factors; paternal factors
parental imprinting 21–2
paternal factors 266–73
  adiposity 270
  alcohol consumption 266, 267, 269–70, 273
  birthweight 270–1
  body mass index 266, 270
  cigarette smoking 269, 270
  cognitive development 271
  diabetes mellitus 266
  diabetes mellitus type 2, 272
  drug use 269–70
  environmental exposure 268–9, 272
  fetal metabolic health 270–1
  intake guidelines 272–3
  micronutrients 267
  nutritional factors 266–7
  obesity 266
  occupational exposures 268–9, 272
  pre-conception 266–70
  pre-conception polycyclic aromatic
    hydrocarbons exposure 238–9
  pregnancy outcomes 270–2
  see also male fertility
PCBs see polychlorinated biphenyls (PCBs)
peanut allergy 227
pellagra 68
penicillins 301–2
per cent daily value (%DV) 31
peripheral neuropathy
  vitamin D deficiency 109
  vitamin E deficiency 134
pernicious anaemia see megaloblastic
    (pernicious) anaemia
pesticides 236–7
  exposure during breastfeeding 300
  paternal factors 268
phenolic acids 129
phenotype 20
phosphatidylcholine 102, 104, 105
phosphatidylethanolamine
    *N*-methyltransferase 102
  enzymatic pathway 103–4
phosphoenolpyruvate decarboxylase 204
phospholipase C 174
phosphorus
  infant formulas 304t
  recommended dietary allowance 280t
photophobia 48
phthalates 268
phylloquinone (vitamin K$_1$) 122–3
physical activity/exercise see exercise
physiology
  calcium 141–2
  exercise 221
phytates 6
  iron absorption inhibition 168

zinc deficiency 197
zinc intake 200
phytotoxins 228–9
pica 242–4
  Africa 243
  amylophagia 243
  pagophagia 243
  USA 243
  see also geophagia
PIH see pregnancy-induced hypertension
    (PIH)
PIVKA-II (protein induced by vitamin K
    absence or antagonist-II) 122
PL (pyridoxal) 71
placenta
  abruption in iodine deficiency 153–4
  antioxidant enzymes 127–8
  blood flow 18
  cigarette smoking effects 242
  exercise effects 221
  iron requirements 163–4
  macronutrient transfer 33
  nutrient transport see placental transport
  vasoconstriction by caffeine 233
  weight in iron deficiency 165
placental hormones 8
placental transport
  vitamin B$_2$ (riboflavin) 64
  zinc 198
planned weight loss see dieting (planned
    weight loss)
plasma levels
  choline 102–3
  homocysteine 83
  see also serum levels
plasma membrane, zinc 196
platelet activating factor (PAF) 102
PLP see pyridoxal-5'-phosphate (PLP)
pollutants
  birth defects 285
  cognitive development 234
  free radicals 127
  see also specific pollutants
polychlorinated biphenyls (PCBs)
  oily fish 45
  predatory fish 229–30
polycyclic aromatic hydrocarbons
    (PAH) 238–9
  paternal factors 268
  see also cigarette smoking
polyphenols (flavonoids) 127, 129–30
  herbal tea 228–9
  iron absorption inhibition 168
  as pro-oxidants 130
polyunsaturated fatty acids (PUFAs) 40–6
  allergies 44
  atopic disorders 44
  Australia 41, 44

brain development  40, 43
breast milk composition  41–2, 44, 295
cognitive development  43
eczema  44
effects of  42–4
 *see also specific effects*
essentiality  6, 40
fetal growth and development  42–3
glucose intolerance  35
intake guidelines  39, 45
maternal mental health  42
middle/late pregnancy  290
in pregnancy  41–2
respiratory disease  44
sources  41
transport  33
visual development  43
*see also* omega-3 polyunsaturated fatty acids;
 omega-6 polyunsaturated fatty acids
population differences, fetal growth  15
porphyria  63
postnatal growth  17
postpartum depression
 maternal breastfeeding benefits  293
 polyunsaturated fatty acids effects  42
postpartum weight retention  293
potassium  184–6
 blood pressure  185, 186
 breast milk composition  185–6
 dairy products  185
 deficiency  184, 185
 diabetes mellitus type 2, 185
 excess  184
 function  184
 infant formulas  304t
 intake guidelines  185–6
 low blood levels  184
 magnesium  174
 in pregnancy  185
 recommended dietary allowance, 186b
 sources  185
poverty *see* socioeconomic status
PPOX (protoporphyrinogen IX oxidase)  63
pre-adipocyte development  43
prebiotics  209–11
 adiposity  211
 atopic disorders  210
 breast milk composition  209
 definition  209
 eczema  209, 210
 Finland  211
 glucose  210–11
 infant formulas  210
 intake guidelines  211
 sources  209
 weaning  210, 211
 *see also* probiotics
pre-conception behaviour  13, 83, 277–86

adolescent pregnancies  13
advice  277
alcohol consumption  277
bodyweight *see* pre-conception bodyweight
developmental effects  23
diabetes mellitus  285–6
dietary guidelines  286, 286t
exercise  284
exposures  284–5
ionizing radiation exposure  285
iron intake guidelines  173
iron supplementation  166–7
nutrition  278–84
obesity  284
recommended intakes  279–81t
supplementation  278–84
vitamin B$_9$ (folate) supplements  83
vitamin B$_{12}$ (cobalamin) supplements  88–9
pre-conception bodyweight  215–16, 283–4
 guidelines  220
 obesity  216, 277
predatory fish  229–30
pre-eclampsia
 amylophagia  243
 antioxidants  128
 calcium  144, 145, 151
 carotenoids  130
 choline  104
 diabetes mellitus type 1, 128
 energy balance  10
 exercise  221, 222, 226
 fibre intake  37
 gestational weight gain  217, 219
 homocysteine levels  97
 hyper-homocystinaemia  72
 magnesium effects  177, 179, 181
 maternal age effects  262
 maternal diet  12, 17
 obesity pre-conception  216
 oxidative stress  128
 pre-pregnancy obesity  216
 risk of  10
 stress management  222
 vitamin B$_6$ (pyridoxine)  72
 vitamin B$_9$ (folate)  84, 288
 vitamin B$_{12}$ (cobalamin)  97
 vitamin C (ascorbic acid) deficiency  131, 140
 vitamin C/D supplementation trials  137–8
 vitamin D deficiency  111, 112, 119, 140
 zinc  199
pregnancy complication avoidance  12
pregnancy guidelines. *see* guidelines for
 pregnancy
pregnancy-induced hypertension (PIH)
 calcium deficiency  145
 magnesium effects  177
 maternal age effects  262
 stress management  222

pregnancy-induced nausea and vomiting *see* morning sickness
prelacteal feeds 251
premature rupture of membranes (PROM)
vitamin C (ascorbic acid) deficiency 131
vitamin C/D supplementation trials 138–9
premenopausal breast cancer 293
prescription drugs 301–2
breastfeeding 300–1
paternal factors 266
pre-conception guidelines 285
vitamin B$_{12}$ (cobalamin) deficiency 95
*see also specific drugs*
preterm birth/labour
adolescent pregnancies 263–4
calcium 145–6
cigarette smoking 242
copper deficiency 193
exercise 223, 225
food risks 11
herbicides 238
homocysteine levels 72, 97
iodine deficiency 153–4
iron deficiency 164–5
magnesium 177, 178, 181
maternal stress 258
obesity pre-conception 216
selenium deficiency 189
stress management 223
urinary tract infections 254
vitamin B$_9$ (folate) 85
vitamin C (ascorbic acid) deficiency 131
vitamin C/D supplementation trials 138–9
vitamin K deficiency 124
zinc 199
preterm infants
docosahexaenoic acid supplements 295
excess iron 170
iron supplementation 167–8
pro-angiogenic factors 221
probiotics 209–11
atopic disorders 210
breast milk composition 209
definition 209
gestational diabetes mellitus 210–11
glucose 210–11
immune system 210
intake guidelines 211
sources 209
*see also* prebiotics
processed foods, calcium 148
pro-inflammatory cytokines 245
PROM *see* premature rupture of membranes (PROM)
propionyl-CoA carboxylase 77
propolis 253
protease inhibitors 255
protein

adiposity 34
breastfeeding requirements 295–6
dairy products 34
fetal growth 34
infant formulas 305
intake guidelines 34–5, 37, 39
magnesium 180
middle/late pregnancy 290
recommended dietary allowance 279t
vitamin B$_3$ (niacin) deficiency 68
protein C 122
protein hydrolase 302
protein induced by vitamin K absence or antagonist-II (PIVKA-II) 122
protein leverage hypothesis 8, 8f
protein S 122
prothrombin *see* factor II (prothrombin)
prothrombin times 136
protoporphyrinogen IX oxidase (PPOX) 63
provitamin A carotenoids 47
sources 52
psychomotor development 156
PTH *see* parathyroid hormone (PTH)
PUFAs *see* polyunsaturated fatty acids (PUFAs)
pulmonary hypertension, neonatal 229
purine nucleotide biosynthesis 81
pyridine nucleotide coenzymes 67
pyridoxal (PL) 71
pyridoxal-5'-phosphate (PLP) 71
dependent enzymes 74
vitamin B$_6$ (pyridoxine)status indicator 72
pyridoxamine 71
pyridoxamine-5'-phosphate 71
pyridoxine *see* vitamin B$_6$ (pyridoxine)
pyridoxine-5'-phosphate 71
sources 75
pyrimidine nucleotide biosynthesis 81
pyrrolizidine alkaloids 229

**R**
RA (retinoic acid) 47
RAEs *see* retinoid activity equivalents (RAEs)
Ramadan 250–1
randomized controlled trials (RCTs)
extreme exercise effects 225
pre-pregnancy iron supplementation 166
vitamin B$_9$ (folate) and neural tube defects 85–6
raspberry 255
RCOG *see* Royal College of Obstetricians and Gynaecologists (RCOG)
RCTs *see* randomized controlled trials (RCTs)
RDAs *see* recommended dietary allowance (RDAs)

reactive oxygen species (ROS) 127
  excess iron 170
  male fertility 267–8
ready-to-eat foods 231
recommended dietary allowance (RDAs) 29,
    30t, 294
  *see also specific nutrients*
recommended nutrient intake (RNI) 29, 30,
    279–81t
recreational drugs 266
recurrent apnoea 193
reduced IQ 154
renin 142
respiratory disease
  acute lower tract infections 199
  polyunsaturated fatty acids 44
  vitamin C/D supplementation trials 139
respiratory distress syndrome 189
respiratory insufficiency, neonatal 50
retinal (retinaldehyde) 47
retinaldehyde (retinal) 47
retinal outlet access 12
retinoic acid (RA) 47
retinoic acid receptors 47
retinoid (preformed vitamin A) 47
retinoid activity equivalents (RAEs) 52
  intake guidelines 53
  vitamin A 54
retinoids 47
retinoid X receptor 47
retinol 47
  sources 52
retinol binding protein 47
retinopathy 189
retinyl esters 52
rheumatoid arthritis 72
rhodopsin 48
riboflavin *see* vitamin B$_2$ (riboflavin)
rickets
  calcium deficiency 147
  in neonates 116
  vitamin D deficiency 109, 110
risk accumulation 13, 14t
RNA
  non-coding RNAs 21
  synthesis 81
RNI (recommended nutrient intake) 29
ROS *see* reactive oxygen species (ROS)
Royal College of Obstetricians and
    Gynaecologists (RCOG)
  alcohol intake 241
  exercise guidelines 225–6
  hairdyes/skincare products 246
  magnesium intake guidelines 182
  vitamin B$_{12}$ (cobalamin) supplements
    92–3
  vitamin E 136
*RUNX3* transcription factor 90

**S**
salicylic acid 246
*Salmonella enterica* infection 231
salt iodization programmes 158
schizophrenia 271
SCOPE study 270
scurvy
  infantile 132
  vitamin C (ascorbic acid) deficiency 5
seaweed 157
secondary hyperparathyroidism 108
seizures 74
selenium 187–91
  alcohol consumption 188
  antioxidants 127, 186, 188
  breastfeeding 189–90
  dairy products 190
  deficiency 187, 188–9
  diabetes mellitus type 2, 190
  excess 190
  fertility 188
  functions 187
  infant formulas 304t
  intake guidelines 190–1
  male fertility 267, 272–3
  in pregnancy 188–90
  recommended dietary allowance 188,
    189b, 280t
  sources 190
  status 187
  upper intake level 191, 191b
self-feeding 309
semen quality
  dairy products 268
serotonin 73–4
serum levels
  calcium in vitamin D excess
    117–18
  calcium measurement 142
  ceruloplasmin 192
  copper 192
  glucose, hepatic gluconeogenesis 7
  manganese 204–5
  soluble transferrin receptor 163
  vitamin B$_{12}$ (cobalamin) status 95
  *see also* plasma levels
serving size, labelling 31
servings per container, labelling 31
sex ratio, maternal stress 260
sexual development 228
  zinc deficiency 197
shoulder dystonia 216
sickle-cell anaemia 184
'sitting month' 251
skincare products 246–7
skin conditions *see* dermatitis
*SLC39A2* gene mutations 200
*SLC39A4* gene mutations 199–200

small-for-gestational-age infants
  homocysteine levels 97
  vitamin E deficiency 135
smooth muscle cell proliferation 134
social–emotional behaviour 165
Society of Obstetricians and Gynaecologists
  of Canada 92
socioeconomic status
  heart disease 25
  pica 243
  vitamin $B_1$ (thiamine) deficiency 59
  zinc 200
sodium
  calcium bioavailability 148
  infant formulas 304t
soluble transferrin receptor (sTfR) 162–3
solvents 268–9
South Africa 65
  magnesium supplements 178
Southampton Women's Survey 246
  vitamin D deficiency 114
soy infant formulas 302
Spain 155
sperm aneuploidy 267
spermatogenesis 23
sphingomyelin 102, 104, 105
sphingophosphorylcholine 102
sphingosine 71
spontaneous abortion
  herbicides 238
  iodine deficiency 153–4
  lead effects 234
  selenium deficiency 188
  vitamin K deficiency 124
Sri Lanka 251
sTfR (soluble transferrin receptor) 162–3
stillbirth, obesity pre-conception 216
St John's Wort *(Hypericum perforatum)*, 254–5
stress
  antioxidants 140
  management 223
  maternal *see* maternal stress
stress hormones 259
stromal cell proliferation 221
sunshine, vitamin D 114–15
superoxide dismutase 204
supplementation
  pre-conception behaviour 278–84
  *see also specific nutrients*
Swedish Birth Registry 262
swimming pool risks 224

**T**
T3 (tri-iodothyronine), iodine 152, 153
T4 (thyroxine), iodine 152, 153
Taoism 250
teratogens
  birth defects 124, 228

  definition 228
  vitamin A 50
tetracyclines 302
tetrahydrofolate (THF) 62
Thailand 251
T-helper cell type 1:2 ratio (Th1/Th2
  ratio), 210
T-helper cell type 2 (Th2) 129
theophylline 233
THF (tetrahydrofolate) 62
thiamine *see* vitamin $B_1$ (thiamine)
thiamine diphosphate levels 57, 58t
thiazide diuretics 184
thioglycolic acid 246
thioredoxin reductases 187
thromboembolism
  maternal age effects 262
  obesity pre-conception 216
thyroid hormones
  iodine 152
  selenium 187
  thyroxine (T4) 152
  tri-iodothyronine (T3) 152, 153
  vitamin D interaction 47
thyroid metabolism, iron deficiency 165
thyroid-stimulating hormone (TSH) 153
thyroxine (T4), iodine 152, 153
tissue deposition 18
tobacco smoking 12
  *see also* cigarette smoking
tolerable upper intake level 30t
  definition 30
topical hair removal products 246
toxoplasmosis 231
traditional remedies *see* herbal remedies
traffic light system, labelling 32
transcobalamin 94
transcription factors, vitamin D 108
transferrin 162
transketolase 57–8, 58t
tretinoin 246
Trier Social Stress Test 259
tri-iodothyronine (T3), iodine 152, 153
trisomy 21 (Down's syndrome) 263, 271
trophoblastic cell proliferation 221
tryptophan 68–9
Turkey
  iodine deficiency 158
  postpartum food practices 251
type 1 diabetes mellitus *see* diabetes mellitus
  type 1
type 2 diabetes mellitus *see* diabetes mellitus
  type 2

**U**
ubiquitation of DNA 20
UK Centre for Maternal and Child
  Enquiries 92–3

UL *see* upper intake level (UL)
ultrasound 15
ultraviolet B (UVB) 107, 114–15
undercooked meats 232t
   toxoplasmosis 231
under-nutrition
   China 10
   at conception 215
   cultural practices 219
   energy balance 10
   fetal effects 25, 220
   maternal stress 257
   obesity with 9
   pre-conception 277
underweight at conception 215
UNICEF 159, 161
UNIMAP (UN Multiple Micronutrient
   Preparation) 167
United Kingdom (UK)
   calcium deficiency 148
   food labelling 31–2
   herbal remedies 256
   iron intake in pregnancy 172
   nutrient intake guidelines 31t
   obesity pre-conception 216
   selenium intake guidelines 190
   vitamin A intake guidelines 56
United Nations Environment Program 247
UN Multiple Micronutrient Preparation
   (UNIMAP) 167
unpasteurized cheese 11
unplanned pregnancies 13
upper intake level (UL) 30, 30t
urinary excretion
   calcium 142
   iodine 152–3
   vitamin $B_1$ (thiamine) 57, 58t
   vitamin $B_2$ (riboflavin) 63
   vitamin $B_3$ (niacin) 67
   vitamin $B_7$ (biotin) 77
urinary tract infections 254
USA
   calcium deficiency 148
   food labelling 31
   fructose 36
   maternal stress 258
   organochlorine chemicals 230
   pica 243
   selenium intake guidelines 190
   vitamin D deficiency 112
US National Health and Nutrition
   Examination Survey
   cigarette smoking 133
   vitamin $B_{12}$ (cobalamin) status 95
US Preventive Services Task Force 92
US Standing Committee on Nutrition 158
uterine blood flow 257
uterine fibroids 261

**V**
valerian 253
vascular disorders, vitamin $B_9$ (folate) 81, 84
vasculopathy 164
vasoconstriction 142
vegans
   vitamin $B_2$ (riboflavin) supplements 66
   vitamin $B_{12}$ (cobalamin) 95–6, 98, 100
vegetables
   middle/late pregnancy 290
   pre-conception intake guidelines 286t
   washing/peeling 231
vegetarian diets
   deficiencies 278
   iron 169, 171–2
   protein intake 295–6
   vitamin A 52
   vitamin $B_2$ (riboflavin) supplements 66
   vitamin $B_{12}$ (cobalamin) 98
   zinc 200, 201
vinclozolin 236
vinyl chloride 268
VIP trial 138
viral transmission 189
visual system 48
   polyunsaturated fatty acids 43
   vitamin $B_{12}$ (cobalamin)–vitamin $B_6$
      (pyridoxine) interactions 96
vitamin A 47–56
   Africa 290
   alcohol consumption 52, 53
   breastfeeding 51, 297
   breast milk composition 54, 297
   conversions 54, 54b
   craniofacial malformations 281
   dairy products 290
   deficiency *see* vitamin A deficiency
   definition 47
   early pregnancy 56, 287–8
   excess 52–3, 228
   infant formulas 303t
   malnutrition, in 53
   maternal stores 49
   metabolism 52
   middle/late pregnancy 290
   precursors 48f
   in pregnancy 49–51
   safe band 7
   sources 52
   storage 47
   supplementation *see* vitamin A
      supplementation
   *see also* retinoids; *specific retinoids*
vitamin A deficiency 48–9, 278
   birth defects 49, 50, 281
   developing countries 50
   India 49
   infertility 48

vitamin A deficiency (*continued*)
  iron mobilization 51
  neonatal respiratory insufficiency 50
  supplementation 50
  weaning 51
vitamin A intake guidelines 53–6, 285
  adolescent pregnancies 54
  Europe 56
  pre-conception guidelines 281
  recommended dietary allowance 52, 55b,
    279t, 281
  upper intake level 53, 54, 55b, 281
vitamin A supplementation 50
  anaemia 51
  India 56, 290
vitamin B₁ (thiamine) 57–61
  alcohol consumption 58
  anorexia 59
  breastfeeding and infancy 59–60
  breast milk composition 59–60
  as cofactor 5
  deficiency *see* vitamin B₁ (thiamine)
    deficiency
  excess 60
  function 57
  infant formulas 303t
  intake guidelines *see* vitamin B₁ (thiamine)
    intake guidelines
  in pregnancy 59
  sources 60
  status indicators 57–8, 58t
vitamin B₁ (thiamine) deficiency 58
  Asia 58
  infant formulas 59–60
vitamin B₁ (thiamine) intake guidelines 60–1
  adolescent pregnancies 60
  recommended dietary allowance 60, 61b,
    279t
  recommended nutrient intake 60, 61
  upper intake level 60
vitamin B₂ (riboflavin) 62–6
  breastfeeding 64–5
  breast milk composition 64–5
  dairy products 63, 64, 65, 66
  deficiency *see* vitamin B₂ (riboflavin)
    deficiency
  functions 62–3
  infant formulas 303t
  intake guidelines 65–6
  in pregnancy 64
  recommended dietary allowance 66, 66b,
    279t
  recommended nutrient intake 70
  sources 65
  status indicators 63
  upper intake level 65
vitamin B₂ (riboflavin) deficiency 63–4, 65
  Africa 63, 65

Asia 63
Gambia 64
weaning 64
vitamin B₃ (niacin) 67–70
  alcohol consumption 68
  anticonvulsant drugs 83, 92
  breast milk composition 68
  Canada 70
  dairy products 69
  deficiency 68
  excess 69
  functions 67
  intake guidelines 69–70
  pregnancy and breastfeeding 68
  recommended dietary allowance 69–70,
    69b, 279t
  sources 68–9
  status indicators 67–8
  supplementation in infant formulas 69
  synthesis 62
vitamin B₅ (pantothenic acid) 303t
vitamin B₆ (pyridoxine) 71–6
  Africa 75
  anaemia 73
  atopic disorders 90
  brain development 73
  breastfeeding 74, 297–8
  breast milk composition 74, 76
  in conception 73
  deficiency 72, 75
  diabetes mellitus type 1, 72
  excess 75
  fetal brain development 73–4
  functions 71
  infant formulas 303t
  intake guidelines 75–6
  metabolism 74–5
  nausea and vomiting 73
  pre-eclampsia 72
  in pregnancy 72–4
  recommended dietary allowance 74, 76b,
    279t
  sources 74–5
  status indicators 72
  supplements 74, 298
  synthesis 62
  upper intake level 75
  vitamin B₁₂ (cobalamin) interactions 96–7
  in weaning 308
vitamin B₇ (biotin) 77–80
  breastfeeding 78
  breast milk composition 79
  dairy products 78
  deficiency 77–8
  excess 79
  functions 77
  infant formulas 303t
  intake guidelines 79–80

pre-conception intake guidelines 283
in pregnancy 78
recommended dietary allowance 79, 79b
sources 78
status indicators 77
vitamin B$_9$ (folate) 81–93
  Africa, intake guidelines 90
  alcohol consumption 83, 93
  anaemia 83, 87
  anticonvulsant drugs 92
  atopic disorders 90
  birth defects 278
  choline interactions 87–8, 103–4
  deficiency *see* vitamin B$_9$ (folate) deficiency
  early pregnancy 288
  excess 89–90
  food fortification 88–9
  functions 81, 83
  genetics 87
  high intakes 7
  intake guidelines *see* vitamin B$_9$ (folate)
    intake guidelines
  pre-conception supplements 278, 281
  pre-eclampsia 288
  in pregnancy 84–6
  sources 88
  status indicators 83
  supplements *see* vitamin B$_9$ (folate)
    supplementation
  vitamin B$_{12}$ (cobalamin) interactions 87–8
vitamin B$_9$ (folate) deficiency 83–4, 86
  birth defects 85
  neural tube defects 7, 83, 84, 85–6, 87, 88–9,
    90–1, 92, 93, 278, 288
vitamin B$_9$ (folate) intake guidelines 90–3
  Canadian recommendations 90
  recommended dietary allowance 91–2, 91b
  upper intake level 89
vitamin B$_9$ (folate) supplementation 85–6, 89,
    265, 288
  asthma 90
  Australia 85
  China 85
vitamin B$_{12}$ (cobalamin) 94–101
  alcohol consumption 95
  anaemia 96, 98
  binding proteins 94
  birth defects 97–8
  brain development 73
  breastfeeding 97–8, 298
  breast milk composition 97, 98, 100, 298
  deficiency 95–6, 97–8
  early pregnancy 287, 288
  equivalents conversion, 91b
  excess 99
  functions 94
  infant formulas 303t
  neonates 98

pre-eclampsia 97
in pregnancy 97–8
recommended amounts 98
sources 98–9
status indicators 95
supplements *see* vitamin B$_{12}$ (cobalamin)
    supplements
vitamin B$_6$ (pyridoxine) interactions 96–7
vitamin B$_9$ (folate) interactions 87–8
in weaning 308–9
*see also* methylcobalamin
vitamin B$_{12}$ (cobalamin) intake guidelines
    99–101
  adolescent pregnancies 99
  Canada 98, 105
  pre-conception 281
  recommended dietary allowance 96, 100b,
    279t
  upper intake level 99
vitamin B$_{12}$ (cobalamin) supplements 99
  India 96–7
vitamin C (ascorbic acid) 127, 130–4
  breastfeeding 131–2
  breast milk composition 132
  deficiency 5, 131, 140
  excess 132–3
  functions 131
  half life 6
  infant formulas 303t
  iron absorption 168
  lead protection 235
  male fertility 268
  metabolism 132
  middle/late pregnancy 291
  in pregnancy 131–2
  sources 132
  supplementation trials 137–9
  supplements 128, 130–1, 132
  weaning 132
vitamin C (ascorbic acid) intake
    guidelines 133–4
  Australia 134
  New Zealand 134
  recommended dietary allowance 133, 133b,
    279t
  upper intake level, 133b
vitamin D 107–21
  Africa 119
  atopic disorders 112–13
  bone mineral density (BMD) 116
  breastfeeding 116–17, 296–7
  breast milk composition 116, 120, 296
  calcium intake *vs.,* 143
  dairy products 115, 282
  deficiency *see* vitamin D deficiency
  early pregnancy 287, 288
  excess *see* vitamin D excess
  extra-skeletal effects 110

vitamin D (*continued*)
functions 107–8
glucose, effects on 107, 109
infant formulas 303t
infertility 114
intake guidelines *see* vitamin D intake
guidelines
metabolism 108f
middle/late pregnancy 290
in pregnancy 110–14, 116
sources 108f, 114–15
supplements *see* vitamin D supplements
thyroid hormone interaction 47
*see also* 1,25-hydroxyvitamin D (calcitriol)
vitamin D₂ (ergocalciferol) 107, 115
vitamin D₃ (cholecalciferol) 107, 115
vitamin D deficiency 108–10
Asia 112, 119
asthma 109
birthweight 113–14
body coverings 13
calcium deficiency 147
definition 109–10
diabetes mellitus type 1, 109
eczema 113
gestational diabetes mellitus 113
hypertension 109
India 112
infection 113
overweight 113–14
pre-eclampsia 112, 119, 140
in pregnancy 111–12
USA 112
vitamin D excess 117–18
appetite 175
asthma 113
eczema 112
vitamin D intake guidelines 118–21
adiposity 111
New Zealand 120
pre-conception 282
recommended dietary allowance 118–19,
118b, 279t
upper intake level 115, 118b, 119
vitamin D supplements 112, 116, 117, 120–1,
287, 288, 297
Africa 118
infant formulas 115, 120
vitamin E 127, 130, 134–7
breastfeeding 135
breast milk composition 136
deficiency 134
excess 136
forms 134–5
functions 134
infant formulas 303t
intake guidelines *see* vitamin E intake
guidelines

male fertility 268
metabolism 135–6
in pregnancy 135
sources 135–6
supplementation trials 137–9
supplements 128, 130–1
vitamin E intake guidelines 136–7, 140
adolescent pregnancies 136
Australia 136
recommended dietary allowance, 137b
279t
upper intake level 136, 137b
vitamin K 122–6
breast milk composition 123, 297
dairy products 124
deficiency *see* vitamin K deficiency
excess 125
functions 122
half-life 124
infant formulas 123, 303t
intake guidelines *see* vitamin K intake
guidelines
metabolism 124
in pregnancy 123–4
sources 124
status indicators 122–3
supplements 123
vitamin K₁ (phylloquinone) 122–3
vitamin K₂ (menaquinone) 124
vitamin K deficiency 123
anticonvulsant drugs 92
Asia 124
birth defects 124
vitamin K epoxide reductase 122
vitamin K intake guidelines 125–6, 297
adolescent pregnancies 125
Europe 124
recommended dietary allowance 125,
125b
upper intake level 125
vomiting
potassium loss 185
vitamin B₁ (thiamine) deficiency 59
*see also* nausea and vomiting

**W**
warfarin embryopathy 124
water *see* drinking water
weaning 8, 306–10
calcium 147
diabetes mellitus type 2, 307
flavour learning 309–10
food preferences 309–10
nutrient requirements 307–8
*see also specific nutrients*
prebiotics/probiotics 210, 211
timing of 306–7
vitamin A deficiency 51

vitamin B$_2$ (riboflavin) deficiency 64
vitamin C (ascorbic acid) 132
*see also* complementary foods
weight
  fibre intake 37
  metabolic control 8
  planned loss 250–1
  postpartum retention 293
  pre-conception *see* pre-conception
    bodyweight
weight gain
  in pregnancy *see* gestational weight gain
  weaning timing 307
weight loss, planned *see* dieting (planned
    weight loss)
weight-to-length ponderal index 17
Wernicke–Korsakoff syndrome 58
Wernicke's encephalopathy 58
Western diets
  Asia 129
  iron 168
  male fertility 268
  oxidative stress 129
  zinc 200
whey:casein ratio, infant formulas 305
World Health Organization (WHO)
  calcium and preterm delivery trials 145–6
  calcium intake guidelines 150
  complementary foods 309
  iodine breastfeeding requirements 299
  iodine deficient areas 158
  iodine intake guidelines 159, 161
  iodine upper intake level 158
  iron deficiency 164
  iron intake in pregnancy 171
  lifestyle risks 247
  manganese intake guidelines 207
  polyunsaturated fatty acids intake
    guidelines 45–6
  pre-pregnancy iron supplementation 166
  selenium intake guidelines 191
  vitamin A deficiency 48
  vitamin A intake guidelines 55
  vitamin B$_1$ (thiamine) intake guidelines 60,
    61
  vitamin B$_3$ (niacin) intake guidelines 70
  vitamin B$_6$ (pyridoxine) intake guidelines 75
  vitamin B$_7$ (biotin) intake guidelines 79
  vitamin C/E supplement trials 137–8
  vitamin D intake guidelines 119–20
  zinc intake guidelines 202

**X**
X chromosome inactivation 22
xenobiotic agents 268
xerophthalmia 48
X-ray exposure 272

**Y**
yeast supplements 66
yoga 223
  maternal stress 222

**Z**
zinc 196–203
  antioxidant properties 127
  bioavailability 200–1
  breastfeeding 199–200, 299
  breast milk composition 199–200, 201–2,
    203, 299
  copper deficiency 193
  dairy products 200
  deficiency *see* zinc deficiency
  excess 201
  functions 196
  gestational hypertension 199
  infant formulas 199–200, 304t
  intake guidelines 201–3
  male fertility 267, 272–3
  middle/late pregnancy 291
  pica 243
  pre-conception intake guidelines 283
  pre-eclampsia 199
  in pregnancy 198–9
  recommended dietary allowance 198, 202b,
    280t
  sources 200–1
  status indicators 196
  upper intake level 201, 202, 202b
  in weaning 309
zinc deficiency 196–8
  adolescent pregnancies 201
  Africa 197, 291
  alcohol consumption 197, 198, 201
  anorexia 197
  Asia 197, 291
  cognitive development 197–8
  growth 197
  immune function 197
  iron supplementation 169–70
  malnutrition 196–7
  neurological development 197–8
zinc transporter gene mutations 199–200

ML        7-16